AF899113

The Neural Basis of Behavior

The Neural Basis of Behavior

Edited by

Alexander L. Beckman, Ph.D.

Senior Research Scientist
Alfred I. duPont Institute
Wilmington, Delaware

MTP PRESS LIMITED
International Medical Publishers

Based on the Symposium on the Neural Basis of Behavior, June 7–8, 1979, Alfred I. duPont Institute, Wilmington, Delaware

Published in the UK and Europe by
MTP Press Limited
Falcon House
Lancaster, England

Published in the US by
SPECTRUM PUBLICATIONS, INC.
175-20 Wexford Terrace
Jamaica, N.Y. 11432

Copyright © 1982, Spectrum Publications, Inc.
Softcover reprint of the hardcover 1st edition 1982

All rights reserved. No part of this book may be reproduced in any form, by photostat, microform, retrieval system, or any other means without prior written permission of the copyright holder or his licensee.

ISBN-13: 978-94-011-6304-0 e-ISBN-13: 978-94-011-6302-6
DOI: 10.1007/978-94-011-6302-6

Contributors

HUDA AKIL, Ph.D.
Department of Psychiatry
Mental Health Research Institute
University of Michigan School of Medicine
Ann Arbor, Michigan

ALEXANDER L. BECKMAN, Ph.D.
Alfred I. duPont Institute
Wilmington, Delaware
and
Department of Physiology
School of Life and Health Sciences
University of Delaware
Newark, Delaware

THOMAS J. CAREW, Ph.D.
Department of Psychiatry
Division of Neurobiology and Behavior
College of Physicians and Surgeons
Columbia University
New York, New York

KENNETH L. CASEY, M.D.
Departments of Physiology and Neurology
University of Michigan School of Medicine
and
Neurology Service
Veterans Administration Medical Center
Ann Arbor, Michigan

VALERIE B. DOMESICK, Ph.D.
Biological Research Laboratories
McLean Hospital
Belmont, Massachusetts

PAUL J. FRAY, Ph.D.
Research Associate
Cambridge University
Cambridge, England

SUSAN D. IVERSEN, Ph.D.
Department of Experimental Psychology
Cambridge University
Cambridge, England

ERIC R. KANDEL, M.D.
Departments of Physiology and Psychiatry
Division of Neurobiology and Behavior
College of Physicians and Surgeons
Columbia University
New York, New York

MANFRED L. KARNOVSKY, Ph.D.
Department of Biological Chemistry
Harvard University Medical School
Boston, Massachusetts

SEYMOUR S. KETY, M.D.
Department of Psychiatry
Harvard University
Boston, Massachusetts
and
Laboratories for Psychiatric Research
Mailman Research Center
McLean Hospital
Belmont, Massachusetts

HANS W. KOSTERLITZ, M.D., Ph.D.
Unit for Research on Addictive Drugs
University of Aberdeen
Aberdeen, Scotland

KEVIN S. LEE, Ph.D.
Department of Psychobiology
School of Biological Sciences
University of California
Irvine, California

MORRIS A. LIPTON, M.D., Ph.D.
Department of Psychiatry
Biological Sciences Research Center
University of North Carolina School of Medicine
Chapel Hill, North Carolina

PETER T. LOOSEN, M.D.
Department of Psychiatry
University of North Carolina
Chapel Hill, North Carolina
and
Clinical Research Unit
Dorothea Dix Hospital
Raleigh, North Carolina

GARY S. LYNCH, Ph.D.
Department of Psychobiology
School of Biological Sciences
University of California
Irvine, California

ADRIAN R. MORRISON, Ph.D.
Laboratories of Anatomy
School of Veterinary Medicine
University of Pennsylvania
Philadelphia, Pennsylvania

WALLE J.H. NAUTA, M.D., Ph.D.
Department of Psychology
Massachusetts Institute of Technology
Cambridge, Massachusetts
and
Mailman Research Center
McLean Hospital
Belmont, Massachusetts

ARTHUR J. PRANGE, JR., M.D.
Department of Psychiatry
University of North Carolina School of Medicine
Chapel Hill, North Carolina

VICTOR E. SHASHOUA, Ph.D.
Department of Biological Chemistry
Harvard Medical School
Boston, Massachusetts
and
Mailman Research Center
McLean Hospital
Belmont, Massachusetts

ERIC J. SIMON, Ph.D.
Departments of Psychiatry and Pharmacology
New York University Medical Center
New York, New York

TONI L. STANTON, Ph.D.
Alfred I. duPont Institute
Wilmington, Delaware

EDGAR T. WALTERS, Ph.D.
Division of Neurobiology and Behavior
College of Physicians and Surgeons
Columbia University
New York, New York

NORMAN M. WEINBERGER, Ph.D.
Department of Psychobiology
School of Biological Sciences
University of California
Irvine, California

Contents

PART IV PAIN

Preface

The Symposium on the Neural Basis of Behavior, from which this volume was produced, was held at the Alfred I. duPont Institute on June 7 and 8, 1979. It brought outstanding investigators in four fundamental areas of behavioral neurobiology into juxtaposition, there to provide an integrated, multidisciplinary perspective on behaviorally significant brain mechanisms.

Particular emphasis was placed on topics of interest to neurobiologists as well as to clinicians in neurological and psychiatric disciplines. The session on central activity states was selected as an appropriate point of departure because the continuum of brain activity states extending from the natural depression of hibernation through the heightened levels of arousal accompanying learning is such a clear and basic determinant of behavioral output. The papers on learning and memory outlined diverse approaches to understanding the basis of these interrelated CNS capabilities that constitute the neural basis of behavioral adaptation. Finally, the topics of affective states and mechanisms of pain provided a focus of clinically relevant discussion covering multiple levels of functional and anatomical CNS organization.

The success of the symposium bore testimony to the excellence of the presentations and to the symbiosis of their content; both are preserved herein. The support and encouragement of Dr. G. Dean MacEwen, Medical Director of the Alfred I. duPont Institute, is gratefully acknowledged.

Alexander L. Beckman
Wilmington, July 1979

The Neural Basis of Behavior

PART I

Central Activity States

Copyright © 1982, Spectrum Publications, Inc.
The Neural Basis of Behavior

1

Central Activity States: Overview

Adrian R. Morrison

INTRODUCTION

In this section we shall focus our attention on the broad range of integrated neural activity that extends from attentive arousal through the various sleep states to a state of prolonged dormancy, hibernation. Central issues herein are (1) the relationships among the different activity states—how they differ and how they are similar—and (2) the means by which the normal central nervous system is able to switch back and forth among central activity states. Although we will not resolve the second problem here, there are interrelationships among the states which have rarely, if ever, been discussed in open forum before, so we can reasonably expect an increment in our understanding.

For the present discussion I have chosen the daily sleep-wakefulness alternation as a focal point for two reasons. In the first place, there are links between sleep and both extremes of the central activity states included in this session, hibernation and attentive arousal, which should stimulate profitable discussion of the central problem of neural control of state change. Second, this discussion will provide a physiological and psychological counterpoint to Karnovsky's chapter on the biochemical factors associated with sleep.

GENERAL COMMENTS ON SLEEP—WAKEFULNESS CONTROL

A brief review of the systems which have been implicated in the control of sleep and wakefulness will be the first step. Two landmark studies on this topic were the discovery of the reticular activating system by Moruzzi and Magoun (1949) and the ushering in of the modern era of sleep research with the description of the state of rapid eye movement by Aserinsky and Kleitman (1953). Developments following the latter two discoveries have, for reasons to be discussed later, tended to draw attention to the lower brainstem and away from the forebrain mechanisms which had been revealed earlier by electrical stimulation experiments and experimental lesions (Moruzzi, 1972; Sprague, 1967). Yet, as Parmeggiani (1968: 350) has stated, "From a behavioural point of view, sleep in animals shows many features that are typical also of other patterns of behaviour expressing basic instincts....In fact, it is relatively easy to recognize that an appetitive phase prepares the consummatory act of sleep.... In this context it is reasonable to grant that sleep behaviour should be regulated by the intervention of prosencephalic (telencephalic and diencephalic) structures, as in the case of other translations of bodily needs into behaviour. On the other hand, if we disregard the role of the prosencephalon in sleep we are forced to endow the brain stem with an imperative influence and a degree of integrative power that are in contrast with the fact that brain stem integration levels are unable to express full instinctive and adaptive behaviour.... We must therefore assume that prosencephalic influences may regulate brain stem mechanisms in order to cope with the basic needs of the whole organism."

It is fair to say, though, that the region critical for conscious awareness in mammals, the group in which this problem has been most studied, is the reticular core of the brainstem. Moruzzi and Magoun (1949) demonstrated that electroencephalographic arousal resulted from electrical stimulation in the mesencephalic reticular formation at a stimulus intensity lower than that needed to produce the same effect if the laterally lying long ascending pathways were stimulated. Thus, arousal of an organism had to be viewed as involving processes more complex than a simple ebb and flow of the tides of daily sensory inflow directly to the cortex. Lesion experiments by Lindsley et al. (1950) soon verified this conclusion because they demonstrated that only lesions of the reticular core produced sommolence; lateral lesions led to disturbances in sensory responses but did not prevent wakefulness. The prevailing view of sleep, that it was a passive process involving progressive functional deafferentation, remained after these discoveries because of Bremer's (1935) earlier discoveries. He had demonstrated that the electrical activity of the brain rostral to a midbrain transection, his famous "cerveau isole" preparation, consisted of continual low-frequency, high-amplitude EEG waves characteristic of sleep.

The question of the relationship of EEG patterns to behavioral states was vastly complicated, however, by the discovery that there is a stage of sleep during which the EEG is essentially identical to that of alert wakefulness

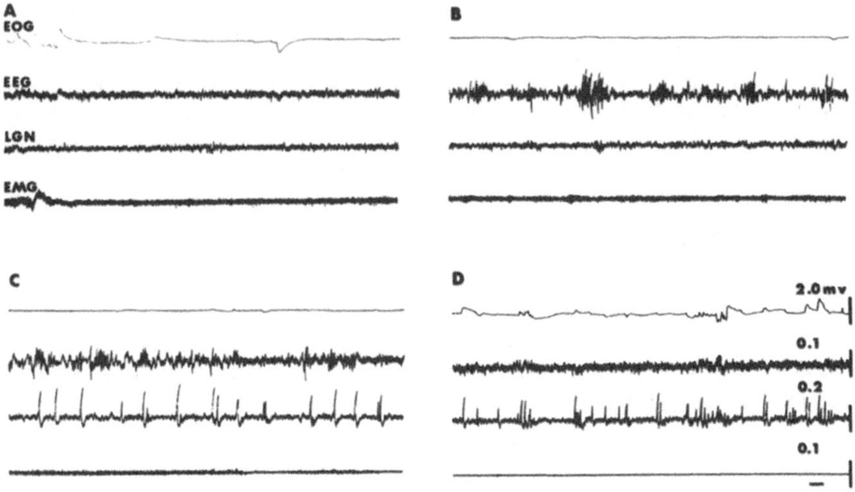

FIG. 1. Characteristics of the behavioral states of (A) quiet wakefulness; (B) slow-wave sleep; (C) transition from slow-wave sleep to paradoxical sleep; (D) paradoxical sleep. EOG, eye movements recorded on the electro-oculogram; EEG, electroencephalogram; LGN, recording of PGO spikes in the lateral geniculate body in C and D, but eye movement potentials practically absent in A; EMG, electromyographic activity of the dorsal cervical muscles which disappears at the end of C and D. Time calibration = 1 second. [Reproduced from Fig. 1, Morrison (1979a), with the permission of Academic Press.]

(Fig. 1). This observation also prompted recognition of the fact that regulation of sleep is an active, complicated process.

Prior to 1953, sleep was characterized as a period during which a typical posture with eye closure and reduced responsiveness was coupled with high-amplitude, low-frequency waves on the EEG. Aserinsky and Kleitman (1953), however, reported that infants exhibited periods during sleep in which there were low-amplitude, high-frequency waves on the EEG and rapid movements of the eyes. These periods were not wakefulness. These episodes have since been demonstrated to be a separate sleep phase which routinely follows the phase of slow wave sleep in cyclic fashion throughout a period of sleep (Jouvet, 1967). The rapid eye movements that typify the former gave rise to a familiar name for this sleep stage, rapid eye movement sleep (or REM sleep) (Fig. 1 D). Another common designation for this state, paradoxical sleep (PS), derives from the fact that mammals, the class in which PS has been unequivocally demonstrated, are paralyzed and in a condition of reduced responsiveness even though the EEG pattern resembles that of wakefulness (compare Fig. 1 A, D) (Jouvet, 1967). Of course, the unusual familiarity of the general public with PS developed with the demonstration that dreams could be identified with this distinct physiological state (Dement and Kleitman, 1957). Though the neural activity immediately producing dream imagery can reasonably be thought to occur in the telencephalon, the mechanisms basically responsible for the onset and maintenance of PS within the sleep cycle reside in the lower brainstem.

PARADOXICAL SLEEP AND ALERT WAKEFULNESS

As a result of a large series of localized lesions and transections, Jouvet (1962) concluded that the pons is the region responsible for generating the basic state of PS. After a transection through the lower midbrain, cats still periodically exhibited the peripheral components of REM sleep: muscle atonia, even in the face of decerebrate rigidity; muscle twitches of the face and extremities especially; and rapid eye movements. This important observation has since been replicated (Villablanca, 1966a), and Bard and Macht (1958) have reported periodic loss of rigidity and lack of head raising in chronic decerebrate cats as well.

Results of attempts to localize the neurons or neuronal groups responsible for the switch from slow wave sleep to PS are much more controversial. There is general agreement, although no direct proof, that the ultimate source of the inhibition of spinal motor neurons responsible for the atonia of PS (Gassel et al., 1965; Morrison and Pompeiano, 1965) is the medullary inhibitory (Magoun and Rhines, 1946) area of the reticular formation (Pompeiano, 1976). The pons, on the other hand, has been regarded as the organizing center for PS. Just how the pons is involved, however, is a matter of conjecture at the moment (Morrison, 1979a). Lesions of the pontine tegmentum, which had been reported to eliminate PS without affecting other states, proved on close analysis (Henley and Morrison, 1974) to have been either nonselective for that state (Carli and Zanchetti, 1965) or to have eliminated only the atonia of PS (Jouvet, 1962). In fact, the latter finding, since replicated (Henley and Morrison, 1974), negates the conclusion (Jouvet, 1962) that absence of atonic episodes following caudal pontine transections provides proof that the mechanisms regulating PS must reside wholly within the pons. There is at least room to consider the medulla in the regulatory mechanism. The theory that a noradrenergic mechanism originating in the locus coeruleus is at the heart of PS, based on effects of locus coeruleus lesions and pharmacological manipulations (Jouvet, 1972), has also been called into serious question by the report that total bilateral destruction of the noradrenergic neurons of the cat's locus coeruleus does not eliminate the PS state (Jones et al., 1977).

At the single-cell level the giant reticular neurons of the pontine tegmentum seemed to be promising candidates for the generating force underlying the switch into PS because they fired selectively at a high rate during PS only (Hobson et al., 1975). A reciprocal interaction between them and cells in the locus coeruleus which fall silent as PS approaches was proposed to underly the switch into and out of PS. Recent studies have shown, however, that in totally unrestrained animals the giant neurons fire in association with movements of principally the head and neck during wakefulness so that they must be regarded as elements involved primarily in motor control (Siegel et al., 1977; Vertes, 1977).

In spite of these problems that have arisen in recent years, it is important to stress that the caudal brainstem, and particularly the pons, is somehow crucially involved in the state-switching process which results in PS. Results with midbrain transections mentioned earlier support this conclusion (Jouvet, 1962; Villablanca, 1966a). Furthermore, several groups have demonstrated that very localized application of cholinomimetic substances within the pontine tegmentum produce a state with all the characteristics of PS (cf. Steriade and Hobson, 1976). Yet, the questions remain, why does the nervous system enter the PS mode and why does PS exhibit the form that it does? Discussion of the myriad of theories of why PS occurs is beyond the scope of this paper, but a reasonable hypothesis for why the state appears in the form that it does—paralysis coupled with activation—can be offered.

First, it is important to stress that PS is a highly activated state in which the brain exhibits many of the phenomena associated with alert wakefulness—activated EEG, hippocampal theta rhythm, and increased brain temperature (Morrison, 1979a). Obvious differences are that in PS animals are less responsive to environmental stimuli, are paralyzed, and have miotic pupils. But studies in our laboratory of the characteristics of ponto-geniculo-occipital (PGO) spikes (Fig. 1C, D), which are recorded as spontaneous potentials with macroelectrodes in the pontine tegmentum, lateral geniculate body, and occipital cortex during PS (Jouvet, 1972), have led to the concept that the brain during PS is constantly in what would be called a state of "orientation" if the animal were interacting with its environment (for experimental details see Bowker, 1979; Bowker and Morrison, 1976). More specifically, these experiments have led us to conclude that the brainstem is in a functional mode normally associated with presentation of novel stimuli and, moreover, that the reticular formation acts as if it were incapable of habituating to novel stimuli although the brain is largely shut off to the outside world. PGO spikes, thought to be spontaneous events of PS, can be elicited by auditory stimulation during slow-wave sleep and PS (Bowker and Morrison, 1976). However, the spikes disappear (habituate) after a few stimulus presentations in slow-wave sleep but occur after more than 60% of the stimuli during PS (Bowker, 1979). This property stems from a lack of serotonergic control by the raphe nuclei during PS (McGinty and Harper, 1976; Simon et al., 1973; Trulson and Jacobs, 1978). During wakefulness, eye movement potentials assume all the properties of PGO spikes for a few seconds whenever a cat is presented with a novel or unexpected stimulus (Bowker and Morrison, 1977). This alerting, or orientation, reaction rapidly habituates.

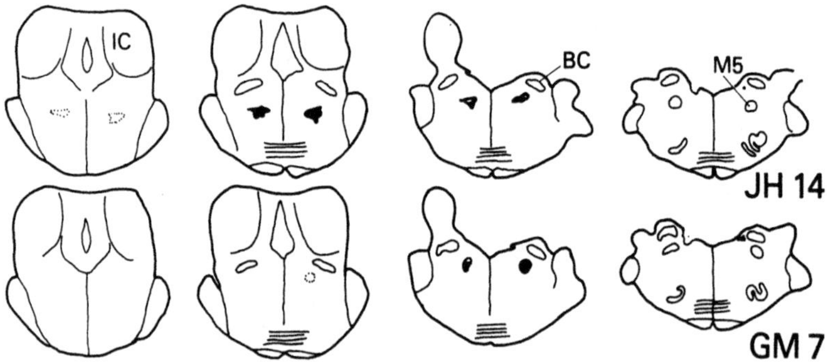

FIG. 2. Lesions which produced paradoxical sleep without atonia. Lesions are denoted by black areas sometimes surrounding areas of cavitation. Dotted circles indicate gliosis. Cross sections are, from left to right, from stereotaxic levels P1 to P4. Both exhibited raising of the head, body righting, searching, and locomotor movements. JH14 also displayed attack. BC, brachium conjunctivum; IC, inferior colliculus; M5, motor nucleus of the trigeminal nerve. [Reproduced from Fig. 4, Morrison (1979b), with the permission of *Acta Neurobiologiae Experimentalis.*]

The relationship of atonia to reticular activation was revealed by cats exhibiting PS without atonia (Jouvet and Delorme, 1965; Henley and Morrison, 1974). Small, bilateral lesions of the pontine tegmentum (Fig. 2) create this phenomenon, which is characterized as follows: After slow wave sleep, when PS with muscle atonia would normally appear, cats raise their heads, make body righting movements, exhibit alternating movements of the limbs, and attempt to stand—sometimes succeeding to the point where we have observed cats walking or trotting with evidence of some impairment of antigravity tone. They exhibit "orienting," "searching," and sometimes "attack" or "rage" behavior. Other characteristics of PS, such as increased brain temperature, hippocampal theta rhythm (both present in alert wakefulness as well) and rapid eye movements are present (Hendricks et al., 1977). Although the pupils are very miotic and the nictitating membranes are generally relaxed, we have recently discovered that the cats will respond to a face or object in the observation window of the recording cage (Mann, Hendricks and Morrison, unpublished observations). This contrasts with an earlier report (Henley and Morrison, 1974) of unresponsiveness to bright floodlights. Never do cats exhibiting PS without atonia have interspersed bouts of normal PS. During wakefulness these cats exhibit alterations in motor control ranging from slight stumbling to more severe cerebellar ataxia. Also, they exhibit an increase (23–127%) in exploratory behavior as measured in an open-field test and also on the basis of general observations (Morrison, 1979b). The conclusion we have reached (Morrison, 1979a) is that the lesions interrupt systems normally facilitating the activity of the medullary inhibitory area (Magoun and Rhines, 1946) and inhibiting a brainstem locomotor area (Shik and Orlovsky, 1976).

Atonia can now be seen to be a natural concomitant of the state of excessive activation that is PS. On the basis of our experiments with cats exhibiting PS without atonia, which show excessive exploratory behavior during wakefulness, we have proposed that the caudal brainstem contains within it a basic control system designed to modulate responses to novel or unexpected stimuli (Morrison, 1979a,b). The response consists of brief hesitation during orientation and analysis of stimulus significance in alert wakefulness (Lynn, 1966), but complete atonia during the tonic unrestrained activation of PS or the hypotonia of tonic immobility (Carli, 1969) when prey animals suddenly encounter a predator at close range (Ratner, 1967). The "final common pathway" from the brainstem for the inhibition of spinal motor neurons would presumably be the caudal medullary inhibitory area (Magoun and Rhines, 1946), which contains neurons capable of inhibiting motor neurons monosynaptically (Peterson, 1979). Recognition of a brainstem linkage between reticular activation and modulation of motor output in wakefulness permits one to view the coupling of extreme tonic activation evidenced by EEG desynchronization and constant PGO spike occurrence with atonia during PS as a natural development of that state. Atonia does not occur so that, in the teleological sense, individuals cannot act out their dreams, which could lead to physical harm; rather, atonia is merely a by-product of a central activity state characterized by excessive reticular activation.

The change from PS to alert wakefulness in normal cats is a profound one in behavioral sense. Essentially, total skeletal muscle paralysis is abruptly reversed; the eyes open, the nictitating membranes retract, the totally miotic pupils widen, and the animal reacts quickly and precisely to stimuli presented to it. Yet the EEG remains essentially the same. Neuronal organization studied at the single cell level, though, is obviously different. Various studies (Steriade and Hobson, 1976) have shown that neurons in different regions tend to fire in long, high-frequency bursts interrupted by periods of silence, unlike in wakefulness. Neurons in particular regions, namely dorsal raphe neurons (Cespuglio et al., 1978a; McGinty and Harper, 1976; Trulson and

Jacobs, 1978) and the caudal locus coeruleus (Hobson et al., 1975) cease firing altogether. Exploration of other areas may well reveal more of the latter type. Thus, the neuronal organization of the brain is quite different when one compares the states of alert wakefulness and PS, even though the EEG patterns are similar and quite complex mental activity, in the form of dreams, occurs in the latter state in humans. Yet, cognitive processing related to events in the external world has been demonstrated to be, at best, at a very low level during PS in humans (Perry et al., 1978); and in spite of the remarkable motor capabilities of cats in PS without atonia, they exhibit greatly reduced awareness. One can only wonder at the location(s) of the switch(es) that reorganizes the nervous system of the organism in PS almost instantly into one capable of the associative learning during attentive wakefulness. That subject is treated in Dr. Weinberger's chapter.

The change from slow-wave sleep to wakefulness is apparently even more profound. In humans, induced awakenings from PS result in performance on a choice reaction-time test not significantly different from waking; they usually lack behavioral confusion and lead to almost immediate reversions of the visual evoked potential to the waking waveform (Broughton, 1975). Arousals from stages 3 and 4 (the deeper stages) of slow-wave sleep, on the other hand, are characterized by varying degrees of confusion, long reaction times that return to working levels only after several minutes, and a parallel slow reversion of the visual evoked potential to the pre-sleep waveform.

SLOW WAVE SLEEP

If the basic cyclicity of PS is expressed by the lower brainstem, just as surely regulation of the onset and maintenance of slow wave sleep is a function of a much wider spectrum of brain structures. This is consonant with the quotation from Parmeggiani (1968). A contrasting viewpoint that stresses the primary role of the brainstem is presented in a review by Jouvet (1972). In this review, involvement of brainstem monoaminergic systems in the regulation of sleep and wakefulness is analyzed and the conclusion is drawn that the serotonergic brainstem raphe neurons play an active primary role in the institution of the slow-wave sleep state and serve a "priming" function in PS onset. These ideas, which have had considerable influence on current thinking about sleep, are based on experiments which have shown that lesions of the raphe nuclei produce insomnia as does administration of serotonin-depleting drugs (Jouvet, 1972). Insomnia is not permanent, however, so that other systems must be involved in the production and maintenance of slow-wave sleep. The picture is further clouded by the fact that dorsal raphe neuronal firing is lower in slow wave sleep than in wakefulness (Cespuglio et al., 1978a; McGinty and Harper, 1976; Trulson and Jacobs, 1978), and localized cooling of this nucleus produced both cortical synchronization and PGO spikes, which is not typical of slow-wave sleep (Cespuglio et al., 1978b). In the nuclei raphe medianus and magnus, Sheu et al. (1974) found lower firing rates in slow-wave sleep than in wakefulness, and Cespuglio et al. (1978a) reported only slight increases in medianus. In view of the many reports of sensitization to various stimuli and enhancement of behaviors during wakefulness as a result of serotonin depletion, McGinty and Harper (1976) proposed that serotonin constrains waking responses and activities that interfere with sleep. The weight of evidence favors this latter view rather than the one (Jouvet, 1972) that states that the raphe serotonergic system generates slow-wave sleep. This conclusion forces us to look further for additional mechanisms which might actively promote sleep onset.

Insomnia has been produced by rostral hypothalamic transections in rats (Nauta, 1946) and preoptic-basal forebrain electrolytic lesions in cats (McGinty and Sterman, 1968). Caudal hypothalamic lesions result in a lethargic syndrome in a variety of species, which can be distinguished from coma because such preparations can be aroused briefly by stimuli and then exhibit some of the preparatory signs of sleep, such as yawning and assuming a comfortable posture (Moruzzi, 1972). A counterpoint to the insomnia-producing effects of preoptic basal forebrain lesions (McGinty and Sterman, 1968) is the report that bilateral basal forebrain stimulation produces EEG synchronization and behavioral signs of drowsiness and sleep with either high or low rates of stimulation and at relatively short latencies (Sterman and Clemene, 1962). In his extensive reveiw Moruzzi (1972) concluded that the sleep-wakefulness rhythm is basic to the hypothalamic area of the brain; because even the chronic "cerveau isole" cat transected through the rostral midbrain (Villablanca, 1965) exhibits alternating periods of cortical synchronization and desynchronization and arousal responses to olfactory stimulation unlike the acute "cerveau isole" (Bremer, 1935). Moruzzi (1972) suggests that the brainstem's role is one of tonic and phasic activation.

If, however, one observes the behavior organized by the structures caudal to a precollicular transection, a high decerebrate preparation, one notes postural and ocular signs of slow wave sleep although the cats tend to collapse in random positions and the pupils of the eyes exhibit fluctuating miosis. The eyelids and nictitating membranes close, however, and the pupils respond with mydriasis to sounds. Periods of extreme miosis and other motoric signs of PS also occur (Villablanca, 1966a). In the previous section it was noted that low decerebrate preparations exhibit peripheral signs of PS as well (Jouvet, 1962; Villablanca, 1966a).

The foregoing forces one to the conclusion, much like that of Villablanca (1966a), that neuronal assemblies in various combinations throughout the extent of the brain are capable of organizing shifts between at least two central activity states, which differ considerably from one another and which resemble what one normally recognizes as sleep and wakefulness to a greater or lesser extent depending upon the degree of behavior the preparation can express. For example, the desynchronized EEG periods of the isolated cerebrum are much more believable as periods of conscious wakefulness if the transection is at the pontomesencephalic junction, so that the preparation can exhibit pupillary dilation during spontaneous EEG activation or with olfactory stimulation (Batsel, 1964; Villablanca, 1966b), or in the pons (the pretrigeminal preparation), so that ocular tracking and visual accomodation occurs (Moruzzi, 1972). Although the high decerebrate cat can express postural and motor criteria of sleep which the "cerveau isole" cannot, its collapse in place lacks the refinement of normal sleep behavior, which includes a search for and often a preparation of a sleeping place, drowsiness, and finally sleep (Parmeggiani, 1968). The decerebrate cat obviously shows a change in activity states, but what can one say about a change in consciousness in such a preparation?

SLEEP, HIBERNATION, AND TEMPERATURE REGULATION

Although sleep and hibernation resemble each other superficially, hibernation is clearly far from sleep in the spectrum of central activity states. Indeed, its apparent reason for being, enforced conservation of energy in homeothermic mammals, dictates a low level of activity in any body system. The nervous system is no exception, as Beckman and Stanton discuss in their chapter. Yet, neural regulation is an absolute necessity for normal entrance into, maintenance of, and arousal from hibernation. At the center of central nervous control of hibernation is the limbic system, particularly the hypothalamus and hippocampus (Beckman and Stanton, this volume). Lowering of body temperature occurs precipitously rather than in modulated steps if the hypothalamus is damaged (Weidler et al., 1974). Also, when the hypothalamus is lesioned, the hibernator is unable to arouse from hibernation and eventually dies while still in torpor (Satinoff, 1970). Although neural activity is essentially absent in vast areas of the brain, the limbic system continues to exhibit low amplitude EEG activity (Beckman, 1978).

In spite of the considerable differences between hibernation and sleep, common ground can be found in the subject of temperature regulation. During each sleep cycle, i.e., from the onset of slow-wave sleep to the termination of the subsequent PS episode, brain temperature follows a predictable course. Temperature falls during slow-wave sleep only to rise again during PS (Parmeggiani, 1977).

Heller and Glotzbach (1977) have suggested that slow-wave sleep and hibernation may be physiologically homologous. They cite evidence that indicates that hibernation begins while the animals are in slow-wave sleep. However, the electrographic pattern soon becomes so reduced in amplitude that this criterion can no longer be used for a point of comparison; in addition, brain temperature drops below the level of normal sleep. The lowering of body temperature that does occur in slow-wave sleep is dependent upon a resetting of central neural controls at a lower level of thermosensitivity, which is characteristic of hibernation, albeit in a much more dramatic fashion. These observations support the suggestion by many (cf. Heller and Glotzbach, 1977) that slow-wave sleep develops for energy conservation. Heller and Glotzbach (1977) view hibernation as a specialized development growing out of a need for lower and lower body temperatures during slow-wave sleep in order to conserve energy, particularly in smaller homeotherms.

Standing apart from these relationships is the peculiar case of PS. Temperature regulation is lacking, so that mammals are essentially poikilothermic whenever they enter this state (Parmeggiani, 1977). This conclusion has been reached on the basis of a variety of data. The work of Parmeggiani and his colleagues (1977) has shown that in cats, shivering ceases at low ambient temperatures before atonia is fully developed and panting is no longer evident at PS onset. Hypothalamic heating, which caused polypnea during slow-wave sleep, had no effect on respiration in PS; only strong heating produced a mild increase in respiratory rate (Parmeggiani et al., 1973). Also, sweating in humans is inhibited (Ogawa et al., 1967). In another species, kangaroo rats, metabolic heat production responses to hypothalamic cooling were lacking during REM sleep (Glotzbach and Heller, 1976). Finally, when maintained in a cool ambient temperature (15°C), cats exhibiting PS without atonia cease shivering, they leave their tightly curled posture and their piloerection subsides. These are profound changes, in view of the fact that these features characterize cat behavior during wakefulness and slow-wave sleep. Hypothalamic temperature, however, follows the same course as in normal cats. Such animals can have almost total postural support so that they should be capable of shivering (Hendricks et al., 1977). Whether the lack of thermoregulation during PS is an example of a behaviorally "meaningless" condition during this state or whether it can be woven into a pattern with the extreme reticular activation remains to be seen.

CONCLUDING REMARKS

This paper has discussed central activity states with the sleep-wakefulness cycle serving as the focal point. This cycle occurs several times during the day and offers the opportunity to study the manner in which the central nervous system organizes fairly dramatic state changes which may bear upon the study of other state changes, such as hibernation. We have not touched on studies of meditative states. Although such studies are frought with technical difficulties (Davidson, 1976), meditative states will quite likely find a legitimate place in the spectrum of brain activity states and may prove to have therapeutic value (Gellhorn and Kiely, 1972). Finally, it is well to note that resolution of the problems of reviving individuals from abnormal state, such as sommolence and coma, and of treating some psychoses depends upon advances in our knowledge of the state-switching and state-maintaining mechanisms in the brain.

ACKNOWLEDGEMENTS

My students, Joan Hendricks, Graziella Mann, and Peter Reiner, assisted greatly in the development of this paper with their keen observations, provocative questions, and bibliographic assistance. I also wish to acknowledge the administrative assistance of my secretary, Caren Greisman. Financial support was provided by N.I.H. Grant, NS 13110.

REFERENCES

Aserinsky, E., and Kleitman, N. Regularly occurring periods of eye mobility, and concomitant phenomena during sleep. *Science* 118, 273–274 (1953).

Bard, P., and Macht, M.B. The behavior of chronically decerebrate cats, in *Neurologic Basis of Behavior,* G.E.W. Wolstenholme and C.M. O'Connor, eds. Little, Brown, Boston (1958), pp. 55–75.

Batsel, H.L. Spontaneous desynchronization in the chronic cat "cerveau isole." *Arch. Ital. Biol.* 102, 547–566 (1964).

Beckman, A.L. Hypothalamic and midbrain function during hibernation, in *Current Studies of Hypothalamic Function 1978*, W.L. Veale and K. Lederis, eds. Karger, Basel (1978), pp. 29–43.

Bowker, R.M. The biological significance of eye movement potentials of wakefulness and the PGO spikes of sleep, Unpublished Ph.D. thesis, University of Pennsylvania (1979).

Bowker, R.M., and Morrison, A.R. The startle reflex and PGO spikes. *Brain Res.* 102, 185–190 (1976).

Bowker, R.M., and Morrison, A.R. The PGO spike: an indicator of hyper-alertness, in *Sleep Research—1976*, W.P. Koella and P. Levin, eds. Karger, Basel (1977), pp. 23–27.

Bremer, J. "Cerveau isole" et physiologie du sommeil. *C.R. Soc. Biol.* 118, 1235–1241 (1935).

Broughton, R.J. Biorhythmic variations in consciousness and psychological functions. *Canad. Psychol. Rev.* 217–239 (1975).

Carli, G. Dissociation of electrocortical activity and somatic reflexes during rabbit hypnosis. *Arch. Ital. Biol.* 107, 219–234 (1969).

Carli, G., and Zanchetti, A. A study of pontine lesions suppressing deep sleep in the cat. *Arch. Ital. Biol.* 103, 751–788 (1965).
Cespuglio, R., Gomez, M.-E., Walker, E., and Jouvet, M. Single unit recordings of the nuclei raphe dorsalis and magnus during sleep-waking cycle. *Sleep Res.* 7, 26 (1978a).
Cespuglio, R., Gomez, M.-E., Walker, E., and Jouvet, M. Effect of localized cooling of the raphe nuclei upon the sleep-waking cycle of the cat. *Sleep Res.* 7, 27 (1978b).
Davidson, J.M. The physiology of meditation and mystical states of consciousness. *Perspect. Biol. Med.* 19, 345–381 (1976).
Dement, W., and Kleitman, N. Cyclic variations of EEG during sleep and their relation to eye movements, body motility, and dreaming. *Electroenceph. Clin. Neurophysiol.* 9, 673–690 (1957).
Gassel, M.M., Marchiafava, P.L., and Pompeiano, O. An analysis of supraspinal influences acting on motoneurons during sleep in the unrestrained cat. Modification of the recurrent discharge of the alpha motoneurons during sleep. *Arch. Ital. Biol.* 103, 25–44 (1965).
Gellhorn, E., and Kiely, W.F. Mystical states of consciousness: Neurophysiological and clinical aspects. *J. Nerv. Ment. Dis.* 154, 339–405 (1972).
Glotzbach, S.F., and Heller, H.C. Central nervous regulation of body temperature during sleep. *Science* 194, 537–539 (1976).
Heller, H.C., and Glotzbach, S.F. Thermoregulation during sleep and hibernation. *Int. Rev. Physiol.* 15, 147–187 (1977).
Hendricks, J.C., Bowker, R.M., and Morrison, A.R. Functional characteristics of cats with pontine lesions during sleep and their usefulness for sleep research, in *Sleep Research — 1976,* W.P. Koella and P. Levin, eds. Karger, Basel (1977), pp. 207–210.
Henley, K., and Morrison, A.R. A re-evaluation of the effects of lesions of the pontine tegmentum and locus coeruleus on phenomena of paradoxical sleep in the cat. *Acta Neurobiol. Exper.* 34, 215–232 (1974).
Hobson, J.A., McCarley, R.W., and Wyzinski, P.W. Sleep cycle oscillation: reciprocal discharge by two brain stem neuronal groups. *Science* 189, 55–58 (1975).
Jones, B.E., Harper, S.T., and Halaris, A.E. Effects of locus coeruleus lesions upon cerebral monoamine content, sleep wakefulness states and the response to amphetamine in the cat. *Brain Res.* 124, 472–496 (1977).
Jouvet, M. Recherches sur les structures nerveuses et les mecanismes responsables des differentes phases du sommeil physioligique. *Arch. Ital. Biol.* 100, 125–206 (1962).
Jouvet, M. Neurophysiology of the states of sleep. *Physiol. Rev.* 47, 117–177 (1967).
Jouvet, M. The role of monoamines and acetylcholine-containing neurons in the regulation of the sleep-waking cycle, in *Ergebnisse der Physiologie: Neurophysiology and Neurochemistry of Sleep and Wakefulness,* Springer-Verlag, New York (1972), pp. 64, 96–117.
Jouvet, M., and Delorme, F. Locus coeruleus et sommeil paradoxal. *C.R. Soc. Biol.* 159, 895–899 (1965).
Lindsley, D.B., Schreiner, L.H., Knowles, W.B., and Magoun, H.W. Behavioral and EEG changes following chronic brain stem lesions in the cat. *Electroenceph. Clin. Neurophysiol.* 10, 483–498 (1950).
Lynn, R. *Attention, Arousal and the Orientation Reaction,* Pergamon, Oxford (1966), pp. 1–118.
Magoun, H.W., and Rhines, R. An inhibitory mechanism in the bulbar reticular formation. *J. Neurophysiol.* 9, 165–171 (1946).
McGinty, D.J., and Harper, R.M. Dorsal raphe neurons: depression of firing during sleep in cats. *Brain Res.* 101, 560–575 (1976).
McGinty, D.J., and Sterman, M.B. Sleep supression after basal forebrain lesions in the cat. *Science* 160, 1253–1255 (1968).
Morrison, A.R. Brainstem regulation of behavior during sleep and wakefulness. *Prog. Psychobiol. Physiol. Psychol..* 8, 91–131 (1979a).

Morrison, A.R. Relationships between phenomena of paradoxical sleep and their counterparts in wakefulness. *Acta Neurobiol. Exper.* 39, 567–583 (1979b).

Morrison, A.R., and Pompeiano, O. An analysis of supraspinal influences acting on motoneurons during sleep in the unrestrained cat. Responses of the alpha motoneurons to direct electrical stimulation during sleep. *Arch. Ital. Biol.* 103, 497–516 (1965).

Moruzzi, G. The sleep-waking cycle, in *Ergebnisse der Physiologie: Neurophysiology and Neurochemistry of Sleep and Wakefulness*, Springer-Verlag, Berlin (1972), pp. 64, 1–165.

Moruzzi, G., and Magoun, H.W. Brainstem reticular formation and activation of the EEG. *Electroenceph. Clin. Neurophysiol.* 1, 455–473 (1949).

Nauta, W.J.H. Hypothalamic regulation of sleep in rats. Experimental study. *J. Neurophysiol.* 9, 285–316 (1946).

Ogawa, T., Satoh, T., and Takagi, K. Sweating during night sleep. *Jap. J. Physiol.* 17, 135–148 (1967).

Parmeggiani, P.L. Telencephalo-diencephalic aspects of sleep mechanisms. *Brain Res.* 7, 350–359 (1968).

Parmeggiani, P.L. Interaction between sleep and thermoregulation. *Waking and Sleeping* 1, 123–132 (1977).

Parmeggiani, P.L., Franzini, C., Lenzi, P., and Zamboni, G. Threshold of respiratory responses to preoptic heating during sleep in freely moving cats. *Brain Res.* 52, 189–201 (1973).

Perry, C.W., Evans, F.J., O'Connell, D.N., Orne, E.C., and Orne, M.T. Behavioral response to verbal stimuli administered during REM sleep: a further investigation. *Waking and Sleeping* 2, 35–42 (1978).

Peterson, B.W. Reticulospinal projections to spinal motor nuclei. *Ann. Rev. Physiol.* 41, 127–140 (1979).

Pompeiano, O. Mechanisms responsible for spinal inhibition during desynchronized sleep: experimental study, in *Narcolepsy—Advances in Sleep Research 3*, C. Guilleminault, W.C. Dement, and P. Passouant, eds. Spectrum, New York (1976), pp. 411–449.

Ratner, S.C. Comparative aspects of hypnosis, in *Handbook of Clinical and Experimental Hypnosis*, J.E. Gordon, ed. MacMillan, New York (1967), pp. 550–587.

Satinoff, E. Hibernation and the central nervous system. *Prog. Physiol. Psychol.* 3, 201–236 (1970).

Sheu, Y.-S., Nelson, J.P., and Bloom, F.E. Discharge patterns of cat raphe neurons during sleep and waking. *Brain Res.* 73, 263–276 (1974).

Shik, M.L., and Orlovsky, G.N. Neurophysiology of locomotor automatism. *Physiol. Rev.* 56, 476–501 (1976).

Siegel, J.M., McGinty, D.J., and Breedlove, S.M. Sleep and waking activity of pontine gigantocellular field neurons. *Exp. Neurol.* 56, 553–573 (1977).

Simon, R.P., Gershon, M.D., and Brooks, D.C. The role of raphe nuclei in the regulation of ponto-geniculo-occipital wave activity. *Brain Res.* 58, 313–330 (1973).

Sprague, J.M. The effects of chronic brainstem lesions on wakefulness, sleep and behavior. *Res. Publ. Assoc. Nerv. Ment. Dis.* 45, 148–188 (1967).

Steriade, M., and Hobson, J.A. Neuronal activity during the sleep-waking cycle. *Prog. Neurobiol.* 6, 155–376 (1976).

Sterman, M.B., and Clemente, C.D. Forebrain inhibitory mechanisms: sleep patterns induced by basal forebrain stimulation in the behaving cat. *Exp. Neurol.* 6, 103–117 (1962).

Trulson, M.E., and Jacobs, B.L. Raphe unit activity in freely moving cats: correlation with level of behavioral arousal. *Brain Res.* 163, 135–150 (1978).

Vertes, R. Selective firing of rat pontine gigantocellular neurons during movement and REM sleep. *Brain Res.* 128, 146–152 (1977).

Villablanca, J. The electrocorticogram in the chronic "cerveau isole" cat. *Electroenceph. Clin. Neurophysiol.* 19, 576–586 (1965)

Villablanca, J. Behavioral and polygraphic study of "sleep" and "wakefulness" in chronic decerebrate cats. *Electroenceph. Clin. Neurophysiol.* 21, 562–577 (1966a).

Villablanca, J. Ocular behavior in the chronic "cerveau isole" cat. *Brian Res.* 2, 99–102 (1966b).

Weidler, D.J., Earle, A.M., Myers, G.G., and Sieck, G.C. Effect of hypothalamic lesions on temperature regulation in hibernating ground squirrels. *Brain Res.* 65, 175–179 (1974).

Copyright © 1982, Spectrum Publications, Inc.
The Neural Basis of Behavior

2

Properties of the CNS During the State of Hibernation

Alexander L. Beckman
Toni L. Stanton

INTRODUCTION

Studies of the properties of the central nervous system (CNS) during hibernation can contribute significantly to the development of our concepts and understanding of the characteristics of central activity states and how they are controlled. This is true for two reasons. First, the hibernating mammalian brain is in a profound state of natural depression and thereby establishes the lower end of the continuum of mammalian brain activity levels. Second, the hibernator displays all the central activity states characteristic of the mammalian brain during its non-hibernating (i.e., euthermic) phase, thereby providing a single model system that is capable of describing the full range of mammalian CNS activity states. Not surprisingly, this wide range of neuronal activity is accompanied by an equally wide behavioral range, extending from the profound inactivity (torpor) of deep hibernation to the complex behavioral patterns observed during euthermia. Determining the properties of CNS function during hibernation and while making the transition between hibernation and euthermia should, therefore, yield important insights into how the brain controls its level of activation. Further, these studies should broaden our understanding of how particular CNS-mediated behavioral and regulatory functions are linked to this control.

GENERAL FEATURES OF MAMMALIAN HIBERNATION

In order to discuss CNS function during hibernation within a more complete perspective, it is worthwhile to consider some of the salient, general features of mammalian hibernation. This is by no means intended to be a comprehensive review of the physiology of hibernation, which is well treated in the literature (Heller, 1979; Hudson and Wang, 1979; Kayser, 1961; Lyman and Chatfield, 1955; Satinoff, 1970; Willis, 1979). Easily, the most apparent and dramatic manifestation of the hibernating state is the striking reduction of body temperature and metabolic rate that commences with the entrance into hibernation and reaches maximum depression during deep hibernation. It is so characteristic a feature that we commonly identify the departure of the euthermic state by the commencement of the fall in these two variables. Thus, whereas during euthermia internal temperature is regulated at approximately 38°C, comparable to that of all other non-hibernating mammals, during hibernation it decreases to levels that closely approach ambient temperature which, under natural conditions, can fall to near 0°C (Wang, 1978). The parallel decline in metabolic rate is equally impressive. For example, in the golden-mantled ground squirrel (*Citellus lateralis*), metabolic rate falls from euthermic values of approximately 0.2 cal/gm/min (Heller et al., 1974) to just 0.002 cal/gm/min during deep hibernation (Hammel et al., 1968; Heller and Colliver, 1974).

In view of this, it is reasonable to assume that a major advantage of the ability to hibernate is the saving of metabolic energy stores. This has been affirmed by Wang (1978), who showed that the total energy consumption of hibernating animals, including that expended during the periodic spontaneous arousals that occur throughout the hibernation season, was 87 percent less than that required by animals who remained euthermic throughout the same period. The value of this energy conserving adaptation is obvious and is an especially impressive strategy for survival when viewed within the context of the natural habitat during winter. It is dominated by two major features, namely, a very scarce food supply and a very low ambient temperature. The latter feature is used to full advantage to counter the challenge of the former, as shown by experiments demonstrating that the energy savings afforded by hibernation increases as ambient temperature falls from 21°C to the low levels normally encountered in the burrow (Baldwin and Johnson, 1941).

The ability to spontaneously increase metabolic rate and body temperature during hibernation despite persisting low ambient temperature, thereby returning to the euthermic state, is an additional characteristic feature of hibernation in mammals. During the hibernation season, these spontaneous arousals occur regularly, so that periods of hibernation are divided into a series of contiguous bouts separated by short intervals [typically 24 hours or less (Torke and Twente, 1977)] of euthermia. The timing of the bouts is cyclical over the season, such that with the onset of the hibernation season in fall, the duration of each bout is short (approximately 2–4 days in *C. lateralis*). The bout length gradually increases to a maximum of 8–12 days by the end of January and then begins to shorten, so that the concluding bouts in early spring once again last 2–4 days (unpublished observations).

During the winter season, therefore, the hibernator cycles in and out of hibernation, with the basic features of each bout being essentially the same. Entrance into hibernation lasts approximately 6–15 hours (Kayser, 1961), during which all physiological parameters gradually decline. In parallel with the reduction of internal temperature and metabolic rate, heart and respiratory rates decline from resting euthermic values of approximately 200 beats/minute and 150 respirations/minute to hibernating values of less than 10 beats, and approximately one or fewer breaths, per minute in ground squirrels (Landau and Dawe, 1958: Steffen and Riedesel, 1979). The level of activity in the CNS also declines dramatically, as indicated by widespread suppression of cortical and subcortical electroencephalographic (EEG) activity during deep torpor (Chatfield et al., 1951; Kayser and Malan, 1963; Shtark, 1970; Strumwasser, 1959b). These conditions remain stable during deep hibernation and then increase to euthermic values during the 2–3 hour period of arousal from hibernation.

Under the natural conditions of hibernation, with internal temperature near 0°C, and heart and respiratory rate at extraordinarily low levels, the hibernator appears outwardly lifeless. Yet, it retains considerable sensitivity and responsiveness to changes in the internal and external environment, clearly indicating the functional integrity of cellular mechanisms in general (Hudson and Wang, 1979; Willis, 1979) and of central and peripheral neuronal mechanisms in particular (Kayser and Malan, 1963; Lyman and O'Brien, 1972; Strumwasser, 1959b; Twente and Twente, 1968).

The maintenance of physiological integrity at such low body temperature clearly requires structural and functional specialization. Neural tissue of hibernators shows greatly increased functional capability at low temperatures over that of non-hibernators. *In vitro* studies comparing hamster and rat tibial nerves showed that hamster nerves (from both hibernating or euthermic animals) continued to conduct action potentials down to 3°C whereas rat nerve failed at 9°C (Chatfield et al., 1948). In both preparations, cooling diminished action potential amplitude, conduction velocity, and excitability in a linear fashion, but these variables decreased at a slower rate in hamsters. Similarly, although cooling increased the duration of the absolute and relative refractory periods for both animals, the effect was less so in hamsters (Chatfield et al., 1948). Peripheral nerve function in ground squirrels (*C. tridecemlineatus*) was comparable to that of hamsters, although nerves from hibernating ground squirrels were excitable at lower temperatures than those from euthermic animals (Kehl and Morrison, 1960).

Synaptic transmission, as demonstrated in peripheral tissues, also maintains functional integrity in hibernators at the low temperatures commonly encountered in deep torpor. Thus, in the phrenic nerve-diaphragm preparation, synaptic transmission in euthermic and hibernating hamsters continued at temperatures of 10° and 5°C, respectively, while that from rats failed at 10°C (South, 1961). In other experiments on hibernating and euthermic hamsters, using the phrenic nerve-diaphragm preparation at a temperature of 20–23°C, the number of acetylcholine (ACh) quanta in the immediately available store of the nerve terminals was found to be the same for animals in each state (Melichar et al., 1973), as was the rate of mobilization of transmitter from the reserve store. Hibernating animals, however, yielded a lower number of ACh quanta in the reserve store, a smaller quantum content of the end-plate potentials, and a lower constant of transmitter synthesis during prolonged stimulation (Melichar et al., 1973).

It is intriguing to consider the possible adaptations that might underlie the remarkable ability of both excitable and non-excitable tissue of hibernators to function at such low temperatures. One current view is that the physical state of cell membranes in hibernators retains its fluid nature at lower temperatures than in non-hibernators, the latter undergoing a lipid phase transition from a more fluid liquid-crystalline form to a more rigid crystalline form at temperatures above the normal range of deep hibernation (Charnock, 1978; Willis, 1979). Such a phase transition would have profound detrimental effects (i.e., increase of activation energy) on the low temperature function of particular enzyme systems, such as those involved in glucose utilization, oxidative phosphorylation, and membrane cation transport (Charnock, 1978; Charnock and Simonson, 1978; Willis, 1979). In this context, it is interesting to note that ground squirrels (*C. lateralis*) undergo a shift in mitochondrial membrane phase transition temperature from 23°C during the euthermic season to below 4°C during the hibernation season (Hudson and Wang, 1979; Willis, 1979).

As noted, improved low temperature membrane fluidity characteristics would aid membrane-bound enzyme systems. Accordingly, Na-K ATPase in hibernating hamster brain exhibits a lower temperature coefficient than that from euthermic animals (Goldman and Albers, 1975), an adaptation that likely results in an improvement in the transport of Na^+ and K^+ across nerve cell membrane at lowered temperature (Goldman and Willis, 1973). Clearly, continued regulation of membrane ion gradients during hibernation is a prime requisite of normal cellular function. Another example of this is found in the red blood cells of ground squirrels. The Na^+–K^+ pump is less inhibited by cooling, and the passive flux of K^+ is more reduced by cooling in these hibernators compared to a non-hibernator (guinea pig) (Willis, 1979).

From the foregoing discussion, it is clear that mammalian hibernation is a highly organized, complex event. As noted, it is a circannual rhythm which has been demonstrated in numerous investigations to be phase-locked with annual cycles of other variables, including sexual behavior, body weight, and behavioral activity (Heller and Poulson, 1970; Mrosovsky, 1978; Pengelley et al., 1976). In the obligate hibernators, exemplified by the golden-mantled ground squirrel, endogenous mechanisms appear to exert predominant control over the timing of these cycles, whereas environmental factors such as photoperiod or temperature are of clear importance in permissive hibernators, such as the edible dormouse (*Glis glis*) (Mrosovsky, 1978).

The internally determined circannual nature of the hibernation season in obligate hibernators suggests that a hormonal mechanism must mediate this long-term process. The work of Dawe and Spurrier (1969, 1972, 1974; Dawe et al., 1979) offers support for this view. They first reported that blood obtained and handled under carefully controlled conditions from winter hibernating animals (woodchucks or ground squirrels) could induce hibernation following injection into euthermic ground squirrels. Blood obtained from winter euthermic animals failed to duplicate these results. Initial attempts to characterize this proposed hibernation-inducing trigger point to an albumin-bound molecule, perhaps a small peptide, whose molecular weight is 5000 daltons or more (Oeltgen et al., 1978). A great deal of further work is needed to complete the identification of this substance (or complex of substances) and to determine its mode of action.

Whereas the seasonal nature of hibernation suggests hormonal control, the timing of the individual hibernation bouts during the season, which last from a few to several days and are separated from each other by euthermic intervals of a few to several hours, must reflect the operation of a short-term neuronal control mechanism. The balance of this chapter will examine some aspects of this neural control. Specifically, we will discuss the elementary information available on what appears to happen in the CNS to cause entrance into hibernation, what is currently known of the functional characteristics of the CNS during this most depressed of central activity states and, finally, what triggers the transition from the hibernating to the active state.

ENTRANCE INTO HIBERNATION: CNS CONTROL

Entrance into hibernation begins during sleep, with the early phase of entry being dominated by slow wave sleep; the periods of slow wave sleep can be interrupted briefly by short periods of paradoxical sleep or wakefulness (Heller and Glotzbach, 1977; South et al., 1969). As the entry progresses below internal temperatures of 25°C, further analysis of sleep state becomes difficult due to the reduction in the amplitude of the EEG (Walker et al., 1977).

Current evidence clearly indicates that the entrance is controlled by the CNS and suggests that this control is manifest by an increase in central inhibitory level. For example, as already mentioned, heart and respiratory rates are depressed during hibernation; however, the decline in the rate of these two variables is not a wholly passive event resulting from the fall in T_b because it is evident during euthermia, prior to any significant decrease in T_b (Lyman, 1958; Strumwasser, 1959a).

In a similar fashion, the amplitude of the EEG also begins to decline before any significant fall in T_b occurs (Wunnenberg et al., 1978). As the entrance into hibernation progresses, further decreases in the amplitude (Shtark, 1970; Strumwasser, 1959a; Walker et al., 1977) and changes in the frequency distribution (Shtark, 1970; South et al., 1969) of the EEG occur with the decline in T_b. Some observations suggest that suppression of EEG activity can take an anatomically stepwise course, being first evident in the cerebral cortex, followed by the midbrain reticular formation (MRF), thalamus, and lastly in areas of the limbic system, notably in the hippocampus and hypothalamus (Shtark, 1970).

Additional evidence for a controlled entry is provided by studies of the CNS regulator of body temperature. During entrance into hibernation, the threshold hypothalamic temperature for activating an increase in metabolic rate was demonstrable at all times, but at increasingly lower levels (Florant et al., 1978; Heller et al., 1977). During smooth entries, the threshold progressively declined so that it remained below actual hypothalamic temperature at all times (Florant et al., 1978; Heller et al., 1977).

DEEP HIBERNATION: CNS EXCITABILITY

Once the animal achieves the resting state of hibernation, the level of electrical activity appears similar to that of the entry phase in that the cortex remains electrically depressed except for varying periods of EEG activity (Shtark, 1970; South et al., 1969; Walker et al., 1977). Likewise, the MRF remains silent for long periods of time that are punctuated by short bursts of spiking activity (Shtark, 1970; South et al., 1969; Strumwasser, 1959b). By contrast, the limbic system (notably the hippocampus, septum, and hypothalamus) displays nearly continuous EEG activity throughout the hibernation bout (Shtark, 1970; South et al., 1969; Strumwasser, 1959b).

This characteristic of limbic structures, contrasted with relative electrical silence in cortical and midbrain areas, has prompted suggestions (South et al., 1972; Beckman and Stanton, 1976) that the proposed increase in central inhibitory level accompanying the transition from the euthermic state to the hibernating mode (Hammel et al., 1973; Luecke and South, 1972) is controlled by neurons within the limbic system. We have adopted this as a working hypotheses in our studies. Taking note of the heavy descending connections between the limbic forebrain structures and the MRF (Crosby et al., 1962; Nauta and Domesick, this volume), some of which are known to be inhibitory in nature (Wang and Aghajanian, 1977; Rabii et al., 1976), we (Beckman and Stanton, 1976) postulated that the MRF would exhibit functional depression during deep hibernation.

In order to test this hypothesis, we implanted bilateral cannula guides into the MRF of euthermic California golden mantled ground squirrels (*C. lateralis*) during late fall to early winter (Beckman and Stanton, 1976). Following recovery from surgery, the animals were placed in a cold room maintained at 5°C wherein they entered hibernation. Following a series of undisturbed hibernation bouts, during which the length of the bouts were measured, individual animals were transferred to an experimental chamber (ambient temperature: 5°C) for study. The experimental protocol consisted of delivering a single, bilateral microinjection (1 μl per side) of ACh at a constant dose during each of the four quarters of the particular animal's current bout and measuring the thermogenic response evoked by each MRF microinjection. We measured changes in interscapular temperature and brain temperature (via a miniature thermistor mounted at the tip of one cannula guide). Interscapular temperature reflects heat production from the axillary brown fat deposits, which serve as a major source of heat during the arousal from hibernation (Hayward and Lyman, 1967; Smith and Horwitz, 1969), and brain temperature serves as a reliable index of internal temperature.

Figures 1 and 2 show two series of these experiments, each using a different concentration of ACh. They show that whereas the responsiveness of the MRF (as reflected by the magnitude of the evoked thermal response) is markedly depressed during hibernation, particularly during the early portions of the bout, it progressively increases as time in the bout elapses. A 200 μg ACh stimulus that evoked a small, transient response when delivered during the final stages of entry into hibernation (Fig. 1, top panel) triggered full arousal when delivered during the fourth quarter of the bout (Fig. 1, bottom panel). The thermal profile of these arousals and the behavior of the animals during the following arousal were comparable to natural, spontaneous arousals, indicating that MRF stimulation activated the natural neuronal trigger process for arousal from hibernation. In parallel with the increased magnitude of the evoked response, response latency decreased as time in the bout elapsed, further illustrating the increase in MRF responsiveness. Lower concentrations of ACh revealed the same profile of increas-

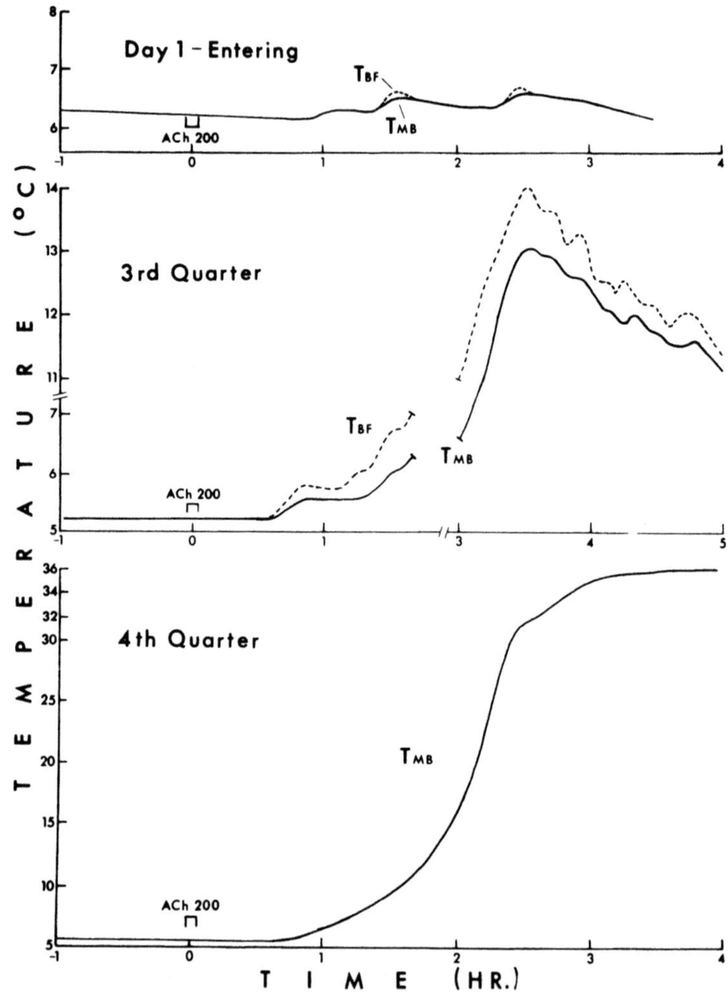

FIG. 1. Increasing responsiveness of MRF during progression of hibernation bout: thermogenic responses evoked by ACh (200 μg/ul). *Top panel*, final phase of entrance: ACh evoked a small magnitude response (0.3°C) with a slow (maximum rate: 0.02°C/min) and variable rising phase following a latency of 56 minutes. *Middle panel*, third quarter of bout: larger response (7.7°) with a smooth, rapidly rising phase (maximum rate: 0.12°C/min) was evoked following shorter latency of 35 minutes. T_{MB} increased continuously during interruption in record. *Bottom panel*, fourth quarter of bout: arousal from hibernation evoked following latency of 38 minutes. Note change in scale of ordinate. T_{MB}: midbrain temperature; T_{bf}: interscapular temperature near brown fat deposits. [From Beckman and Stanton, 1976.]

ing responsiveness (Fig. 2). The lowest concentration tested (50 μg/μl) failed to evoke any change in internal temperature during the first three quarters of the bout; during the fourth quarter, small transient increases in brain

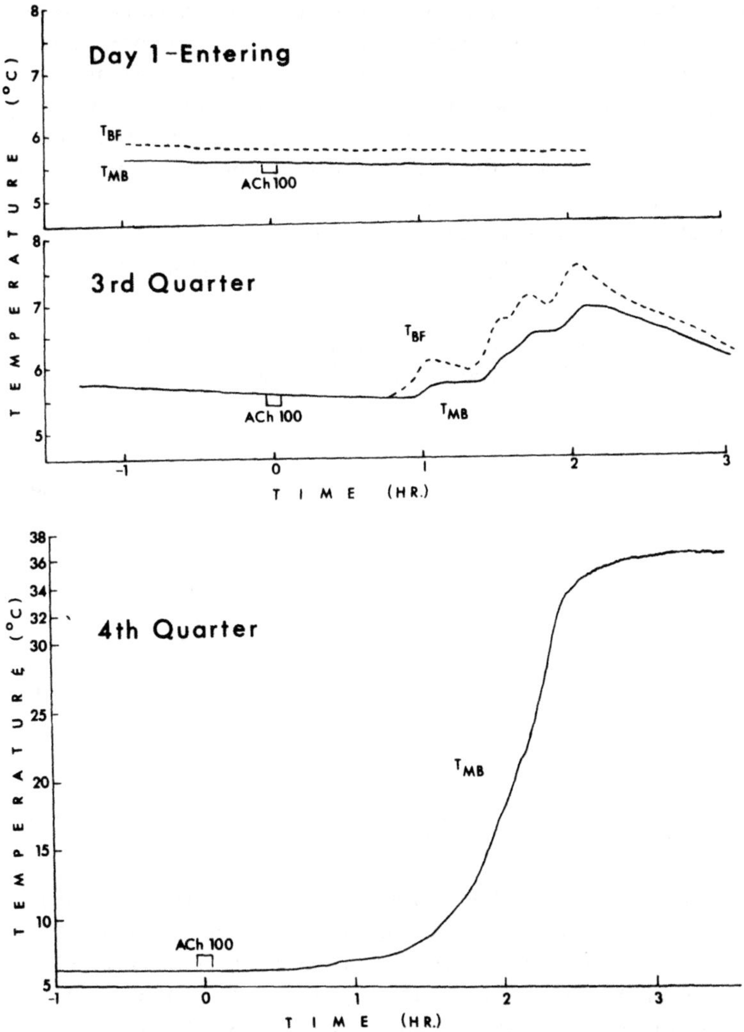

FIG. 2. Increasing responsiveness of MRF during progression of hibernation bout: thermogenic responses evoked by ACh (100 μg/ul). *Top panel*, final phase of entrance: ACh evoked no change in temperature. *Middle panel*, third quarter of bout: ACh evoked a small magnitude response (1.3°C) with a slow (maximum rate: 0.04°C/min) and variable rising phase following a latency of 58 minutes. *Bottom panel*, fourth quarter of bout: arousal from hibernation was evoked following a latency of 33 minutes. Note change of scale in ordinate. T_{MB} and T_{bf} as in Fig. 1. [From Beckman and Stanton, 1976.]

temperature averaging 0.2°C were evoked. Illustrating the overall decline in MRF responsiveness during hibernation, increases in internal temperature averaging 0.48°C were produced by 50 μg microinjections of ACh into the MRF during euthermia (Beckman and Stanton, 1976).

These data from hibernating animals, summarized in Table 1, were subjected to an analysis of covariance which showed that elapsed time in the bout was a significant variable across all treatments. Interestingly, elapsed time in the bout was also a significant treatment factor for control experiments with 0.9 percent NaCl, dramatically indicating that the progressive return in responsiveness in the CNS reached the point in the fourth quarter wherein MRF neurons were sufficiently sensitive to the ancillary effects of microinjection (e.g., transient decrease in pH and brief mechanical stimulation associated with volume change) to activate a thermogenic response.

Table 1. Changes in Temperature Following Chemical Stimulation in MRF during Hibernation

Stimulus	Quarter of Bout			
	First	*Second*	*Third*	*Fourth*
Isotonic saline	0 (2)	0 (2)	0 (3)	0.07 (3)
ACh, 50 μg	0 (2)	0 (3)	0 (2)	0.20 (2)
ACh, 100, μg	0 (3)	0.08 (4)	0.35 (4)	0.15 2 FA (4)
ACh, 200 μg	0.01 (3)	1.84 1 FA (5)	7.70 1 FA (2)	1 FA (1)

Temperatures are mean values, °C. Values in parentheses are number of observations. FA, full arousal. [From Beckman and Stanton, 1976.]

We believe that the initial dramatic decline in MRF responsiveness associated with entry into hibernation, followed by the progressive return in responsiveness during the bout, serves as a gating mechanism. This function would control the flow of input through the MRF that originates from peripheral sources and converges upon the MRF as it proceeds rostrally to innervate, among other structures, the hypothalamus and hippocampus.

The importance of such a mechanism to the maintenance of the bout is illustrated by subsequent experiments which have demonstrated that the hypothalamus, specifically the preoptic/anterior area (POA), and the hippocampus are more sensitive to direct chemical modulation than is the

MRF during hibernation, which renders these two structures much more potent sites for activating arousal from hibernation (Stanton and Beckman, 1977; Stanton et al., 1980).

Figure 3 illustrates two experiments in the POA that reveal an increase in responsiveness to ACh as time in the bout elapsed, which was similar to that observed in the MRF. There were, however, two important differences in the POA, compared to the MRF. The first is that the strength of the ACh stimulus that was adequate to evoke arousal from hibernation was much

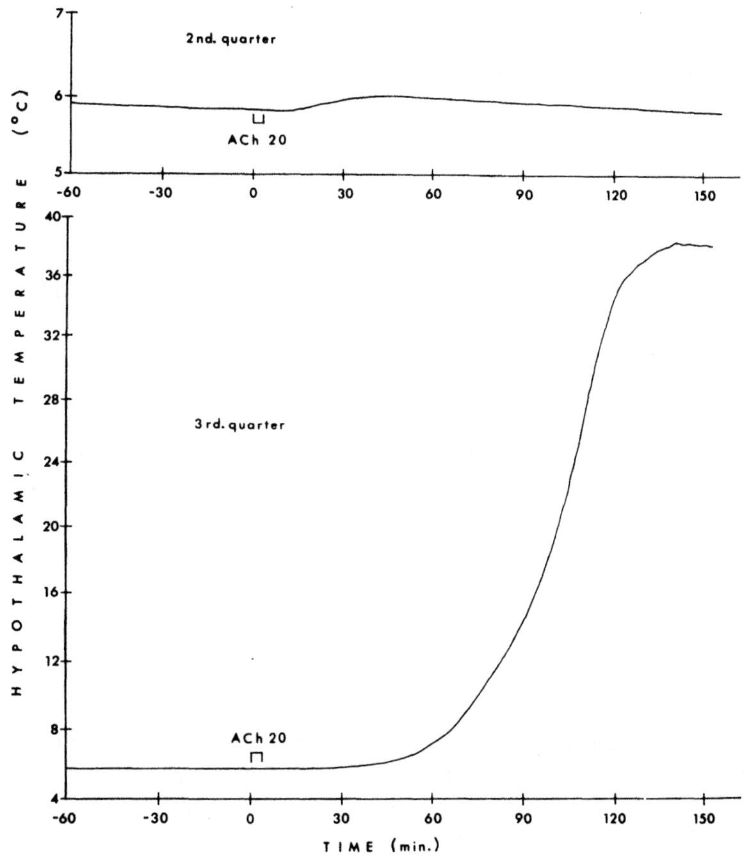

FIG. 3. Increasing responsiveness of POA during progression of hibernation bout: thermogenic responses evoked by ACh (20 μg/ul). *Top panel*, second quarter of bout: small response (0.2°C) was evoked following latency of 13 minutes. *Bottom panel*, third quarter of bout: arousal from hibernation evoked following a latency of 23 minutes. [From Stanton and Beckman, 1977.]

lower in the POA than in the MRF. Whereas in the MRF, concentrations of 50–200 μg were needed to demonstrate arousal from hibernation, in the POA, concentrations of 20–50 μg were sufficient. This dose range (20–50 μg) was similarly effective in evoking thermal responses when microinjected into both structures during euthermia, indicating that the POA is less suppressed during hibernation than is the MRF. The second difference is that although the magnitude of the thermogenic responses evoked by the POA was reduced during the early portion of the bout (relative to euthermia) and increased as time in the bout elapsed, the shift in responsiveness of the POA was much more rapid around the 50 percent point of the bout. This was in contrast with the slower, more progressive increase in the MRF. As a result of this rapid shift, the percentage of experiments (across all concentrations) that resulted in an evoked thermal response increased from 27 percent in the first half of the bout (in which only transient increases in temperature occurred) to 71 percent in second half (in which the majority were full arousals) (Table 2).

Table 2. Thermogenic Responses and Arousal from Hibernation Produced by Intrahypothalamic ACh during First vs. Second Half of the Hibernation Bout

	First half of bout			Second half of bout		
Stimulus	No change in T_{HY}	Transient↑ in T_{HY}	Full arousal	No change in T_{HY}	Transient↑ in T_{HY}	Full arousal
ACh, 10 μg	1	0	0	3	1	1
ACh, 20 μg	6	2	0	1	3	3
ACh, 50 μg	1	1	0	0	0	2
Total	8	3	0	4	4	6

Values represent number of observations. Total number tests: 11 (first half); 14 (second half). [From Stanton and Beckman, 1977.]

These results indicate that the POA is more sensitive to direct stimulation (ACh application) during hibernation compared with the MRF. This could be a reflection of the difference in bioelectric activity in these two sites during hibernation, wherein the MRF is relatively quiescent and the hypothalamus exhibits near constant activity (Shtark, 1970; South et al., 1969; Strumwasser, 1959b). Taken together, these observations are consistent with the hypothesis that the level of inhibition in the POA is less than that in the MRF during hibernation, particularly in the second half of the bout. This characteristic would render the POA more sensitive to potentially arousing stimuli that would be free to ascend through the brainstem in the absence of the gating function of the MRF.

Stanton et al. (1980) have shown that the hippocampus (HPC) may be a more potent site yet for triggering arousal from hibernation. Using the endogenous neuropeptide thyrotropin releasing hormone (TRH), we demonstrated thermogenic responses and arousal from hibernation following bilateral microinjection of concentrations as small as 0.1 ng (Fig. 4).

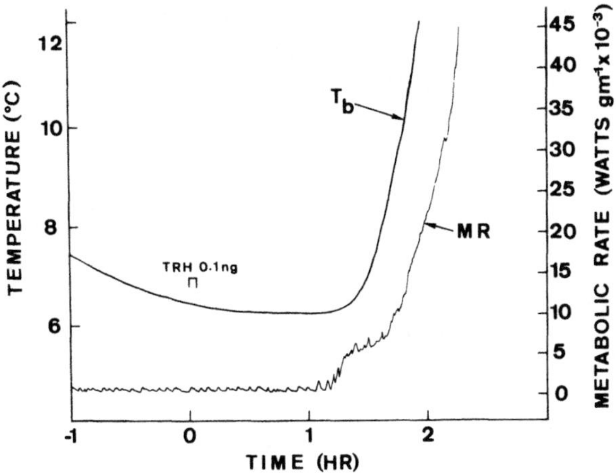

FIG. 4. Arousal from hibernation evoked by TRH action in the dorsal hippocampus. Record shows early stage of arousal evoked by 0.1 ng of TRH microinjected during final phase of entrance into hibernation. Latency of response, 68 minutes. MR: metabolic rate; T_b: brain temperature measured in cortex; ambient temperature: 4°C. [From Stanton et al., 1980.]

Microinjection of much higher concentrations (up to 1 μg/μl) into sites outside the HPC (cortex and in preliminary experiments, POA) were without observable effect. These experiments are of interest for two reasons. First, they establish the extreme sensitivity of the hibernating HPC to direct action of an endogenous neuropeptide and its apparent supreme potency, compared to the POA and MRF, in activating the trigger process for arousal from hibernation. Second, they lend support to the proposed function of the HPC as a source for the inhibitory control that appears to dominate the hibernating brain (Stanton et al., 1980). Whereas the effect of TRH on the activity of individual hippocampal neurons in hibernating *C. lateralis* has not been established, the predominant effect of the direct application of TRH to single neurons in another rodent's brain (rat) is one of potent inhibition (Dyer and Dyball, 1974; Renaud and Martin, 1975; Winokur and

Beckman, 1978). Assuming a similar effect in the ground squirrel, it would appear that intrahippocampal microinjection of TRH activates arousal from hibernation by suppressing the ongoing hippocampal inhibitory control.

The results of EEG (Shtark, 1970; South et al., 1969; Wunnenberg et al., 1978) and POA thermal stimulation studies (Florant et al., 1978; Heller et al., 1977) during entrance into hibernation, together with our neurotransmitter microinjection studies in the MRF (Beckman et al., 1976a,b; Beckman and Stanton, 1976), POA (Beckman and Satinoff, 1972; Stanton and Beckman, 1977), and HPC (Stanton et al., 1980) during deep hibernation, suggest a tentative description of the neuronal control of the hibernating brain that is summarized in the scheme depicted in Fig. 5.

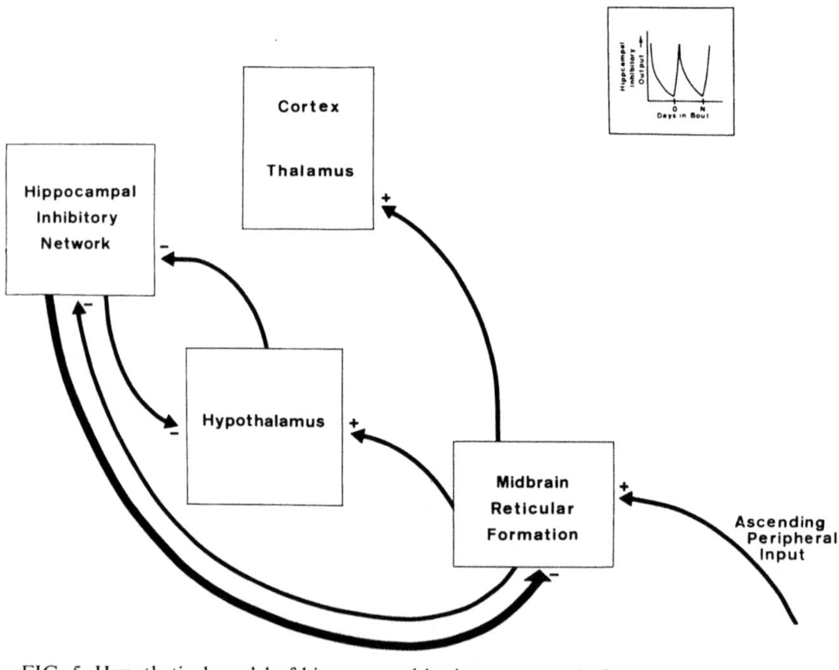

FIG. 5. Hypothetical model of hippocampal-brainstem control of central activity state during hibernation. *Inset*: oscillation of hippocampal inhibitory output; N is length of hibernation bout. See text for further explanation.

According to this working hypothesis, which will undoubtedly undergo modifications with the addition of new data, the HPC contains an inhibitory network that rhythmically oscillates from high through low levels of activity with a period that corresponds to a bout of hibernation (Fig. 5, inset). The descending outflow of this network exerts a major suppressive influence on the excitability of the MRF, and a lesser one on that of the hypothalamus. As a result, the inhibitory activity projecting into the MRF creates a gating mechanism therein for controlling (restricting) the flow of neural traffic that normally ascends through the MRF during the euthermic state from peripheral sources to hypothalamic, hippocampal, thalamic, and cortical areas. Hippocampal suppresion of hypothalamic excitability serves to reduce the functional level of physiological systems under major hypothalamic control, such as those concerned with energy balance, cardiovascular, and endocrine function. It also serves to reduce the ascending suppressive hypothalamic input to the hippocampal inhibitory network.

The rapid increase in hippocampal inhibitory outflow, therefore, is responsible for the entrance into hibernation. As time in the bout elapses, the inhibitory outflow progressively decreases, permitting the excitability of the MRF and rostral structures to increase. As a consequence, increasing amounts of peripheral input are permitted to ascend through the MRF, contributing further to an increased excitability of the MRF and POA, and an increased suppression of hippocampal inhibitory activity. When the magnitude of these effects reaches the threshold for adequate suppression of hippocampal inhibitory control, transition to the euthermic state (i.e., arousal from hibernation) occurs. The rate of reduction of the hippocampal inhibitory outflow, therefore, determines the length of each hibernation bout. Maintenance of the euthermic state is achieved by the now unhindered flow of neural impulses ascending through the MRF that predominantly activates diencephalic and cortical structures and suppresses the hippocampal inhibitory network itself. Entry into the subsequent hibernation bout begins when the rising phase of the inhibitory network output once again reduces the excitability of the MRF.

Adopting the terminology used by Morrison in this volume, this hippocampal-brainstem gating mechanism (Fig. 5) is viewed as being responsible for switching between the hibernating and euthermic central activity states.

Whereas this hypothesis is largely untested, salient features of the model are well supported by numerous observations in non-hibernating and hibernating species. For example, the proposed periodic oscillation of the hippocampal inhibitory output should be reflected in a rhythmic change in hippocampal excitability. This has been reported by Barnes et al. (1977), who described rhythmic, circadian changes in hippocampal excitability in rats and monkeys. Moreover, hippocampal suppression of hypothalamic and MRF electrical activity is well documented (Feldman, 1962; MacLean, 1975; Rabii et al., 1976; Van Hartesveldt, 1975; Vinogradova, 1975), as is the reduction of hippocampal neuronal excitability by the MRF (Finch and Babb, 1976; Grantyn, 1970; Vinogradova, 1975). Considering the role of the MRF, it has been shown to receive widespred peripheral input (Bell et al., 1964; Kadjaya and Narikashvili, 1966) that ascends to innervate hypothalamus (Boulant and Hardy, 1974; Feldman, 1962; Feldman and Dafny, 1968), hippocampus (Segal, 1974; O'Keefe and Dostrovsky, 1971), thalamus (Crosby et al., 1962; Edwards and de Olmos, 1976), and cortex (Cordeau et al., 1963; Crosby et al., 1962). The importance ascribed in the model to changes in the excitability of the MRF in controlling the level of CNS arousal is supported by a report (Toth, 1976) correlating increases in the level of MRF neural activity with increases in the level of arousal of hibernating *C. lateralis*. Finally, the notion that the reduction of hippocampal inhibitory outflow can be accelerated by an increase in peripheral input, thereby shortening the duration of the hibernation bout, is supported by data showing that bout duration of *C. lateralis* shortens with increased ambient temperature (Twente and Twente, 1965).

DEEP HIBERNATION: CNS CONTROL

The foregoing discussion has established that, in comparison to the euthermic state, the essential difference in the central activity state of hibernation is one of a dramatic downward resetting of functional level. The rate, magnitude, and duration of the change in functional level defines what might be termed the "profile" of hibernation. The electrophysiological and thermoregulatory characteristics of the entrance phase, as well as the progressive and regionally distinct recovery of brain excitability that occurs during the deep phase and that culminates in arousal from hibernation, support the concept that the shape of the profile is determined by CNS control.

To extend our understanding of the characteristics of the hibernation state, it is important to ask whether the profile is actively maintained in the face of potentially disruptive stimuli. Two approaches to this problem have been taken, one involving thermal stimulation and the other direct synaptic stimulation of the MRF by ACh. The results of experiments within each context suggest that the state of hibernation is, in fact, actively defended by CNS mechanisms against spurious disruption.

With regard to defense against thermal disruption, it is clear that the CNS thermoregulatory mechanism remains functionally intact following its downward resetting during entrance into hibernation. Numerous experiments have shown that a gradual decline in either ambient or resting hypothalamic temperature (by means of local cooling with indwelling thermodes) below a threshold value evokes an increase in metabolic rate (Hammel et al., 1968; Heller and Colliver, 1974; Heller and Hammel, 1972; Mills and South, 1972) that is proportional to the magnitude of the stimulus (Heller and Colliver, 1974). Internal temperature is thereby prevented from following the slow decline in ambient temperature below a lower limit and the hibernating state is preserved intact. The level of this threshold for increased metabolic heat production (T_{MHP}) appears to decline slowly during the initial portion of deep hibernation and then increase near the end of the bout (Florant and Heller, 1977). Average values of T_{MHP} have been reported to be between 1.2 and 12.5°C during deep hibernation, with variation commonly occurring between animals and within animals across different hibernation bouts (Florant and Heller, 1977; Heller and Colliver, 1974). The limit of the thermoregulatory system's ability to defend the hibernation state against thermal disruption is apparently defined by the nature of the imposed sustained fall in temperature. If it is too rapid or large, the hibernation state is abandoned with the triggering of arousal from hibernation (Hammel et al., 1968; Heller and Colliver, 1974; Heller and Hammel, 1972; Lyman and O'Brien, 1972; Lyman and O'Brien, 1974).

Experiments in our laboratory have provided evidence for the abrupt activation in *C. lateralis* of a neural mechanism that inhibits arousal from hibernation when the accompanying increase in internal temperature reaches a threshold, or ceiling, temperature (Beckman et al., 1976b). In these studies, we observed two types of thermogenic responses during hibernation that occurred spontaneously or following either a brief handling stimulus or ACh microinjection into the MRF. These responses, which we termed type I or type II, are illustrated in Fig. 6. Type I responses were characterized by small magnitude and a slow (mean rate: 0.03°C/min), variable rising phase. Type II responses were characterized by a smooth, rapid rising phase (mean rate: 0.11°C/min) and by an abrupt reversal of the rising phase within a restricted ceiling temperature band (mean value: 9.4°C).

The striking aspect of these experiments was the relatively constant temperature at which evoked or spontaneous increases in body temperature reversed within a given animal, irrespective of the starting temperature at which the increase began. This is illustrated in the experiment shown in Fig. 7. Here, an animal hibernating at an ambient temperature of 6°C was given a microinjection of ACh (200 $\mu g/\mu l$) into the MRF at each of three points within a 4-hour period. The first microinjection evoked an increase in resting internal temperature (measured in the midbrain, T_{MB}) of 2.8°C, with a maximum rate of increase of 0.13°C/min. Following spontaneous reversal at 9.7°C, T_{MB} began to decline toward the resting hibernation baseline. (Note that changes in interscapular temperature, reflecting brown fat thermogenesis [T_{bf}], preceded all changes in T_{MB}, indicating the role of this heat source as a major thermogenic after during hibernation.) A second microin-

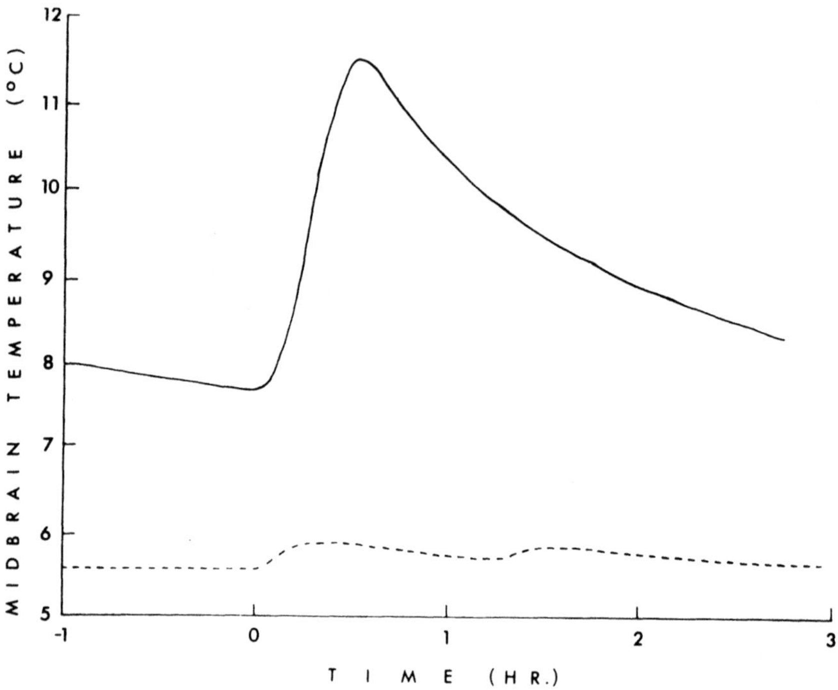

FIG. 6. Spontaneously evoked type I and type II responses. Solid line is type II response; record begins during final phase of entrance into hibernation. Continuous increase in T_{mb} began at 7.7°C and lasted 30 minutes, raising T_{mb} to 11.3°C before reversing. Maximum rate of increase, 0.18°C/min. Dashed line shows type I response with a magnitude of 0.3°C and a maximum rate of increase of 0.04°C/min. Ambient temperature: 6°C, upper record; 5°C, lower record. [From Beckman et al., 1976.]

jection of ACh was delivered at a T_{MB} of 8.8°C and this evoked an increase in T_{MB} of 0.11°C/min that reversed at 10.2°C. Following reversal, T_{MB} declined for 12 minutes, whereupon it began to increase spontaneously. The spontaneous increase began at a T_{MB} of approximately 9.8°C, reached a maximum rate of 0.05°C/min and reversed once again at 10.2°C. The third microinjection was given 1.3 hours after the second, during which brown fat thermogenic activity was greater than in the interval separating the first and second microinjections. This final stimulus was thus given during a period of activated hibernation and was sufficient to trigger full arousal from hibernation. It is striking that the three peaks of these type II responses were within 0.5°C of each other, despite widely different starting temperatures. Likewise, those of T_{bf} reversed within an even narrower band of 0.3°C, clearly suggesting the activation of a mechanism that prevents increasing temperature from exceeding a hibernation ceiling threshold.

These experiments also demonstrated that the characteristics of the rising phase of type II responses (i.e., profile and rate) were equivalent to those of the duplicate portion of full arousals. It may be that a common neural sequence, which functions as the trigger for arousal from hibernation, is responsible for producing both the type II responses as well as the corresponding phase of full arousals. The results of experiments such as those shown in Fig. 7 therefore suggest that the reversal of type II responses at the ceiling level represents the inhibition of the trigger process for arousal from hibernation. Experimental manipulation of hypothalamic temperature during the early stage of arousal, discussed in the following section on arousal from hibernation, supports this hypothesis.

In preliminary experiments, Beckman (1978) has begun to examine the characteristics of the presumed neural components of this trigger inhibiting mechanism. Using unanesthetized, hibernating *C. lateralis*, he recorded the spontaneous extracellular activity of individual hypothalamic neurons with five-barrel micropipettes during periods of thermogenic activity. The working assumption underlying these studies is that the activation of the trigger inhibiting mechanism should be characterized by appropriate changes in single unit activity that occur in conjunction with the reversal of type II

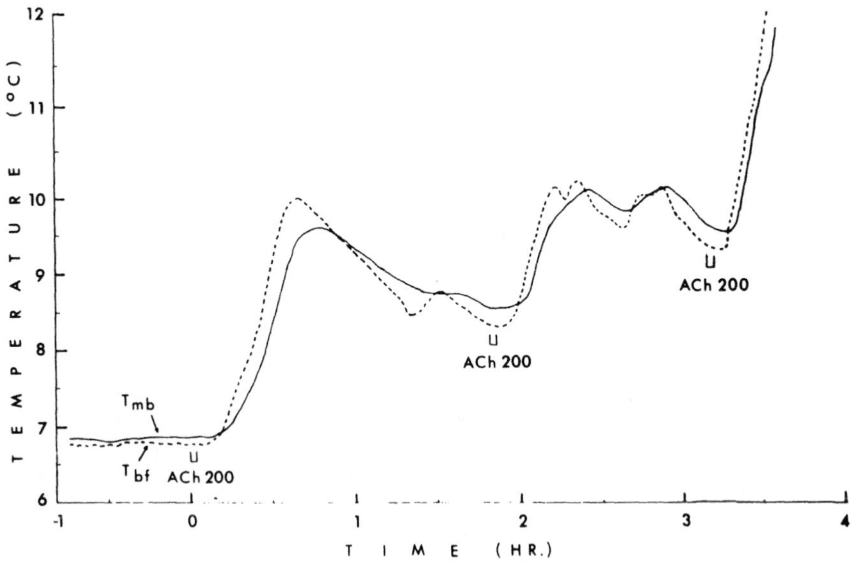

FIG. 7. Repeated reversals of increasing temperature at hibernation ceiling level. T_{mb} (*solid line*) reversed at 9.7°C and 10.2°C after first and second microinjection ACh (200 μg) into the MRF, given at starting temperatures of 6.9°C and 8.8°C, respectively. Third peak of T_{mb}, after a spontaneous increase of thermogenesis, reversed at 10.2°C. [From Beckman et al., 1976.]

responses. Figure 8 illustrates an experiment in which a hypothalamic neuron behaved in this fashion. Here, rapidly increasing hypothalamic temperature (top panel) had been evoked by previous physical disturbance of the animal. The rise in hypothalamic temperature (T_{HY}) abruptly reversed at approximately 14°C and subsequent oscillations at this ceiling level continued for 26 minutes before full arousal began. Records of the discharge of this cell (bottom panel) showed an increase in firing rate during periods of decreasing T_{HY} and decreased activity during periods of increasing temperature. Such behavior is compatible with a role of this cell in a network which, when activated, inhibits the trigger process and its associated rise in body temperature.

The purpose of a mechanism for inhibiting the arousal process is evidently to prevent the spontaneous increases in regional neural activity that occur during hibernation (Kayser and Malan, 1963; Shtark, 1970; South et al., 1969; Strumwasser, 1959b) from resulting each time in a full arousal. The arousal process is metabolically costly, consuming approximately 20 percent of the energy budget for the hibernation season (Wang, 1978). Inhibiting spurious arousals thereby contributes to the adaptive value of the strategy of hibernation by increasing the stability of the hibernating state and, as a result, maximizing the saving of metabolic energy stores.

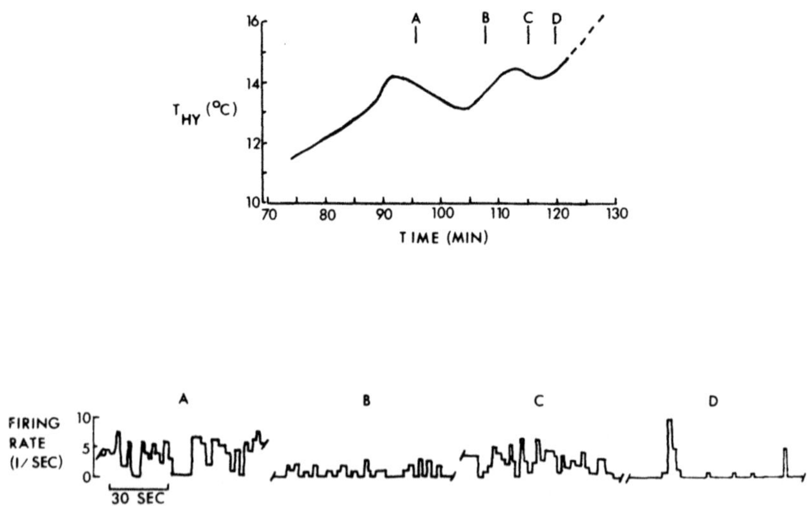

FIG. 8. Spike activity of hypothalamic neuron during reversals of increasing temperature at hibernation ceiling level. *Upper panel*: record of spontaneous changes in hypothalamic temperature. *Bottom panel*: excerpts of spontaneous activity of neuron during periods of decreasing (A and C) and increasing (B and D) temperature. Beginning of arousal from hibernation is shown by dashed portion of curve. [From Beckman, 1978.]

AROUSAL FROM HIBERNATION

Studies of regional EEG activity during hibernation and the beginning of arousal from hibernation indicate that the arousal process is initiated by increases in electrogenic activity in the hippocampus and hypothalamus (Chatfield and Lyman, 1954; Shtark, 1970; South et al., 1969). Other areas of the limbic system and brainstem then become increasingly active in conjunction with the characteristic rapid increase in thermogenesis (Shtark, 1970). Although simultaneous measurements of activity in widespread areas of the arousing brain have not been made, it would appear from the data on hand that as the intensity of hippocampal and hypothalamic neuronal activity increases, these structures begin to activate other areas of the brainstem that, in turn, activate the rest of the brain. Our studies on the spontaneous inhibition of the trigger process suggest that once increasing brain temperature exceeds the ceiling level, the arousal becomes irreversible. Changes in CNS, cardiovascular, and metabolic parameters then continue until euthermic levels are reached.

In this context, it is interesting that the CNS thermoregulator appears to remain in the hibernating mode during the initial stages of arousal followed by an abrupt change to the euthermic mode, possibly when increasing temperature exceeds the ceiling level. Evidence for this is derived from experiments in which arousals were initiated by cooling the POA of *C. lateralis* with indwelling thermodes (Heller and Hammel, 1972). If the POA was then heated to a temperature of 11–12.5°C (i.e., the ceiling band) within 15 minutes after the beginning of the cooling-induced thermogenesis, the arousal could be reversed. However, if the arousal progressed beyond 15–30 minutes before POA heating was begun, it could not be reversed. In this latter case, T_{HY} had to be heated to the euthermic level before the rate of thermogenesis could be reduced (Heller and Hammel, 1972).

We have recently begun to study changes in the activity of single neurons during the arousal process. Preliminary evidence supports the concept that the hibernating brain is under inhibitory control and that, as suggested by EEG observations (Chatfield and Lyman, 1954; Shtark, 1970; Stanton and Beckman, unpublished observations), the arousal is mediated by a powerful and progressive recruitment of neural activity. We have observed neurons that were silent during deep torpor or during the early stages of arousal, but which responded readily to iontophoretically applied ACh (Fig. 9). As the arousal progressed, the cells then became spontaneously active, rapidly reaching their euthermic levels of baseline activity (Fig. 9). The threshold at which spontaneous activity ensued varied in different cells, as shown in the experiment depicted in Fig. 10. This neuron was essentially silent until brain temperature reached approximately 33°C, at which spontaneous activity abruptly increased. Throughout the arousal period, however, the cell responded to ACh, indicating that the natural inactivity was not due to an inability to fire at low brain temperature. Most likely, as noted above, it is due to either direct inhibition or inhibition of its sources of input.

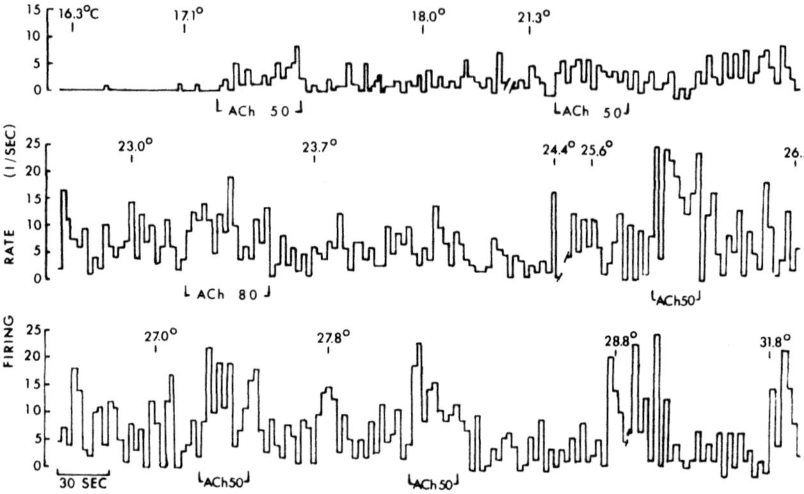

FIG. 9. Onset of continuous spontaneous firing of hypothalamic neuron during arousal from hibernation. Below T_{HY} of 17°C, cell was silent and was acquired by continuous iontophoretic application of ACh. Continuous spontaneous firing began at T_{HY} 17°C and increased to maximum firing levels by T_{HY} 23°C. Cell retained responsiveness to ACh throughout period of observation. ACh applied at brackets; numerical value is iontophoretic current intensity in nanoamperes. [From Beckman, 1978.]

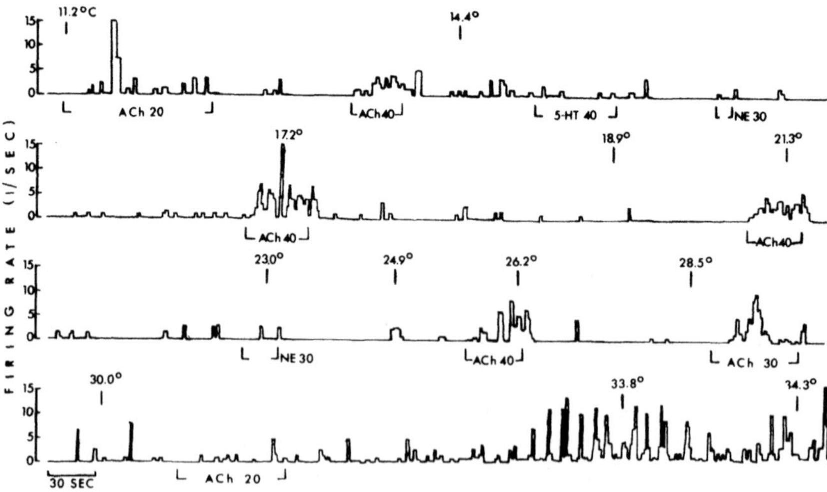

FIG. 10. Onset of continuous spontaneous firing of thalamic neuron during arousal from hibernation. Below brain temperature of 11°C, cell was silent and was acquired by continuous iontophoretic application of ACh. Continuous firing began at approximately 33°C. Notation as in Fig. 9.

CONCLUSIONS

The hibernating CNS is a truly remarkable mammalian neuronal system. It exists in a mode of profound depression, yet remains responsive to the internal and external encironment, actively maintaining and defending the hibernation state against disruption.

Studies of the full range of its characteristics lie ahead of us. For example, we have yet to explore the range of behavioral control that may exist in this state. We do know that animals in deep torpor exhibit such simple behaviors as postural adjustments, orienting responses to auditory stimuli, and vocalization (Strumwasser, 1959a, b). Complex behavioral heat-loss responses, elicited by experimentally raising T_{HY} to the ceiling temperature range, have also been observed (Mills and South, 1972). Embedded in the realm of behavioral control are questions pertaining to the characteristics of sensory systems and of the capabilities for learning and memory. Exploring the answers to these questions in this unique mammalian state promises to enrich our understanding of these fundamentals of the neural basis of behavior.

ACKNOWLEDGEMENTS

The authors wish to thank Darlene Langille and Susan Keenan for their work in preparing the typescript of this chapter, and Gretchen Mercer for her valuable artwork and photographic contributions.

This research was supported by grants from the National Institutes of Health (NS 10597) and the National Science Foundation (BNS 77-11352 and BNS 78-19002), and by the Alfred I. duPont Institute of the Nemours Foundation.

REFERENCES

Baldwin, F.M., and Johnson, K.L. Effects of hibernation on the rate of oxygen consumption in the thirteen-lined ground squirrel. *J. Mammal* 22, 180–182 (1941).

Barnes, C.A., McNaughton, B.L., Goddard, G.V., Douglas, R.M., and Adamec, R. Circadian rhythm of synaptic excitability in rat and monkey central nervous system. *Science* 197, 91–92 (1977).

Beckman, A.L. Preliminary observations of hypothalamic single unit activity in arousing and unanesthetized authermic ground squirrels. *J. Thermal Biol.* 3, 93 (1978).

Beckman, A.L., and Satinoff, E. Arousal from hibernation by intrahypothalamic injections of biogenic amines in ground squirrels. *Am. J. Physiol.* 222, 875–879 (1972).

Beckman, A.L., Satinoff, E., and Stanton, T.L. Characterization of midbrain component of the trigger for arousal from hibernation. *Am. J. Physiol.* 230, 368–375 (1976a).

Beckman, A.L., and Stanton, T.L. Changes in CNS responsiveness during hibernation. *Am. J. Physiol.* 231, 810–816 (1976).

Beckman, A.L., Stanton, T.L., and Satinoff, E. Inhibition of the trigger process for arousal from hibernation. *Am. J. Physiol.* 230, 1018–1025 (1976b).

Bell, C., Sierra, G., Buendia, N., and Segundo, J.P. Sensory properties of neurons in mesencephalic reticular formation. *J. Neurophysiol.* 27, 961 (1964).

Boulant, J.A., and Hardy, J.D. The effect of spinal and skin temperatures on the firing rate and thermosensitivity of preoptic neurones. *J. Physiol.* 240, 639–660 (1974).

Charnock, J.S. Membrane lipid phase-transitions: a possible biological response to hibernation?, in *Strategies in Cold: Natural Torpidity and Thermogenesis.* L.C.H. Wang and J.W. Hudson, eds. Academic Press, New York (1978), pp. 417–460.

Charnock, J.S., and Simonson, L.P. Variation in ($Na^+ + K^+$)-ATPase and Mg^{2+}-ATPase activity of the ground squirrel brain during hibernation. *Comp. Biochem. Physiol.* 59B, 223–229 (1978).

Chatfield, P.O., Battista, A.F., Lyman, C.P., and Garcia, J.P. Effects of cooling on nerve conduction in a hibernator (golden hamster) and non-hibernator (albino rat). *Am. J. Physiol.* 155, 179–185 (1948).

Chatfield, P.O., and Lyman, C.P. Subcortical electrical activity in the golden hamster during arousal from hibernation. *Electroenceph. Clin. Neurophysiol.* 6, 403–408 (1954).

Chatfield, P.O., Lyman, C.P., and Purpura, D.P. The effects of temperature on the spontaneous and induced electrical activity in the cerebral cortex of the golden hamster. *Electroenceph. Clin. Neurophysiol.* 3, 225–230 (1951).

Cordeau, J.P., Moreau, A., Beaulnes, A., and Laurin, C. EEG and behavioral changes following microinjections of acetylcholine and adrenaline in the brain stem of cats. *Arch. Ital. Biol.* 101, 34–47 (1963).

Crosby, E.C., Humphrey, T., and Lauer, E.W. *Correlative Anatomy of the Nervous System.* Macmillan, New York (1962), pp. 266–309, 412–501.

Dawe, A.R., and Spurrier, W.A. Hibernation induced in ground squirrels by blood transfusion. *Science* 163, 298–299 (1969).

Dawe, A.R., and Spurrier, W.A. The blood-borne trigger for natural mammalian hibernation in the 13-lined ground squirrel and the woodchuck. *Cryobiology* 9, 163–172 (1972).

Dawe, A.R., and Spurrier, W.A. Summer hibernation of infant (6 wk old) 13-lined ground squirrels, *Citellus tridecemlineatus. Cryobiology* 11, 33–43 (1974).

Dawe, A.R., Spurrier, W.A., and Armour, J.A. Summer hibernation induced by cryogenically preserved blood "trigger." *Science* 168, 497–498 (1979).

Dyer, R.G., and Dyball, R.E. Evidence for a direct effect of LRH and TRH on single unit activity in the rostral hypothalamus. *Nature (Lond.)* 252, 486–488 (1974).

Edwards, S.B., and de Olmos, J.S. Autoradiographic studies of the projections of the midbrain reticular formation: asecending projections of nucleus cuneiformis. *J. Comp. Neurol.* 165, 417–432 (1976).

Feldman, S. Neurophysiological mechanisms modifying afferent hypothalamo-hippocampal conduction. *Exp. Neurol.* 5, 269–291 (1962).

Feldman, S., and Dafny, N. Acoustic responses in the hypothalamus. *Electroenceph. Clin. Neurophysiol.* 25, 150–159 (1968).

Finch, D.M., and Babb, T.L. Effects of mesencephalic and pontine brain stem stimulation on hippocampal neuronal activity in cats. *Soc. Neurosci. Abs.* 2, 385 (1976).

Florant, G.L., and Heller, H.C. CNS regulation of body temperature in euthermic and hibernating marmots (*Marmota flaviventris*). *Am. J. Physiol.* 232, R203–R208 (1977).

Florant, G.L., Turner, B.M., and Heller, H.C. Temperature regulation during wakefulness, sleep, and hibernation in marmots. *Am. J. Physiol.* 235, R82–R88 (1978).

Goldman, S.S., and Albers, R.W. Cold resistance of the brain during hibernation. Temperature sensitivity of the partial reactions of the Na^+, K^+-ATPase. *Arch. Biochem. Biophys.* 169, 540–544 (1975).

Goldman, S.S., and Willis, J.S. Cold resistance of the brain during hibernation. I. K^+ transport in cerebral cortex slices. *Cryobiology* 10, 212–217 (1973).

Grantyn, A. An intracellular study of hippocampal responses to reticular stimulation. *Brain Res.* 22, 409–412 (1970).

Hammel, H.T., Dawson, T.J., Abrams, R.M., and Andersen, H.T. Total colorimetric measurements on *Citellus lateralis* in hibernation. *Physiol. Zool.* 41, 341–357 (1968).

Hammel, H.T., Heller, H.C., and Sharpe, F.R. Probing the rostral brainstem of anesthetized, unanesthetized, and exercising dogs and of hibernating and euthermic ground squirrels. *Federation Proc.* 32, 1588–1597 (1973).

Hayward, J.S., and Lyman, C.P. Nonshivering heat production during arousal from hibernation and evidence for the contribution of brown fat, in *Mammalian Hibernation III*. K.C. Fisher, A.R. Dawe, C.P. Lyman, E. Schönbaum, and F.E. South, eds. Oliver and Boyd, Edinburgh (1967), pp. 86–96.

Heller, H.C. Hibernation: neural aspects. *Ann. Rev. Physiol.* 41, 305–321 (1979).

Heller, H.C., and Colliver, G.W. CNS regulation of body temperature during hibernation. *Am. J. Physiol.* 227, 583–589 (1974).

Heller, H.C., Colliver, G.W., and Anand, P. CNS regulation of body temperature in euthermic hibernators. *Am. J. Physiol.* 227, 576–582 (1974).

Heller, H.C., Colliver, G.W., and Beard, J. Thermoregulation during entrance into hibernation. *Pflugers Arch.* 369, 55–59 (1977).

Heller, H.C., and Glotzback, S.F. Thermoregulation during sleep and hibernation, in *International Review of Physiology, Environmental Physiology II*, Volume 15. D. Robertshaw, ed. University Park Press, Baltimore (1977), pp. 147–188.

Heller, H.C., and Hammel, H.T. CNS control of body temperature during hibernation. *Comp. Biochem. Physiol.* 41, 349–359 (1972).

Heller, H.C., and Poulson, T.L. Circannian rhythms—II. Endogenous and exogenous factors controlling reproduction and hibernation in chipmunks (*Eutamius*) and ground squirrels (*Spermophilus*). *Comp. Biochem. Physiol.* 33, 357–383 (1970).

Hudson, J.W., and Wang, L.C.H. Hibernation: endocrinologic aspects. *Ann. Rev. Physiol.* 41, 287–303 (1979).

Kadjaya, D. and Narikashvili, S.P. Topography of electrical responses to different peripheral stimuli in the mesencephalic reticular formation of the cat. *Physiol. Behav.* 1, 209–213 (1966).

Kayser, C. *The Physiology of Natural Hibernation*, Pergamon Press, New York (1961).

Kayser, C., and Malan, A. Central nervous system and hibernation. *Experientia* 19, 441–451 (1963).

Kehl, T.H., and Morrison, P. Peripheral nerve function and hibernation in the thirteen-lined ground squirrel, *Spermophilus tridecemlineatus*. *Bull. Mus. Comp. Zool., Harvard Univ.* 124, 387–403 (1960).

Landau, B.R., and Dawe, A.R. Respiration in the hibernation of the 13-lined ground squirrel. *Am. J. Physiol.* 194, 75–82 (1958).

Luecke, R.H., and South, F.E. A possible model for thermoregulation during deep hibernation, in *Hibernation and Hypothermia, Perspectives and Challenges*. F.E. South, J.P. Hannon, J.R. Willis, E.T. Pengelley, and N.R. Alpert, eds. Elsevier, Amsterdam (1972), pp. 577–604.

Lyman, C.P. Oxygen consumption, body temperature and heart rate of woodchucks entering hibernation. *Am. J. Physiol.* 194, 83–91 (1958).

Lyman, C.P., and Chatfield, P.O. Physiology of hibernation in mammals. *Physiol. Rev.* 35, 403–425 (1955).

Lyman, C.P., and O'Brien, R.C. Sensitivity to low temperature in hibernating rodents. *Am. J. Physiol.* 222, 864–869 (1972).

Lyman, C.P., and O'Brien, R.C. A comparison of temperature regulation in hibernating rodents. *Am. J. Physiol.* 227, 218–223 (1974).

MacLean, P.D. An ongoing analysis of hippocampal inputs and outputs: microelectrode and neuroanatomical findings in squirrel monkeys, in *The Hippocampus, Volume I: Structure and Development*. R.L. Isaacson and K.H. Pribram, eds. Plenum Press, New York (1975), pp. 177–211.

Melichar, I., Brozek, G., Jansky, L., and Vyskocil, F. Effect of hibernation and noradrenaline on acetylcholine release and action on neuromuscular junction of the golden hamster (*Mesocricetus auratus*). *Pflugers Arch.* 345, 107–122 (1973).

Mills, S.H., and South, F.E. Central regulation of temperature in hibernation and normothermia. *Cryobiology* 9, 393–403 (1972).

Mrosovsky, N. Circannual cycles in hibernators, in *Strategies in Cold: Natural Torpidity and Thermogenesis*. L.C.H. Wang and J.W. Hudson, eds. Academic Press, New York (1978), pp. 21–65.

Oeltgen, P.R., Bergmann, L.C., Spurrier, W.A., and Jones, S.B. Isolation of a hibernation inducing trigger(s) from the plasma of hibernating woodchucks. *Preparative Biochem.* 8, 171–188 (1978).

O'Keefe, J., and Dostrovsky, J. The hippocampus as a spatial map. Preliminary evidence from unit activity in the freely moving rat. *Brain Res.* 34, 171–175 (1971).

Pengelley, E.T., Asmundson, S.J., Barnes, B., and Aloia, R.C. Relationship of light intensity and photoperiod to circannual rhythmicity in the hibernating ground squirrel, *Citellus lateralis. Comp. Biochem. Physiol.* 53A, 273–277 (1976).

Rabii, J., Koranyi, L., Carrillo, A., and Sawyer, C.H. Inhibition of brainstem neuronal activity by electrochemical stimulation (ECS) of the dorsal hippocampus in the freely moving rat. *The Physiologist* 19, 332 (1976).

Renaud, L.P., and Martin, J.B. Thyrotropin-releasing hormone (TRH): depressant action on central neuronal activity. *Brain Res.* 86, 150–154 (1975).

Satinoff, E. Hibernation and the central nervous system, in *Progress in Physiological Psychology*. E. Stellar and J. Sprague, eds. Academic Press, New York (1970), pp. 201–236.

Segal, M. Convergence of sensory input on units in the hippocampal system of the rat. *J. Comp. Physiol. Psychol.* 87, 91–99 (1974).

Shtark, M.B. The brain of hibernating animals. NASA Technical Translation TTF-619, Washington, 1972. Translation of *Mozg Zimnespyashchekt* (Nauka Press, Siberian Branch, Novosibirsk, 1970).

Smith, R.E., and Horwitz, B.A. Brown fat and thermogenesis. *Physiol. Rev.* 49, 330–425 (1969).

South, F.E. Phrenic nerve-diaphragm preparations in relation to temperature and hibernation. *Am. J. Physiol.* 200, 565–571 (1961).

South, F.E., Breazile, J.E., Dellmann, H.D., and Epperly, A.D. Sleep, hibernation and hypothermia in the yellow-bellied marmot (*M. flaviventris*), in *Depressed Metabolism*. X.J. Musacchia and J.F. Saunders, eds. Elsevier, New York (1969), pp. 277–312.

South, F.E., Heath, J.E., Luecke, R.H., Mihailovic, L.T., Myers, R.D., Panuska, J.A., Williams, B.A., Hartner, W.C., and Jacobs, H.K. Status and role of the central nervous system and thermoregulation during hibernation and hypothermia, in *Hibernation and Hypothermia, Perspectives and Challenges*. F.E. South, J.P. Hannon, J.R. Willis, E.T. Pengelley, and N.R. Alpert, eds. Elsevier, Amsterdam (1972), pp. 629–633.

Stanton, T.L., and Beckman, A.L. Thermal changes produced by intrahypothalamic injections of acetylcholine during hibernation and euthermia in *Citellus lateralis. Comp. Biochem. Physiol.* 58A, 143–150 (1977).

Stanton, T.L., Winokur, A., and Beckman, A.L. Reversal of natural CNS depression by TRH action in the hippocampus. *Brain Res.* 181, 470–475 (1980).

Steffen, J.M., and Riedesel, M.L. Respiratory tidal volume, expired gas analyses and EKG during hibernation and arousal of golden mantled ground squirrels (*Spermophilus lateralis*). *Federation Proc.* 38, 1226 (1979).

Strumwasser, F. Thermoregulatory, brain and behavioral mechanisms during entrance into hibernation in the squirrel, *Citellus beecheyi. Am. J. Physiol.* 196, 15–22 (1959a).

Strumwasser, F. Regulatory mechanisms, brain activity and behavior during deep hibernation in the squirrel, *Citellus beecheyi. Am. J. Physiol.* 196, 23–30 (1959b).

Torke, K.G., and Twente, J.W. Behavior of *Spermophilus lateralis* between periods of hibernation. *J. Mammal.* 58, 385–390 (1977).

Toth, D.M. Role of the brain stem reticular formation in the modulation of arousability in hibernating ground squirrels. *Soc. Neurosci. Abs.* 2, 955 (1976).

Twente, J.W., and Twente, J.A. Regulation of hibernating periods by temperature. *Proc. Nat. Acad. Sci.* 54, 1058 (1965).

Twente, J.W., and Twente, J.A. Progressive irritability of hibernating *Citellus lateralis. Comp. Biochem. Physiol.* 25, 467–474 (1968).

Van Hartesveldt, C. The hippocampus and regulation of the hypothalamic-hypophyseal-adrenal cortical axis, in *The Hippocampus, Volume I: Structure and Development.* R.C. Isaacson and K.H. Pribram, eds. Plenum Press, New York (1975), pp. 375–391.

Vinogradova, O.S. Functional organization of the limbic system in the process of registration of information: facts and hypothesis, in *The Limbic System, Volume II. Neurophysiology and Behavior.* R.L. Isaacson and K.H. Pribram, eds. Plenum Press, New York (1975), pp. 3–69.

Walker, J.M., Glotzback, S.F., Berger, R.J., and Heller, H.C. Sleep and hibernation in ground squirrels (*Citellus spp.*): electrophysiological observations. *Am. J. Physiol.* 233, R213–R221 (1977).

Wang, L.C.H. Energetic and field aspects of mammalian torpor: the Richardson's ground squirrel, in *Strategies in Cold: Natural Torpidity and Thermogenesis.* L.C.H. Wang and J.W. Hudson, eds. Academic Press, New York (1978). pp. 109–145.

Wang, R.Y., and Aghajanian, G.K. Physiological evidence for habenula as major link between forebrain and midbrain raphe. *Science* 197, 89–91 (1977).

Willis, J.S. Hibernation: cellular aspects. *Ann. Rev. Physiol.* 41, 275–286 (1979).

Winokur, A., and Beckman, A.L. Effects of thyrotropin-releasing hormone, norepinephrine, and acetylcholine on activity of neurons in the hypothalamus, septum, and cerebral cortex of the rat. *Brain Res.* 150, 205–209 (1978).

Wunnenberg, W., Merker, G., and Speulda, E. Thermosensitivity of preoptic neurons and hypothalamic integrative function in hibernators and non-hibernators, in *Strategies in Cold: Natural Torpidity and Thermogenesis.* L.C.H. Wang, and J.W. Hudson, eds. Academic Press, New York (1978), pp. 267–297.

Copyright © 1982, Spectrum Publications, Inc.
The Neural Basis of Behavior

3

Biochemical Factors Associated with the Sleep State

Manfred L. Karnovsky

The questions of why sleep is required by higher animals, and of what instigates sleep, are hardly novel. Though the answers must ultimately be couched largely in chemical terms, biochemical studies of sleep are not very numerous. Recently, however, the tempo of research has quickened and two reviews have appeared within the past three years that offer a glimpse both of the more historical aspects of the field and of recent progress (Guiditta, 1977; Karnovsky and Reich, 1977). Though these reviews were written completely independently of each other, by authors with entirely different fundamental interests, they cover virtually the same ground, and even offer several identical examples from the literature. This one might take as an indication of how small is the number of biochemical laboratories that are engaged in research on sleep.

Most studies of molecular events in the brain during sleep adopt a comparative approach, and present data for waking animals in conjunction with those for sleeping animals. It is clearly recognized that sleep is not a unitary state (Cohen and Dement, 1965; Jouvet et al., 1964; Roldan and Weiss, 1963) so that a definition of the stage of sleep, or of whether slow-wave (SWS) or rapid-eye movement sleep (REM) is being observed, is an essential datum, though one not always offered in every study. Since sleep, generally, is a very difficult state to work with because of its will-'o-the-wisp quality, focusing upon a particular stage of sleep is an objective that is often beyond the grasp of the investigator. This comment is particularly applicable in the case of attempts to focus upon REM sleep in small laboratory animals where its occurrence is sporadic and brief. As a consequence of this, many investigators have taken what one might call an "upside-down" approach to studies of of sleep, and REM sleep in particular. In that approach, waking animals are used after deprivation of total sleep or specifically of REM sleep. Such animals are compared with animals not so deprived. The great benefit is that the experiments are then done with waking animals, and all the uncertainties of entering an experiment with an animal that may inopportunely awaken are eliminated.

Furthermore, the invention of a truly successful technique for depriving animals specifically of REM sleep, the so-called "flower-pot" method, has encouraged numerous investigations of the biochemistry of the brain of animals so deprived (Jouvet et al., 1964; Cohen and Dement, 1965; reviewed by Karnovsky and Reich, 1977). In these experiments, animals are placed on small pedestals surrounded by a "moat" of water. As the animals enter REM sleep, muscle tone is lost and they fall into the water, awaken and climb back onto the pedestal. After perhaps 72 hours of such treatment the actual experimental measurements are made.

The data obtained have then been interpreted as reflecting aspects of the biochemical or physiological abasis of REM sleep. However, as has been sharply emphasized previously (Karnovsky and Reich, 1977), even if the most meticulous care is taken to perform appropriate control experiments, (e.g., Mendelson et al., 1974) the difficulties of controlling for the *stress* of sleep deprivation, in particular, usually renders the deprivation much less than satisfying.

As a consequence, our laboratory has attempted to make biochemical studies of natural, spontaneous slow-wave sleep and wakefulness. The frustrations and difficulties are many, and one must freely admit that problems of artefacts, incomplete controls, etc., are even then not totally eliminated.

This paper will be restricted to a brief mention of biochemical factors that control sleep and wakefulness, and to some aspects of the differentiation, at the molecular level, of the metabolism of the brain during wakefulness from the metabolism of the brain during slow wave sleep.

HUMORAL FACTORS AND THE CYCLE OF SLEEP AND WAKEFULLNESS

Starting in 1910, Legendre and Pieron (1910, 1913; Pieron, 1913) published studies on the effects of a heat stable, non-dialyzable substance in the cerebrospinal fluid of sleep-deprived dogs upon recipient dogs. The latter did respond with increased sleep, but the conditions were severe indeed. In 1939, Schnedorf and Ivy reinvestigated the phenomenon under more reasonable conditions and were able to obtain confirmation, although they manifested some skepticism because of the variability of the results, the hyperthermia that occurred, and the necessity for the lengthy sleep deprivation of donors. Three laboratories, especially, have pursued the question of a humoral factor intensively in more recent years. Monnier and his colleagues have isolated and characterized a nonapeptide form the blood of rabbits maintained asleep by stimulation of the hypothalamus (Monnier and Hosli, 1964; Monnier et al., 1972; Monnier and Schoenenberger, 1973). The structure of this compound, delta sleep-inducing peptide (DSIP), which has been synthesized (Schoenenberger et al., 1978), is:

Trp-Ala-Gly-Gly-Asp-Ala-Ser-Gly-Glu

A different approach was taken by Pappenheimer and his colleagues in Boston (Fencl et al., 1971; Pappenheimer et al., 1975; Krueger et al., 1978). Starting with sleep-deprived goats, this group demonstrated the presence of a sleep-inducing substance in the cerebrospinal fluid, obtained with minimal trauma. Later, the same substance was extracted from the brains of sleep-deprived animals, particularly rabbits. The recipients (test animals) were rats or rabbits, and the phenomenon was followed by measuring locomotor activity and EEG (duration of sleep episodes together with assessment of amplitude of EGG) in the two species, respectively (Pappenheimer et al., 1975; Krueger et al., 1978). The active substance was found to be of apparent molecular weight less than 500 Daltons. It was susceptible to carboxypeptidases A and B, which destroyed the activity.

The third group involved in studies of a humoral sleep-promoting substance is active in Japan. This group has obtained its compound from the brains of rats deprived of sleep in an ingenious automatic maze arrangement (Nagasaki et al., 1974).

The substances under study in the laboratories of the last two groups have points of considerable chemical and physiological similarity. The substance described by Monnier and his colleagues, DSIP, is different in that it is larger and acts physiologically only at levels that are much higher than is true for the substance (Factor S) described by Pappenheimer's group. In addition, the time-course of action is different (Krueger et al., 1978).

It would be interesting to hypothesize that these substances both play a role, perhaps sequentially, with one preceding the other. DSIP is available as a pure synthetic compound; several investigators have had an opportunity to carry out studies without, as yet, any startling results. One provocative observation concerns the cleavage of the peptide by brain extracts. The N-terminal tryptophan is decreased rather rapidly (2.5 μmole gm^{-1} fresh weight). One is much tempted to relate this observation to the work of the Jouvet school, who have implicated serotonin in sleep (e.g., Jouvet, 1972;

reviewed by Karnovsky and Reich, 1977). Could it be that the function of the nona-peptide is to provide tryptophan at the appropriate site, with specificity being conferred by the rest of the nona-peptide that acts to "steer" the tryptophan to the proper place, presumably for conversion to serotonin?

Factor S awaits total elucidation of structure and synthesis. There is every reason to believe that synthesis of this low molecular weight substance labeled with ^{14}C or ^{3}H will not be difficult, nor, hopefully, long delayed. Certainly one would expect a flood of information concerning the instigation of sleep to follow those steps, including identification of specific brain areas involved, the nature of receptor(s), and the fate of the substance in the brain.

METABOLISM OF CARBOHYDRATES IN BRAIN DURING SLEEP

A number of attempts have been made to examine the carbohydrate metabolism of brain in sleep compared with wakefulness (Richter and Dawson, 1948; Shimizu et al., 1966; Cocks, 1967; Van den Noort and Brine, 1970; Reich et al., 1972). In addition, the energy balance of the brain has been considered by determining phosphorylated intermediates and nucleotides (reviewed by Karnovsky and Reich, 1977). The studies cited examined slow-wave sleep and were done under very different conditions including induction of sleep in rats by bright light, the use of long periods of exercise on a treadmill, and spontaneous sleep. The data show considerable variability when one compares the various studies. Thus, a clear recognition of the metabolic characteristiscs of SWS remains elusive.

In the case of studies on REM sleep, one already cited (Mendelson et al., 1974) came closest to yielding definitive results though, as mentioned, it utilized deprivation rather than natural sleep.

CEREBRAL GLYCOGEN

No published studies of natural slow-wave sleep include measurements of brain glycogen. On the other hand, numerous studies on deprivation of REM sleep have examined cerebral glycogen (e.g., Karadzik and Mrsulja, 1969; reviewed by Karnovsky and Reich, 1977). In general, it appears that the small amount of cerebral glycogen is rather labile, falling about 50 per cent (though variably, in different structures) during REM deprivation and rising to normal levels during "recuperative" sleep of up to nine hours.

These studies, despite our expressed criticisms, together with the non-existence of data for natural slow-wave sleep, stimulated our interest. Further, the fact that during such sleep, the mean rate of neuronal discharge in all of nine structures studied declined slightly compared with waking (reviewed in Steriade and Hobson, 1976) suggests that slow-wave sleep is a period of rest for many brain regions and that energy supplies might be recouped. Cerebral A-V oxygen differences and cerebral oxygen consumption did not change in slow-wave sleep compared with wakefulness, though blood flow increased in 10 of 25 regions studied (Reivich et al., 1968). In contrast, during REM sleep the mean rate of neuronal discharge increased markedly as did blood flow in all 25 regions studied (Steriade and Hobson, 1976; Reivich et al., 1968). It is against this backdrop of possible decreased energy demand during slow-wave sleep, and unchanged fuel supply, that one views the possibility of increased macromolecule synthesis and remodeling, in our case with special reference to glycogen.

We have, therefore, performed some rather simple experiments to find out whether cerebral glycogen levels rise during normal spontaneous slow-wave sleep. The animals (rats) were operated upon for installation of EEG and EMG electrodes (Reich et al., 1973) and monitored for sleep or wakefulness. They were placed in the observation cage at 9 a.m. Between 11 a.m. and 12 noon, we frequently observed significant periods of slow-wave sleep. The periods of sleep were recorded and the animals that slept were compared with animals that did not sleep, or were prevented from sleeping. In a further series of studies, sleeping animals were killed by immersion in liquid nitrogen without awaking and their levels of cerebral glycogen were compared with those of animals that had spontaneously awakened after a significant sleep period and were allowed to remain awake for a measured period of time prior to being killed. Some of these data are given in Table 1. It appears that cerebral glycogen rapidly builds up during slow-wave sleep to a level about 50 per cent above the waking level. Upon spontaneous

Table 1. Effect of Slow-Wave Sleep on Rat Brain Glycogen

	Duration (minutes)	*n*	*Brain Glycogen ($n\,mol \cdot mg^{-1}$ protein)*
(A)	0	7	15.7 ± 1.3
Sleep	5–11	4	26.7 ± 0.9
	17–55	6	23.6 ± 0.8
(B)	2–5	5	15.9 ± 2.0
Wakefulness	10–20	4	15.0 ± 1.6

A. Animals were permitted to sleep between 11 A.M. and noon. They were frozen within 30 seconds after waking.

B. Animals awoke spontaneously from a period of sleep greater than 15 minutes (at the same time of day as above). After a measured period of time they were frozen.

awakening, the additional glycogen is discharged within a few minutes and the normal waking level is reestablished.

During the daylight hours rats undergo many periods of slow-wave sleep. Animals killed while awake in the early morning exhibited normal waking levels of cerebral glycogen. Animals killed while asleep in the afternoon (4 p.m.) exhibited the same level of cerebral glycogen manifested by the sleeping rats of Table 1, i.e., no higher than the short-term sleeping levels, despite many repeated sleep periods. One must assume, then, that the brain glycogen of rats rises and falls with the sleep and waking periods through the daylight hours. In none of the above circumstances was any sleep-related change in liver glycogen observed.

These findings are in concert with the "rest theory" of slow-wave sleep; i.e., that is, neurons in some structures "recuperate" during slow-wave sleep, permitting, in this case, accumulation of an energy reserve which may be used in the early period of waking that might require a source of rapidly available "fuel."

GLUCOSE-6-PHOSPHATASE

In 1967, Reich et al. demonstrated that in weanling rats, sleep was accompanied by an increase in the incorporation of administered ^{32}P-inorganic orthophosphate into what appeared to be a phosphoprotein (Fig. 1). The phosphate moiety could be removed from the macromolecule with hot acid. The livers showed no effect, and the blood radioactivity was the same for sleepers and wakers.

In these experiments, monitoring by EEG was not feasible, and the use of immature rats that had been mildly sleep-deprived left some degree of uncertainty. In a new series of experiments with adult rats equipped with EEG and EMG leads, and to which the phosphate was administered intraventricularly, the observation was confirmed (Reich et al., 1973). The putative phosphoprotein, which was insoluble, was shown to be cleavable by pronase to yield the affected organic phosphate in soluble form. The pronase products were subjected to paper-chromatography, and the phosphate of interest was observed to be associated with a ninhydrin positive entity. An observation whose significance was not appreciated fully at the time was the fact that the phosphoprotein was solubilized by sodium dodecyl sulfate or deoxycholate (as would be expected for glucose-6-phosphatase; see below).

The phosphoprotein affected by slow-wave sleep was identified by Anchors and Karnovsky (1975). The attack on the problem was as follows. Rats were equipped with monitoring electrodes and ventricular cannulas, as before. Each rat was administered $^{32}P_i$ or $^{33}P_i$ and allowed to sleep, or kept awake by very mild stimulation (rustling of paper, movement in the room, soft conversations between personnel). Each waker was matched to a sleeper for weight, date of operation, time of administration of isotope, and duration of the period from administration of isotope to killing by immersion in liquid nitrogen (Anchors and Karnovsky, 1975). The brains of matched sleepers and wakers were worked up together. Dilipidation with lipid solvent, extraction of the resulting lipid-free material with sodium dodecyl sulfate and polyacrylamide gel electrophoresis permitted both recognition of the sleep-affected substance and its isolation on a scale large enough to conduct various chemical procedures.

It seemed probable that the polypeptide that showed the "sleep-effect" and which was isolated as above was part of a larger biologically active entity. In a second series of experiments, the protein was obtained by non-denaturing means (removal of myelin by centrifugation; gel-filtration of the deoxycholate-solubilized protein of the delipidized pellet on Sephadex-G-

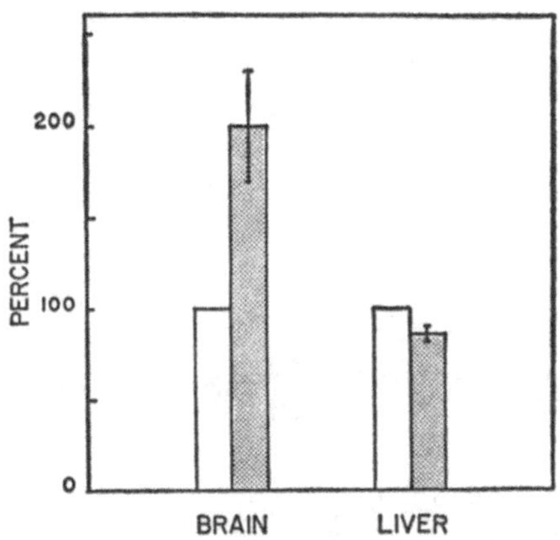

FIG. 1. Effect of sleep on incorporation of $^{32}P_i$ into an acid labile fraction of the brains of 20 day-old rats. Littermates were kept awake for 90 minutes and then injected with orthophosphate-32P in the tail vein (4 μCi per gram of body weight). The letters were then divided into two groups of equal number. One group (S) was placed in quiet cages where the animals fell asleep spontaneously in two to three minutes. The other group (W) was kept awake by gentle manual stimulation. After about 30 minutes the animals were decapitated and the brains were extracted with chloroform-methanol (2:1). The residue was washed three times at room temperature with 95 percent ethanol, once with water at 4°C, and three times with 2.5 percent trichloroacetic acid at 4°C; it was then extracted with 5 percent trichloroacetic acid at 90°C for 30 minutes. Data are given for the hot TCA extract. Shaded bars are sleepers; open bars are wakers set at 100 percent for 45 pairs of animals, brain data for sleepers and wakers differed with $p<0.001$. Hot TCA released inorganic phosphate from phosphoprotein. No other fractions showed differences.

100; chromatography on DEAE-Sephadex). The final product was recognized as the enzyme glucose-6-phosphatase, and a summary of properties is given in Table 2.

Table 2. Characteristics of the Phosphoprotein Involved in Slow-Wave Sleep (Reich et al., 1973; Anchors and Karnovsky, 1975)

1. Insoluble in salt solutions or non-ionic detergents; solubilized by sodium dodecyle sulfate or sodium deoxycholate.
2. Cleaved by pronase, but trypsin cleaves only after pronase treatment.
3. Molecular weight, 28,000 Daltons (Polyacrylamide gel electrophoresis with sodium dodecyl sulfate). The native substance (sodium deoxycholate, chromatography on Sephadex G-200) had a molecular weight < 70,000 Daltons. This, on polyacrylamide gel electrophoresis, yields only the single polypeptide above.
4. Both products above were homogeneous. On the limited amounts available, amino acid composition was: Ala 18; Arg 4–6; Asp 16–18; Cys 0; Glu 32–34; Gly 46–47; His 2; Ileu 6; Leu 9–12; Lys 18–21; Met 1; Phe 3–5; Pro 9–14; Ser 32–38; Thr 5–9; Tyr 1; Val 8.
5. NH^2 terminal is isoleucine.
6. Phosphate is attached to histidine.
7. Native protein is enzymatically active, as glucose-6-phosphatase-acting as phosphohydrolase and phosphotransferase. Level: 4.8 nmols · min^{-1} mg^{-1} protein (after sonication).
8. Present in all parts of brain examined, in neuronal membranous subsellular fractions.

RELEVANCE OF INCREASED LABELING OF GLUCOSE-6-PHOSPHATASE TO SLEEP

The phosphoprotein isolated as described above is apparently the enzyme intermediate (Enz-P) in the following reactions:

$$X\text{–P}+\text{Enz}=\text{Enz–P}+X \qquad \text{(i)}$$
$$\text{Enz–P}+Y=Y\text{–P}+\text{Enz} \qquad \text{(ii)}$$

Nordlie (1971; 1974) has shown that glucose-6-phosp-ohatase is a multifunctional enzyme and may act as a phosphotransferase as well as a phosphohydrolase. Thus X above may be glucose and Y water, in which case the hydrolysis of glucose-6-phosphate is described. On the other hand, X may be ATP or carbamyl phosphate or inorganic pyrophosphate, for example, and Y may be glucose or mannose, in which case a phosphotransferase function is described. One should note also that glucose-6-phosphatase has long been known to have pyrophosphatase activity.

The following questions may be raised with reference to the observations that the labeling of Enz-P is grossly elevated (by almost an order of magnitude; Anchors and Karnovsky, 1975) in slow-wave sleep:

(a) Is the specific activity of the phosphate of the nucleotide pool, and in turn that of glucose-6-phosphate, elevated? This would lead to increased label in Enz-P without, necessarily, augmented activity of the enzyme.

The specific activity of the phosphate of the cerebral nucleotide pool did not appear to be increased during slow-wave sleep (Anchors and Karnovsky, 1975).

(b) Was the actual enzyme activity of glucose-6-phosphatase enhanced? The enzyme was extracted from the brains of *8* pairs of sleeping or waking rats and analyzed by standard means *in vitro* (Zakim and Vessy, 1973) (Dr. Bessie Lee, unpublished experiments). We found that the enzyme titer per brain showed only a small increment, 15±7 percent ($p<0.05$), after a period of slow-wave sleep of about 15 minutes.

The difficulty with this approach is that the standard conditions of extraction and assay (cations, pH, etc.) might counteract the conditions *in vivo* which give rise to the labeling effect, if that is dependent upon increased activity of the enzyme *in vivo.*

(c) In which direction is the enzyme operating (hydrolase or phosphotransferase)? We have made two separate approaches to this question. In the first, we examined several cultured cell lines of neural origin as well as cerebral capillaries, brain slices, and liver slices, *in vitro.* All the preparations manifested glucose-6-phosphatase, pyrophosphate-glucose phosphotransferase, and hexokinase. Liver, as expected, had fifty-fold more of the first activity than brain. The cultured cells of neural origin (transformed) had an order of magnitude more activity in this context than brain. The phosphotransferase activity was always about one-quarter to one-third that of the hydrolase activity. Brain exhibited fifteen to seventy-five fold more hexokinase that the other preparations (Anchors, et al., 1977). Against this backdrop, the transport of glucose into the cells was evaluated using ^{14}C-2-deoxyglucose as the indicator. In three of the cell lines and brain slices, uptake was more rapid than phosphorylation; in three other cell lines of neural origin and in cerebral capillaries, phosphorylation was at least as rapid as uptake. None of the preparations was able to phosphorylate 3-0-methylglucose (which is not a substrate for hexokinase, but is one for glucose-6-phosphatase in its phosphotransferase function). The indications were thus that glucose-6-phosphatase was not acting to phosphorylate glucose, and that phosphorylation was not obligatory for entry of glucose into the cells.

Further, studies of efflux of 2-deoxyglucose yielded no evidence that that enzyme was active vectorially to transport glucose to the outside of cells. That is, the glucose moeity of glucose-6-phosphate was not preferentially conveyed to the exterior of the cells compared with free intracellular glucose. However, intracellular glucose-6-phosphate *was* hydrolyzed, presumably by glucose-6-phosphatase, prior to release of glucose to the exterior in nervous tissue (brain slices) and cells of neuronal origin, as well as by liver slices, in which tissue such action is certainly expected.

These observations left conventional hydrolytic action of glucose-6-phosphatase as the function that is probably enhanced in the brain during slow-wave sleep.

A series of experiments was performed to test this *in vivo*. The procedure was based on the observations of Sokoloff et al. (1977). In the latter work, it was shown that tracer doses of ^{14}C-2-deoxyglucose administered to rats reaches a virtual plateau in the brain after 45 minutes. Sokoloff and his colleagues have employed the first 45 minutes after administration of the labeled glucose analogue (i.e., the period during which brain structures are accumulating label) to demonstrate neural pathways (visual, olfactory, etc.) that depend upon enhanced demand for glucose and consequent accumulation of ^{14}C-2-deoxyglucose-6-phosphate, which is neither anabolized to glycogen nor catabolized by glycolysis (Kennedy et al., 1975). The phosphorylated analogue is, however, cleaved by glucose-6-phosphatase (Hawkins and Miller, 1978). Presumably, this activity is minimal in the conscious rat's brain. During slow-wave sleep, however, the indications are that this hydrolase activity increases markedly.

In our experiments, ^{14}C-2-deoxyglucose was given to rats by the tail vein. After 45 minutes (when a virtual plateau of radioactivity, as ^{14}C-2-deoxyglucose-6-phosphate, had been reached in the brain) animals were permitted to sleep, or were kept awake, for 15–20 minutes. All data were collected on matched sleepers and wakers, monitored by EEG, as outlined previously. The animals were then killed and the brains extracted. The phosphorylated ^{14}C-2-deoxyglucose and the free sugar were measured. There was a marked decrease in the levels of both forms in the brains of sleepers (Fig. 2). It should be noted that these data represent substrate disappearance, as in an enzyme assay *in vitro*. The 35 per cent diminution of 2-deoxyglucose-6-phosphate during slow-wave sleep compared to wakefulness does not indicate a mere one-third increase in the enzyme's activity, but may reflect an increase of an order of magnitude or more, the substrate being in excess.

As a matter of interest one may consider the following:

(a) Normal level of glucose-6-phosphate in conscious rat brain = 156 nanomoles $\cdot$ gm^{-1} fresh weight (Veech and Hawkins, 1974).

(b) Then, in about 15 minutes of sleep one-third is lost (see above = 52 nanomoles $\cdot$ gm^{-1} fresh weight.

(c) Rat brain has an enzyme content that can hydrolyze 4.8 nanomoles of glucose-6-phosphate $\cdot$ $min^{-1} \cdot mg^{-1}$ protein. This is roughly 7,000 nanomoles $\cdot$ gm^{-1} fresh weight in 15 minutes.

Thus, even during the stimulation of activity in slow-wave sleep, the enzyme is functioning at only about 1 percent of its capacity. The calculation yields a *minimum value;* it does not take account of possible changes in the level of glucose-6-phosphate due to changes in hexokinase activity (see below). Furthermore, 2-deoxyglucose-6-phosphate, through an effective substrate, may not be able to *reach* the enzyme *in vivo* (Arion et al., 1972), since it may not cross the membrane of the endoplasmic reticulum (see below). Whatever the level, it seems clear that the enzyme is acting as a hydrolase *in vivo* with consequent diminution of its substrate, at least as indicated by 2-deoxy-D-glucose-6-phosphate, which has no other fate.

d. What controls the glucose-6-phosphatase? This enzyme is subject to numerous inhibitors and effectors (Nordlie, 1971; 1974). However, some recent observations of Nilsson and his collaborators (1978), and of our own, raise speculations concerning regulation that have, perhaps, unusual appeal. It appears that in intact miscrosomes, which reflect the structure of the endoplasmic reticulum form which they derive, the hydrolase is located on the lumenal side of the membrane. On the microsome exterior (cytoplasmic side of the endoplasmic reticulum) is a protein that transports the substrate to the interior. Though the hydrolase functions toward mannose-6-phosphate roughly as well as toward glucose-6-phosphate, the transport function is specific for glucose-6-phosphate. Nilsson et al. (1978) recently observed that diazotized sulfanilate, a nonpenetrating reagent with respect to biological membranes, attacks the transport protein of intact liver microsomes, which then do not hydrolyze glucose-6-phosphate. Rupture of the treated microsomes with deoxycholate or by sonication restores much of the activity. In our hands, the nonpenetrating reagent DIDS (4,4′ di-isothiocyanostilbene-2,2′-disulfonic acid), a blocking agent for anion channels in red cells (Cabantchik et al., 1978), was found to be a potent inhibitor of glucose-6-phosphatase activity of liver microsomes at 50 μM. Destruction of

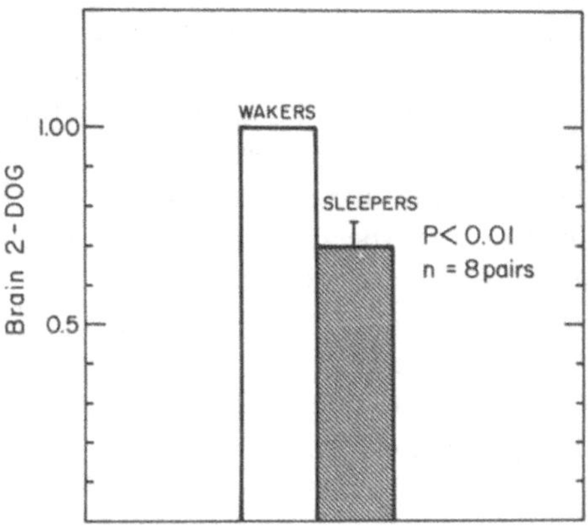

FIG. 2. Diminution of cerebral ^{14}C-2-deoxyglucose-6-phosphate during slow-wave sleep (ca. 15 minutes). Wakers and sleepers were paired; the brains were extracted and the free and phosphorylated forms of the sugar separated by ion exchange chromatography. About 80 percent of the label was present as the phosphate; no sleep-related difference in proportion of free and phosphorylated sugar was found. The cerebral ^{14}C-2-deoxyglucose-6-phosphate is shown. (See text for details).

microsomal integrity with deoxycholate restored full activity—i.e., the hydrolase protein itself was unaffected by DIDS. The most important observation was that glucose-6-phosphate, *but not mannose-6-phosphate*, if present when the DIDS was applied, could block the action of that substance toward microsomes virtually completely. That is, it could protect the transport protein specifically (M. Zoccoli, unpublished observations).

A number of matters require clarification. For example, why is DIDS so successful a blocking agent in this case? It cannot be purely by virtue of its anion-binding site-seeking ability, since mannose-6-phosphate does not protect. It is also not clear that the transport protein and the hydrolase protein are completely distinct entities. However, the hypothesis that the former exerts control over the activity of the latter is one that certainly merits more detailed investigation. In particular, transfer of the findings to brain microsomes is important. One cannot be certain that brain microsomes behave exactly like liver microsomes nor that the enzyme in brain is completely limited to the endoplastic reticulum (Sephens and Sandborn, 1976). The nature of the factors that "relax" the barrier between the hydrolase and its substrate during sleep must be determined; this is central to the thesis that the transport protein mentioned plays a role in cerebral carbohydrate metabolism during sleep.

CONCLUSION

A brief review has been given of the biochemistry of factors that induce slow-wave sleep, and of metabolic changes that occur during slow-wave sleep. In the latter context only a very few aspects, and then only of carbohydrate metabolism, were touched upon. Information concerning, for example, protein, amino acid, and nucleic acid metabolism has indeed been obtained and is reviewed by Guiditta (1977) and Karnovsky and Reich (1977).

In our own work we have attempted to study only spontaneous, natural slow-wave sleep as far as is possible. The pitfalls and uncertainties that arise by studying sleep deprivation more than balance the difficulties of trying to obtain periods of natural sleep. This has been specially emphasized in the case of REM sleep where deprivation studies are more prevalent.

We have observed that cerebral glycogen builds up early in SWS and dissipates rapidly upon awakening. It is possible that the extra glycogen is available for the increased metabolic demand that underlies increased electrical activity upon awakening. In the same context, i.e., of providing instant energy, the augmented activity of glucose-6-phosphatase may be one leg of a substrate cycle (Fig. 3). Such cycles have been discussed intensively recently; they are a means of providing rapid adaptability and control for metabolic pathways (Newsholme and Crabtree, 1978; Katz and Rognstad, 1976). Much greater detail is necessary to evaluate the situation in slow-wave sleep, including adequate quantitative measurements. In particular, studies are

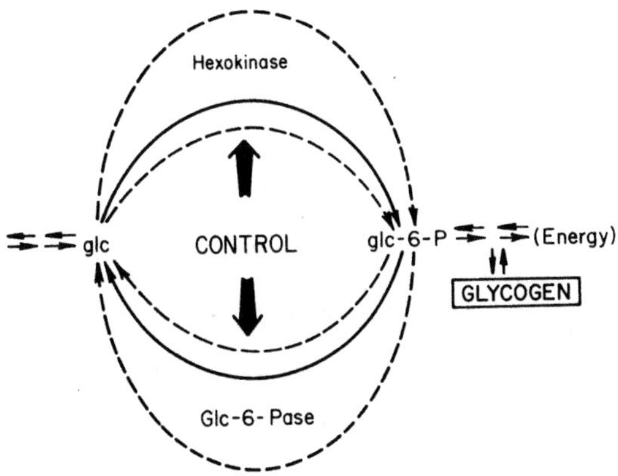

FIG. 3. Summary of possible roles of glucose-6-phosphatase and increased cerebral glycogen in the cycle of slow-wave sleep and waking. The dashed lines indicate limits between which enzyme activity may be modulated by effectors or other factors such as transport of substrate (see text). The substrate cycle is a sensitive means of regulating flow of metabolites [Newsholme and Crabtree (1978); Katz and Rognstad (1976)]. Another immediate source of energy is provided by the increased glycogen stored during the first few minutes of slow-wave sleep (see text).

urgently needed that deal with the individual structures of the brain—studies such as those that are carried out by the ^{14}C-2-deoxyglucose technique, that yield both qualitative and quantitative information on each brain region with a high degree of resolution (Kennedy et al., 1975; Sokoloff et al., 1977). These are now in progress.

ACKNOWLEDGEMENTS

This work was performed with support from U.S.P.H.S. Grant NS 07484-05 and a contract with the Office of Naval Research No. N00014-77-C-0774.

REFERENCES

Anchors, J.M., Haggerty, D.F., and Karnovsky, M.L. Cerebral glucose-6-phosphatase and the movement of 2-deoxy-D-glucose across cell membranes. *J. Biol. Chem.* 252, 7035–7041 (1977).

Anchors, J.M., and Karnovsky, M.L. Purification of cerebral glucose-6-phosphatase. An enzyme involved in sleep. *J. Biol. Chem.* 250, 6408–6416 (1975).

Arion, W.J., Wallin, B.K., Carlson, P.W., and Lange, A.J. The Specificity of glucose-6-phosphatase of intact liver microsomes. *J. Biol. Chem.* 247, 2558–2565 (1972).

Cabantchik, Z.I., Knauf, P.A., and Rothstein, A. The anion transport system of the red blood cell: The role of membrane protein evaluated by the use of probes. *Biochem. Biophys. Acta* 515, 239–302 (1978).

Cocks, J.A. Change in the concentration of lactic acid in the rat and hamster brain during natural sleep. *Nature* 215, 1399–1400 (1967).

Cohen, H.B., and Dement, W.C. Sleep: changes in threshold to electroconvulsive shock in rats after deprivation of "paradoxical phase." *Science* 150, 1318–1319 (1965).

Feldman, F., and Butler, L.G. Protein bound phosphoryl histidine: A probable intermediate in the microsomal glucose-6-phosphatase/inorganic pyrophosphatase reaction. *Biochem. Biophys. Acta* 268, 698–710 (1972).

Fencl, V., Koski, G., and Pappenheimer, J.R. Factors in cerebrospinal fluid from goats that affect sleep and activity in rats. *J. Physiol.* 216, 565–589 (1971).

Giuditta, A. The biochemistry of sleep, in *Biochemical Correlates of Brain Structure and Function.* A.N. Davison, ed. Academic Press, London (1977), pp. 293–337.

Hawkins, R.A., and Miller, A.L. Loss of radioactive 2-deoxy-D-glucose-6-phosphate from brains of conscious rats: Implications for quantitative autoradiographic determination of regional glucose utilization. *Neuroscience* 3, 251–258 (1978).

Jouvet, M. The role of monoamines and acetyl-choline-containing neurones in the regulation of the sleep-waking cycle. *Ergeb. Physiol.* 64, 166–307 (1972).

Jouvet, D., Vimont, P., Delorme, F., and Jouvet, M. Etude de la privation selective de la phase paradoxale de sommeil chez le chat. *C. R. Soc. Biol.* (Paris) 158, 456–759 (1964).

Karadzik, V., and Mrsulja, B. Deprivation of paradoxical sleep and brain glycogen. *J. Neurochem.* 16, 29–34 (1969).

Karnovsky, M.L., and Reich, P. Biochemistry of sleep, in *Advances in Neurochemistry.* B.W. Agranoff and M.H. Aprison, eds. Plenum Press, New York (1977), Vol. 2, pp. 213–275.

Katz, J., and Rognstad, R. Futile cycles in the metabolism of glucose, in *Current Topics in Cellular Regulation.* B.L. Horecker and E.R. Stadtman, eds. Academic Press, New York (1976), Vol. 10, pp. 237–289.

Kennedy, C., Des Rosiers, M.H., Jehle, J.W., Reivich, M., Sharpe, F., and Sokoloff, L. Mapping of functional neuronal pathways by autoradiographic survey of local metabolic rate with ^{14}C-deoxyglucose. *Science* 187, 850–853 (1975).

Krueger, J.M., Pappenheimer, J.R., and Karnovsky, M.L. Sleep-promoting factors: purification and properties. *Proc. Nat. Acad. Sci.* 75, 5235–5238 (1978).

Legendre, R., and Pieron, H. Des resultats histo-physiologiques de l'injection intra-occipito atlantodienne des liquide insomniques. *C. R. Soc. Biol.* (Paris) 68, 1108–1109 (1910).

Legendre, R., and Pieron, H. Recherches sur le besoin de sommeil couse cutif a une veille prolongee. *Z. Allg. Physiol.* 14, 235–262 (1913).

Mendelson, W., Guthrie, R.D., Guynn, R., Harris, R.L., and Wyatt, R.J. Rapid eye movement (REM) sleep deprivation, stress, and intermediary metabolism. *J. Neurochem.* 22, 1157–1159 (1974).

Monnier, M., Hatt, A.M., Cueni, L.B., and Schoenenberger, R.A. Humoral transmission of sleep VI. Purification and assessment of a hypnogenic fraction of "sleep dialysate" (factor delta). *Pflugers Arch.* 331, 257–265 (1972).

Monnier, M., and Hosli, L. Dialysis of sleep and waking factors in blood of the rabbit. *Science* 146, 796–798 (1964).

Monnier, M., and Schoenenberger, G.A. Erzeugung, Isolierung und Charakterisierung eines physiologische Schlaffaktors "Delta." *Schweiz. Med. Wochenschr.* 103, 1733–1743 (1973).

Nagasaki, H., Iriki, M., Inoue, S., and Uchizono, K. The presence of a sleep-promoting material in the brain of sleep-deprived rats. *Proc. Japan. Acad.* 50, 241–246 (1974).

Newsholme, E., and Crabtree, B.: Substrate cycles in the control of energy metabolism in the intact animal, in Symposium Al *Regulatory Mechanisms of Carbohydrate Metabolism*. V. Esmann, ed. Federation of European Biochemical Societies, 11th meeting, Copenhagen, Pergamon Press, New York (1978), Vol. 42, pp. 285–295.

Nilsson, O.S., Arion, W.J., DePierre, J.W., Dallner, G., and Ernster, L. Evidence for the involvement of a glucose-6-phosphate carrier in microsomal glucose-6-phosphatase activity. *Eur. J. Biochem.* 82, 627–638 (1978).

Nordlie, R.C. Glucose-6-phosphatase, hydrolytic and synthetic activities, in *The Enzymes* P.D. Boyer, ed. Academic Press, New York (1971), Vol. 4, pp. 543–605.

Nordlie, R.C. Metabolic regulation by multifunctional glucose-6-phosphatase, in *Current Topics in Cellular Regulation*. B.L. Horecker and E.R. Stadtman, eds. Academic Press, New York (1974), Vol. 8, pp. 33–117.

Pappenheimer, J.R., Koski, G., Fencl, V., Karnovsky, M.L., and Krueger, J. Extraction of sleep-promoting Factor S. from cerebrospinal fluid and from brains of sleep-deprived animals. *J. Neurophysiol.* 38, 1299–1311 (1975).

Passonneau, J.V., and Lauderdale, V.R. A comparison of three methods of glycogen measurement in tissues. *Anal. Biochem.* 60, 405–412 (1974).

Pieron, H. *Le probleme physiologique du sommeil*. Masson, Paris (1913).

Reich, P., Driver, J.K., and Karnovsky, M.L. Sleep: effects on incorporation of inorganic phosphate into brain fractions. *Science* 157, 336–338 (1967).

Reich, P., Geyer, S.J., and Karnovsky, M.L. Metabolism of brain during sleep and wakefulness. *J. Neurochem.* 19, 487–497 (1972).

Reich, P., Geyer, S.J., Steinbaum, L., Anchors, J.M., and Karnovsky, M.L. Incorporation of phosphate into rat brain during sleep and wakefulness. *J. Neurochem.* 20, 1195–1205 (1973).

Reivich, M., Isaacs, G., Evarts, E., and Kety, S.S. The effect of slow-wave sleep and REM sleep on regional cerebral blood flow in cats. *J. Neurochem.* 15, 301–306 (1968).

Richter, D., and Dawson, R.M.C. Brain metabolism in emotional excitement and in sleep. *Am. J. Physiol.* 154, 73–79 (1948).

Roldan, E., and Weiss, T. Neural mechanisms underlying sleep cycle in rodents. *Bol. Inst. Estud. Med. Biol. Mex.* 24, 467–483 (1963).

Schnedorf, J.G., and Ivy, A.C. An examination of the hypnotoxin theory of sleep. *Am. J. Physiol.* 125, 491–505 (1939).

Schoenenberger, G.A., Maier, P.F., Tobler, H.J., Wilson, K., and Monnier, M. The delta EEG (sleep)-inducing peptide (DSIP) XI. Amino acid analysis, sequence, synthesis and activity of the nonapeptide. *Pflugers Arch.* 376, 119–129 (1978).

Shimizu, H., Tabushi, K., Hishikawa, Y., Kakimoto, Y., and Kaneko, Z. Concentrations of lactic acid in rat brain during natural sleep. *Nature* 212, 936–937 (1966).

Sokoloff, L., Reivich, M., Kennedy, C., Des Rosiers, M.H., Patlak, C.S., Pettigrew, K.D., Sakuroda, O., and Shinohara, M. The ^{14}C-deoxyglucose method for the measurement of local cerebral glucose utilization: Theory, procedure and normal values in the conscious and anesthetized albino rat. *J. Neurochem.* 28, 897–916 (1977).

Stephens, H.R., and Sandborn, E.B. Cytochemical localization of glucose-6-phosphatase activity in the central nervous system of the rat. *Brain Res.* 113, 127–146 (1976).

Steriade, M., and Hobson, J.A. Neuronal activity during the sleep-waking cycle. *Prog. Neurobiol.* 6, 155–376 (1976).

Van den Noort, S., and Brine, K. Effect of sleep on brain labile phosphates and metabolic rate. *Am. J. Physiol.* 218, 1434–1439 (1970).

Veech, R.L., and Hawkins, R.A. Brain blowing: a technique for *in vivo* study of brain metabolism, in *Research Methods in Neurochemistry*. N. Marks and R. Rodnight, eds. Plenum Press, New York-London (1974), Vol. 2, pp. 171–182.

Zakim, D., and Vessy, P.A. Techniques for the characterization of UDP-glucuronyltransferase, glucose-6-phosphate, and other tightly bound microsomal enzymes, in *Methods in Biochemical Analysis*. D. Glick, ed. John Wiley and Sons, New York (1973), Vol. 21, pp. 1–37.

Copyright © 1982, Spectrum Publications, Inc.
The Neural Basis of Behavior

4

Effects of Conditioned Arousal on the Auditory System

Norman M. Weinberger

INTRODUCTION

Central activity states have several manifestations. Dr. Beckman has addressed the topic of hibernation while Drs. Morrison and Karnovsky have been concerned with the neural substrates of different aspects of sleep. There is yet another aspect of central activity states, namely the state of arousal. Each of these states may be characterized by its moment-to-moment variance or fluctuations. We have seen that even hibernation is a dynamic state, in which state fluctuations do occur. Of course, it is well known that the general state of sleep is characterized by shifts from one state to another; the time course of such changes is apparently more rapid than for hibernation. The state of arousal is characterized by even more numerous fluctuations in level, the duration of which may be as short as one or two seconds, as during habituation of arousal (Sharpless and Jasper, 1956) or as long as minutes, as during a sustained attention task in which a high level of performance is maintained throughout (Mirsky and Pragay, 1970). The fact that the state of arousal includes numerous instances of increments and decrements in level during the course of a period of non-sleep is undoubtedly related to the fact that most of an animal's transactions with its environment occur during wakefulness, and environmental conditions are often highly variable. For example, novel, unexpected or sudden stimuli elicit an increment in arousal level as a major component of the orienting reflex (see, for example, Sokolov, 1963, 1975).

We have also seen that hibernation and sleep are highly regulated states. This is also true for the state of arousal. Thus, both forebrain and hindbrain mechanisms are able to "deactivate" an organism by limiting the activity of neural substrates of arousal (Dell et al., 1961). In turn, deactivating mechanisms themselves can be damped under conditions requiring sudden increments in arousal and readiness to deal with or react to environmental and also to internal demands (Lindsley, 1970; Moruzzi, 1972). The net effect of these counterbalancing forces is to yield a level of arousal, which at any moment is appropriate to the performance of adaptive behavior. The regulation of arousal has been termed "reticular homeostasis," and the adaptive result of such regulation is a level of arousal which provides for "critical reactivity" (Dell, 1963).

If changes in arousal level provide for critical reactivity or "vigilance" only in response to novel or strong environmental stimulation, organisms would be more like reflex machines than they actually are—unable to prepare for or anticipate such stimulation. Fortunately, adjustments in arousal level can precede the actual occurrence of an event, such as an intense stimulus, which "demands" an increment in arousal as an antecedent to mobilization for behavior (e.g., flight). The process of learning provides for anticipatory adjustments in arousal level (see, for example, Champion, 1969). It is this aspect of stimulus control of arousal, the role of learning in controlling arousal, that I will address. As it happens, investigation of this topic also provides a particularly good opportunity to investigate the neuronal bases of learning as well. I will return to this point shortly.

The issue that I will address may be posed in the following way. It is agreed that neuronal changes must underly behavioral learning. Studies have shown that there are widespread electrophysiological changes in the brain during learning (John, 1961; Morrell, 1961; Thomas, 1962; Galeano, 1963; Thompson et al., 1972). But it is not known whether or not all neurons are capable of active participation in learning. That is, do all neurons have the inherent property of developing a plastic change (as evidenced in their discharge characteristics) due to associative learning? If not, then by definition there are two broad classes of neurons; those which do develop a change and those which do not change as a function of learning. For convenience, I will refer to these simply as "learning" and "non-learning" cells, respectively.

If neurons can be classified as learning or non-learning types, there should be some distinguishing characteristics, possibly some predisposing features, which would provide clues about general principles and mechanisms of neuronal learning. Thus, one might record from many neurons during conditioning procedures, classify the cells as learning or non-learning types, measure many characteristics of each cell (e.g., initial responsiveness to stimuli, rate of spontaneous discharge, perhaps even morphological factors), and compare the features of two types. Those features which are common to both learning and non-learning cells could not explain their different learning capabilities, while those features which are different might help explain cellular "learnability." For example, some workers have reported that learning cells are predisposed to respond to both conditioned and unconditioned stimuli (e.g., Yoshii and Ogura, 1960; Bures and Buresova, 1965; O'Brien and Fox, 1969a,b; Ben-Ari and LaSalle, 1972). Others have emphasized the importance of the background ("spontaneous") rate of discharge (Kotlyar and Mayorov, 1971).

The general strategy of comparing the physiological characteristics of learning and non-learning neurons appears quite reasonable. However, before progress along this line can occur, it is necessary to be cognizant of two factors, one logical, the other empirical.

First, it is logically possible that some (types of) neurons are inherently non-plastic; that is, can't change as a function of learning. However, one can never prove that some neurons cannot learn, although this is a biological possibility. It could always be argued that the cells in question *would* learn, given the appropriate circumstances (e.g., type of training, etc.); but it is impossible to run an infinite number of conditioning experiments. Nonetheless, experiments can be done to determine the variety of circumstances under which a particular set of neurons learns, so that it is possible to evaluate the *relative* plasticity of cells during associative learning.

Second, there is an empirical problem of interpreting data from non-learning cells. Thus, in the past, neurons that don't learn have been classified simply as "non-learning" cells. But negative data might also be obtained from a "substandard" preparation, that is, from an animal which, for whatever reason, was incapable of forming associative conditioned responses at the time of testing. Physiologists are quite familiar with "poor preparations" while psychologists may refer to these simply as "stupid subjects." Unfortunately, previous experiments have not included an independent assessment of animals' learning ability as they were confined to recording single cell discharges only. A concurrent analysis of behavioral conditioning is necessary to determine the adequacy of the preparation to learn. If a negative finding is obtained in a subject which simultaneously develops a behavioral conditioned response, then the preparation was not substandard; in this case, the cell can be considered, at the very least, to be *relatively less plastic* than some other neurons. However, if a behavioral conditioned response is *not* elaborated, one may reasonably conclude that the animal was in some way substandard, and the data from such an animal cannot be readily interpreted.

In light of these considerations, the following steps are appropriate to determine whether or not neurons differ in learning ability, and if so, the mechanisms responsible for this difference:

1. Establish a behavioral conditioned response that allows for concurrent and continuous recording of discharges from individual neurons.

2. Locate learning cells, and perhaps non-learning cells.
3. Compare characteristics of the two types of cells (e.g., predisposition to respond to the conditioned and unconditioned stimuli, rate of spontaneous discharge, perhaps even morphological features).
4. Focus on *different* characteristics to formulate hypotheses about mechanisms underlying different cellular learning ability.
5. Determine that the learning cells are actually the site of active learning processes rather than sites that secondarily reflect learning processes occurring elsewhere; if so, test the hypotheses.

All of these steps have not been achieved yet in the case of associative learning. However, I will relate our progress to date, and the essential role played by the central activity state of arousal.

CONDITIONED AROUSAL

Given the need for a concurrent behavioral index of learning, it is interesting that neurophysiological approaches to conditioning have focused on specific somatic responses, e.g., limb flexion, extension of the nictitating membrane, and eyeblink. Such motor responses are quite *specific* to the nature of the unconditioned stimulus (US), i.e., flexion (withdrawal) to pawshock, and eyeblink to airpuff delivered to the eye. However, these conditioned responses are acquired slowly, so that generally it has not been feasible to record single neuron discharges throughout the course of training. But, behavioral conditioning is also evident in the modification of autonomic and non-specific somatic responses, e.g., heart rate, galvanic skin response, change of blood pressure, pupillary dilation, change in general muscle tone, and respiration. Such conditioned responses are *not specific* to the nature of the unconditioned stimulus; they are generally elicited by almost all unconditioned stimuli and also by initial presentation of neutral or novel stimuli. These characteristics of non-specific responses, particularly autonomic responses, often have led them to be regarded with disdain or simple neglect in studying brain mechanisms underlying associative learning.[1] It has even been alleged that autonomic conditioned responses are artefacts resulting from performance of specific somatic responses (Smith, 1954). This is false because autonomic conditioned responses develop quite well in curarized animals (e.g., Gerall and Obrist, 1962; Black, 1965). Actually, the shoe may be on the other foot, for non-specific conditioned responses develop more quickly than specific somatic conditioned responses.

[1] However, see Cohen, 1974.

Table 1 provides a summary of the rates at which various responses develop stable changes during classical conditioning; the experiments selected generally include proper controls for sensitization and pseudoconditioning. Granted that the rate of learning is influenced by a host of variables (e.g., temporal parameters, stimulus intensity, etc.), nevertheless, over a variety of subjects, stimuli, and test situations, autonomic responses and non-specific somatic responses express conditioning sooner than do specific somatic responses.

A second key point is that the constellation of non-specific responses comprises a picture of heightened behavioral excitability, of increased arousal. These responses surely indicate a change in central activity state. Systematic changes in non-specific responses due to the association of two

Table 1. Rates of Classical Conditioning of Various Response Systems

Response System	*Rate (Trials)**	*Subject*	*References***
"Non-Specific"			
GSR	5–10	Cat	van Twyver and King, 1969
	5–10	Rat	Holdstock & Schwartzbaum, 1965
Pupil	5–12	Cat	Ashe et al., 1976, 1978 Gerall and Obrist, 1962 Oleson et al., 1972
Blood Pressure	10–15	Rabbit	Yehle et al., 1967
Non-Specific Motor	10–15	Rat	deToledo and Black, 1966 Parrish, 1967
Respiration	5–10	Lizard	Davidson and Richardson, 1970
	10–15	Rabbit	Yehle et al., 1967
Heart	5–10	Lizard	Davidson and Richardson, 1970
	10	Rabbit	Yehle et al., 1967
	11–20	Pigeon	Cohen, 1974
	24–36	Rat	deToledo and Black, 1966
"Specific"			
Nictitating Membrane	70–164	Rabbit	Gormezano et al., 1962
Eyelid (Airpuff)	160–240	Rabbit	Schneiderman et al., 1962
Limb Flexion	125–300	Cat	Bruner, 1969 O'Brien and Packham, 1973
Eyelid (Glabella Tap)	600–900	Cat	Woody and Brozek, 1969

*Earliest consistent CRs. In cases where the authors did not specify the rate of learning, estimates were obtained from the published data or authors' comments.

**References cited are representative and do not constitute an exhaustive list.

stimuli and will be referred to as instances of *conditioned arousal* in the balance of this paper.[2]

We see, then, that conditioned stimuli very quickly develop the ability to modulate the central activity state of arousal, and that this is expressed even before the acquisition of specific somatic conditioned responses. This situation can be exploited to permit the study of single neuron discharge characteristics during the entire course of acquisition of a behavioral response, i.e., the acquisition of conditioned arousal.

PUPILLARY CONDITIONING

As an index of conditioned arousal, we record the pupillary dilation conditioned response in the waking cat under neuromuscular paralysis and artificial respiration. Pupillary behavior is employed as the index of arousal rather than conventional EEG recordings because within the general state of arousal, the EEG may be insensitive to increments of arousal level. For example, contrary to the belief that behavioral inhibition or Pavlovian "internal inhibition" is invariably accompanied by increased electrocortical synchrony (John et al., 1961), the EEG often does not differentiate between an animal which is actively responding to a conditioned stimulus and one which is not responding to a non-reinforced differential stimulus (Weinberger et al., 1967). More sensitive electrophysiological indices are available. Thus, the degree of shift in the cortical steady potential is more sensitive to changes in organismic arousal than is the EEG (Rowland, 1967). So also are the amplitude of thalamically-induced electrocortical recruiting waves (Weinberger et al., 1968). But use of these indices involves highly complex equipment and experimental designs. A second major reason for choosing pupillary behavior is that numerous studies in humans have shown a direct relationship between measures of pupillary size and the degree of arousal present or induced by task demands (Nunnally et al., 1967; Kahneman and Beatty, 1966; Simpson and Hale, 1969). Furthermore, there appears to be a direct relationship between pupillary size and the amount of ongoing information processing (Bradshaw, 1968), and there is good reason to conceive of arousal level in terms of the information processing rate of the central nervous system (Delius, 1970).

We measured pupillary size with the aid of an infrared pupillometer. The pupillary dilation reflex is evoked by sensory stimulation, and habituates to moderate stimulation (e.g., acoustic or tactile stimuli) that later serve as

[2]Conditioned "de-arousal," as indicated by the enhancement of EEG synchrony in the sleeping cat in response to a non-reinforced stimulus, has also been reported (Gluck and Rowland, 1959).

conditioned stimuli (Weinberger et al., 1975). It maintains responsiveness to pawshock, which serves as the unconditioned stimulus. Introduction of pawshock following habituation produces dishabituation, but such sensitization is transient (Oleson et al., 1972). The pupillary dilation reflex exhibits the major classical conditioning phenomena first described by Pavlov: systematic increase in magnitude due to pairing with an unconditioned stimulus (Gerall and Obrist, 1962; Oleson et al., 1972; Ashe et al., 1978b), extinction (Gerall and Obrist, 1962), discrimination between reinforced and non-reinforced stimuli (both between modalities and different stimuli within a single modality) (Oleson et al., 1972, 1975; Ashe et al., 1976, 1978a; Ryugo and Weinberger, 1978), discrimination reversal when the stimulus contingencies are reversed (Oleson et al., 1972, 1975), conditioned inhibition (Weinberger et al., 1973), and inhibition of delay (Oleson et al., 1973). Examples of some of these phenomena are presented in Fig. 1–3.

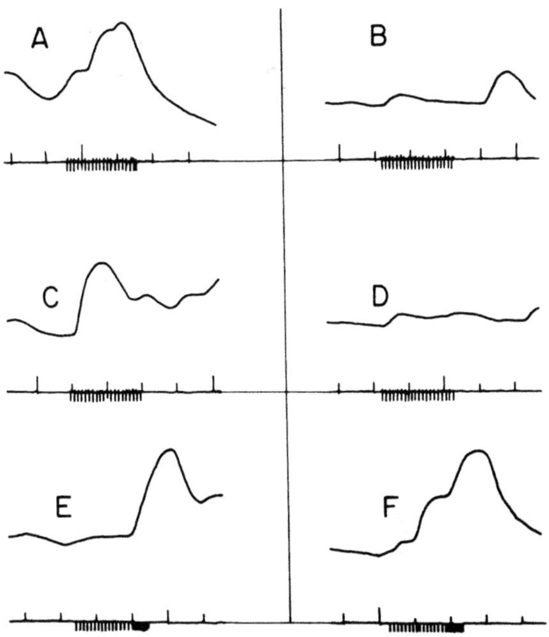

FIG. 1. Single trial pupillary dilation responses to white noise pips for one cat before habituation (A), after habituation (B), during early sensitization (C), after repeated sensitization trials (D), early in conditioning series (E), and after acquisition (F). Upward vertical lines indicate one second marker, downward vertical lines indicate auditory pips and shock. In this and in Fig. 2, a rise in pupillometer write-out indicates increased dilation. In this and Fig. 2, the pupil response may appear to procede the stimulus marker because of the curvilinear nature of the pen writing system.

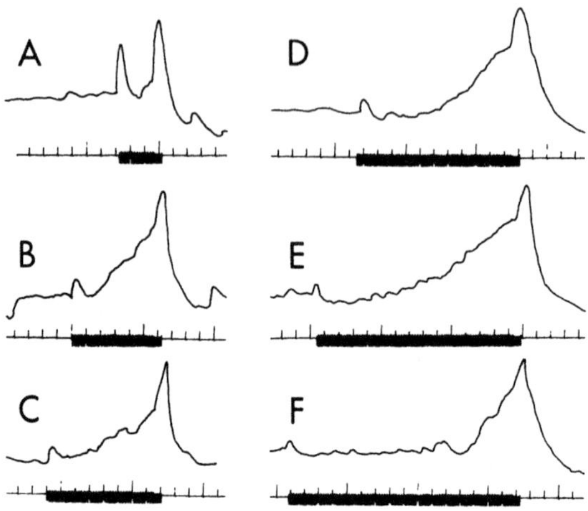

FIG. 2. Single trial pupillary dilation responses to while noise pips for one cat as a function of increasing the CS-US interval from 2.5 seconds (A) to 16 seconds (F). Upward vertical deflections indicate one second marker, downward vertical lines indicate auditory pips and shock (last 0.5 second of marker).

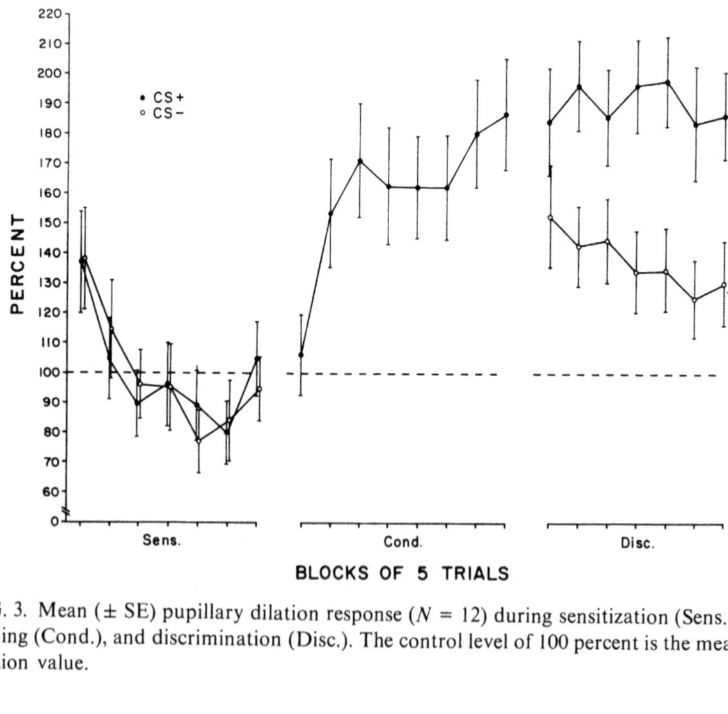

FIG. 3. Mean (± SE) pupillary dilation response ($N = 12$) during sensitization (Sens.), conditioning (Cond.), and discrimination (Disc.). The control level of 100 percent is the mean sensitization value.

In summary, the pupillary dilation conditioned reflex is subject to the same laws of classical (Pavlovian) conditioning as other conditioned responses, including specific somatic conditioned responses. Furthermore, its role as a non-specific response allows it to serve as an index of *conditioned arousal*. Finally, its rapid development is advantageous for concurrent study of neuronal activity during conditioning.[3]

AUDITORY SYSTEM NEURONAL LEARNING

The next step is locating some cells that learn. Certainly, such cells are not confined to one place in the brain—the choice of where to look first is somewhat arbitrary. We began with the auditory system, the system of the conditioned stimulus. Initial neurophysiological studies used the recording of more than one cell at a time (so-called "multiple unit" or "unit cluster" recordings) in order to locate regions within the auditory system in which neuronal learning occurs. This approach is analogous to using a broad-beam searchlight which can indicate the presence of a target quickly but which does not provide detailed information.

Investigation of the lowest and highest levels of the auditory system (the cochlear nucleus and primary auditory cortex, respectively) revealed neuronal learning in both regions (Oleson et al., 1972). (The subjects developed pupillary conditioned reflexes as well). In the auditory cortex, this learning consisted of enhanced response to the conditioned stimulus during pairing of acoustic stimulation and pawshock, relative to a sensitization control period during which the same two stimuli were presented randomly. Additionally, neural discrimination was evident as responses to the reinforced conditioned stimulus were significantly greater than activity evoked by a non-reinforced differential stimulus. Furthermore, when the animals underwent discrimination reversal training one week later, neural discrimination reversal developed. These findings demonstrate that the neural changes are a function of specific stimulus contingencies (associations) and also that the effects of conditioning upon auditory system neuronal activity are not restricted to the particular nature of the acoustic stimuli initially used, but are attributable to the relationship between acoustic stimuli and the unconditioned stimulus.

Changes in evoked neuronal activity within the auditory system during conditioning could in principle be caused by changes in effective stimulus intensity due to movement of the head (Marsh et al., 1962) or pinna (Wiener et

[3] Interestingly, the pupillary dilation conditioned response is not merely a result of activation of the sympathetic control of the iris; rather, inhibition of the parasympathetic innervation serves a critical function (Ashe et al., 1978a,b; Ashe and Cooper, 1978).

al., 1966) relative to the sound source, action of the middle ear muscles (Galambos and Rupert, 1959), or even to masking noise produced by the subject's own movements (Imig and Weinberger, 1970; Irvine and Webster, 1972). However, in the present experiment, these effects are attributable to central neural processes because stimulus constancy was assured by neuromuscular paralysis. Additionally, the within-trial latency of neuronal learning was less than the latency for pupillary dilation, ruling out any possible role for sensory feedback from the pupillary conditioned response itself. Finally, an independent assessment of cochlear function was made by recording the cochlear microphonic response during conditioning. There was no systematic change in the cochlear microphonic, once again ruling out changes in effective stimulus intensity at the receptor (Ashe et al., 1976).

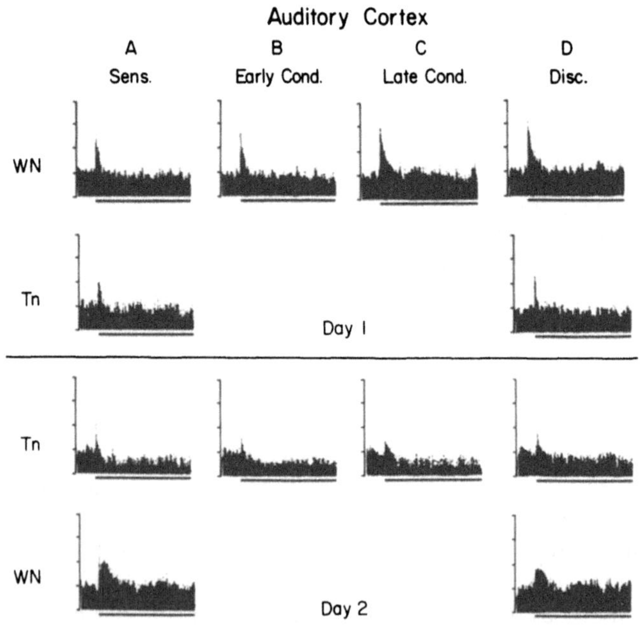

FIG. 4. Average histograms of multiple-unit activity in the auditory cortex of one animal during sensitization (A), early conditioning (trials 1–10), late conditioning (trials 46–55), and discrimination (trials 86–94 for white noise and trials 66–75 for tone for Day 1; vice versa for Day 2). Response to the acoustic stimuli during sensitization on Day 1 consisted of a brief increase in activity followed by sustained discharges below pretrial levels ("inhibition"). Note the increase in the initial discharge and the reduction or abolition of the following inhibition during conditioning and discrimination. On Day 2 (reversal training), the enhanced response to the white noise stimulus, which developed on Day 1, is still evident (Day 2, A). The inhibition to the tone is systematically reduced during conditioning (B,C) and discrimination (D). Calibration: 96 spikes per division. Bar denotes CS presentation; duration: 5 seconds.

COMPARTMENTALIZATION OF NEURONAL LEARNING

In view of the rapid neuronal learning in auditory cortex, it seemed advisable to study its major source of input, the medial geniculate nucleus within the thalamus. The medial geniculate nucleus actually consists of three major subdivisions or compartments: the ventral, the dorsal, and the medial (magnocellular) areas (Morest, 1964). All three regions project to auditory cortex, including primary, secondary, and other auditory cortical fields. It is particularly noteworthy that the ventral region projects only to primary auditory cortex, while the medial region alone projects to *all* areas (Winer et al., 1977). The medial and ventral regions both receive ascending input via the brachium of the inferior colliculus (Moore and Goldberg, 1963, 1966; Jones and Rockel, 1971). A Golgi reconstruction reveals some of the differences (Fig. 5). The ventral region contains so-called tufted cells, charac-

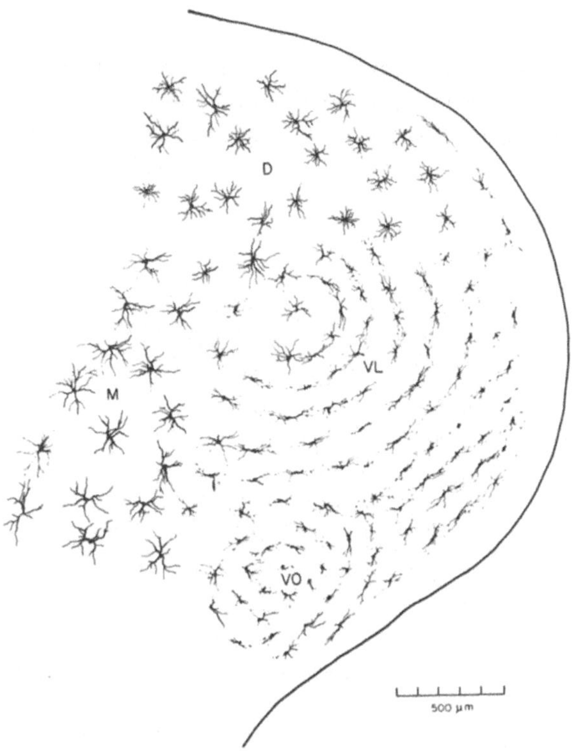

FIG. 5. Camera lucida reconstruction of the MGB from Golgi material. Typical distribution of neuronal types through the middle of the medial geniculate body of the adult cat. Coronal section, Golgi-Cox. Abbreviations: D, dorsal division; M, medial division; VL, ventral division, pars lateralis; VO, ventral division, pars ovoida.

teristic of topographically-organized sensory nuclei (Morest, 1964) laid out in lamina (Morest, 1965a). Each neuron receives the terminals of only a few collicular efferents, and as expected, the ventral region is tonotopically organized (Aitkin and Webster, 1972). The dorsal region is more diffusely organized, with medium sized cells having evenly spaced radiating dendrites (Morest, 1964, 1965b); it has no tonotopic features (Aitkin and Webster, 1972). The medial division is of particular interest; its large neurons have especially long dendrites radiating from the soma, each cell receiving contacts from many ascending auditory fibers (Morest, 1964), no doubt accounting for their broad tuning curves and the absence of tonotopic organization (Aitkin, 1973; Love and Scott, 1969). In short, the medial geniculate nucleus contains regions that appear to be "auditory specific" or lemniscal line (ventral region) and "less specific" or lemniscal adjuncts (medial and dorsal) (see also Graybiel, 1972). Primary auditory cortex receives convergent input from the ventral and medial regions, i.e., from lemniscal line and lemniscal adjunct loci.

An investigation of neuronal plasticity in the medial geniculate during classical conditioning, as indexed by the pupillary dilation response, revealed that neuronal learning is obtained only in the medial subdivision (Ryugo and Weinberger, 1976, 1978). A histological summary denotes learning sites as open circles, non-learning sites as closed circles (Fig. 6). All

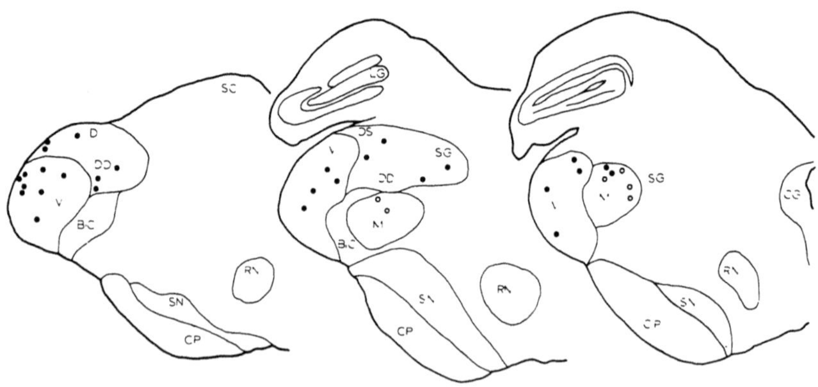

FIG. 6. Histological verification of microelectrode placements in MGB. Solid circles indicate electrode placements where conditioned changes were not detected. Open circles indicate sites of conditioned change. All of the loci which exhibited conditioned changes were confined to MGm. Abbreviations: BIC, brachium of inferior colliculus; CG, central gray; CP, cerebral peduncles; D, dorsal division, DD, deep dorsal nucleus; DS, superficial dorsal nucleus; LG, lateral geniculate body; RN, red nucleus; SC, superior colliculus; SG, suprageniculate nucleus; SN, substantia nigra; V, ventral division.

learning sites are located in the medial subdivision; none are found in the ventral or dorsal regions. Note that there are two non-learning sites in the medial division; we will consider these again momentarily. The differential plasticity within the medial geniculate is underscored by the fact that data from learning sites in the medial division were obtained simultaneously with data from non-learning sites in the other areas, i.e., from within the same subject. Figure 7 shows trial-by-trial learning curves obtained concurrently for the pupil, medial and ventral divisions. In each case, the pupil developed

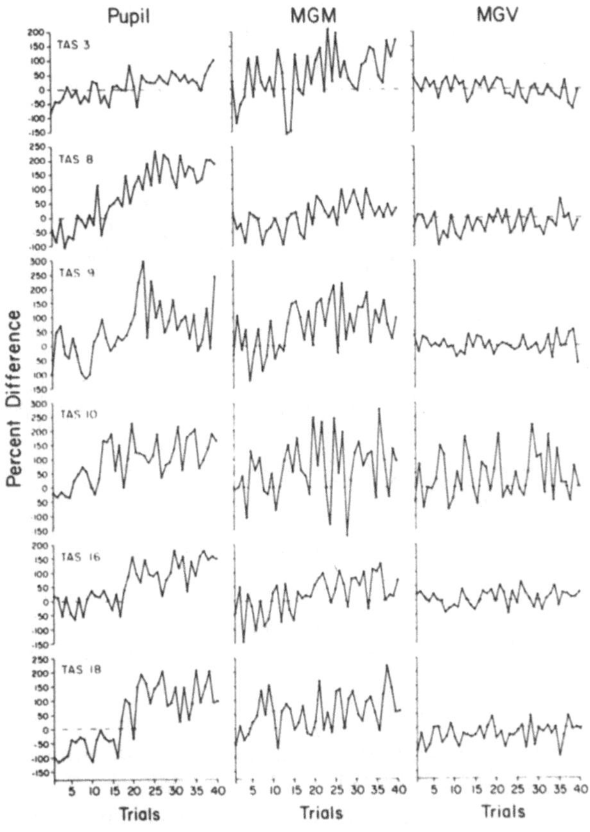

FIG. 7. Trial-by-trial plot of pupillary, MGm, and MGv response changes during conditioning. Each point represents the normalized response to the CS+ during its 1.0 second presentation, expressed as a percent difference score relative to its mean sensitization value (*dashed line*). Both pupil and MGm neuronal activity exhibit a systematic growth of responsivity during conditioning. MGv neuronal activity fails to demonstrate such conditioned response enhancement. Data are from animals that developed pupillary conditioning and had placements in MGm and MGv of the same medial geniculate body.

a conditioned response and so did the medial division. The ventral division functions are in no case significantly greater than control levels obtained during random presentation of the CS and US.[4] This experiment also included discrimination training, with the result that loci in the medial division that developed neuronal learning also developed differential responding between two acoustic stimuli. Neural discrimination did not develop in the ventral or dorsal regions.

As noted above, neural learning is obtained only in the medial division, but two loci in this region did not learn. This raises the question of interpretation of *negative* findings, and the importance of a behavioral index of the adequacy of the preparation, as discussed previously. Pupillary and neural data from these two cases are provided in Fig. 8. Note that the failure

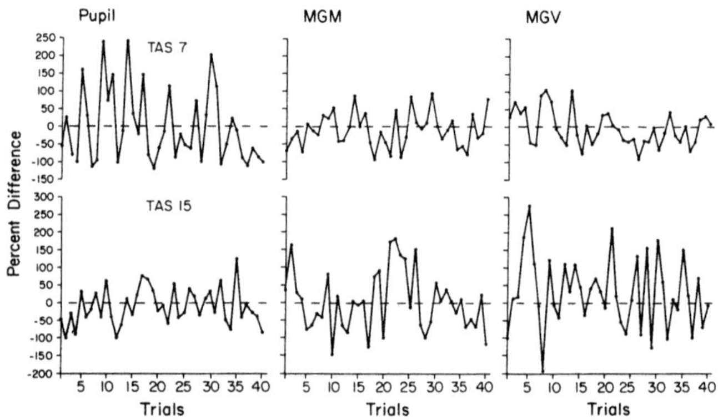

FIG. 8. Trial-by-trial plots of pupillary, MGm, and MGv response changes during conditioning in cats that failed to attain pupillary acquisition criteria. Each point represents the normalized response to the CS+, expressed as a percent difference score relative to its mean sensitization value (*dashed line*). Neither pupil nor neuronal activity exhibit any systematic change in responsiveness during conditioning, indicating that lack of learning in MGm occurs only in behaviorally substandard animals.

of neural learning in these cases occurred in the only two subjects in which a pupillary conditioned response also failed to develop. Therefore, these negative findings cannot be considered cases of non-learning in the medial division as the animals, for whatever reasons, were substandard. These results illustrate the tight coupling between behavioral and neural learning

[4] Functions for the medial division are statistically significant but the slopes are modest. There is good reason to believe that these data represent a mixture of discharges from neurons that learn and neurons that don't learn or that acquire a decreased response to the CS; we will return to this point later.

in the medial division, and underscore the importance of having a behavioral control for interpreting neurophysiological data during learning.

Overall, these findings indicate that neuronal learning within the source of auditory cortex inputs is *compartmentalized*, being restricted to the medial region of the medial geniculate nucleus. As primary auditory cortex is highly plastic, it may be that this character is conferred by projections from the learning medial division while tonotopic information is provided by the non-learning ventral division.

CHARACTERISTICS OF SINGLE NEURON DISCHARGES

The third step is to determine the discharge characteristics of single cells within the medial geniculate nucleus during classical conditioning. In particular, we have been concerned with comparing and contrasting discharge properties that might predict whether or not cells develop enhanced responses to the conditioned stimulus during subsequent training. Extensive observations have been completed for neurons in the magnocellular division and the following data refer only to neurons from this area.

Single cell recordings concurrent with formation of the pupillary dilation conditioned reflex were obtained from 34 cells in 34 cats. As the goal of these experiments was to seek discharge characteristics *predictive* of conditionability, the data from only one cell per animal were suitable. Thus, while it was technically feasible to run a second training series, recording from a second cell after completion of the initial training, the cat was no longer naive; neither were its neurons.[5]

Of 34 cells, 24 (71%) did learn, i.e., develop a significant change in evoked discharge. The total number were divided into four groups: (A) cells with increased response meeting a rigorous criterion ($p < .001$), $n = 8$; (B) cells with increased response meeting a less severe criterion ($p < .05$), $n = 9$; (C) cells failing to meet significance at the 5 percent level ($n = 10$); (D) cells developing a significant decrease in response during conditioning ($n = 7$).

Figure 9 depicts learning curves for these four groups for sensitization (random presentation of the stimuli) and the first twenty trails of conditioning (CS-US pairing).

Group A shows pronounced habituation during the sensitization phase followed by an *increased response* which is clearly present by trials 8 to 10, and which has *not* reached asymptote by the end of the first twenty con-

[5] The possibility of running an extinction session before recording from a second cell fails to take into account the fact that extinction comprises a form of learning rather than erasure, and ignores the very real factor of spontaneous recovery.

ditioning trials. There is no pronounced change in background activity. Group B, which met a less severe statistical criterion, has a less pronounced habituation function but also does exhibit rapid learning. In contrast to

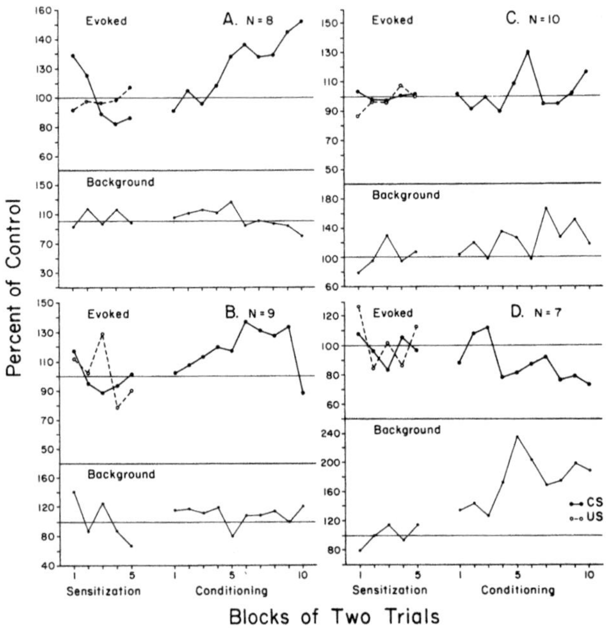

FIG. 9. Learning curves for four cell groups according to learning criteria. See text for details.

Group A, this potentiated evoked discharge reaches asymptote quickly (trial 12) and returns to baseline at the end of twenty trials. Background activity is also more variable for these cells, and there is an indication of a slight increase in background discharges during conditioning. (However, the nature of this increase could not account for the incremental learning curve for evoked activity.) Cells which failed to meet statistical significance (Group C) have a poor habituation function and no clear learning function.[6] Of interest, there is a significant increase in background discharge during conditioning. Cells developing a *decrease* in response to the conditioned stimulus (D) also develop a significant *increase* in background activity. The functions for evoked and background discharges are almost mirror images;

[6] The close relationship between apparent neuronal habituation and conditioning is intriguing, but not considered further due to space limitations.

thus the apparent decremental learning is due to the *increase* in *background activity* rather than to an actual decrease in the number of spikes evoked by the conditioned stimulus. The conditioning procedure has in effect converted cells which initially had little if any response to the CS into cells with an inhibitory response.

The different learning functions of the groups probably account for the modest slopes of learning curves seen in the previous experiment, in which *multiple-unit* recordings were used. Thus, addition of the single unit data from all four groups of neurons would yield only a modest positive slope.

The rate of learning for cells in Groups A and B is extremely rapid, possibly faster than any previously reported. Figure 10 gives data for a cell

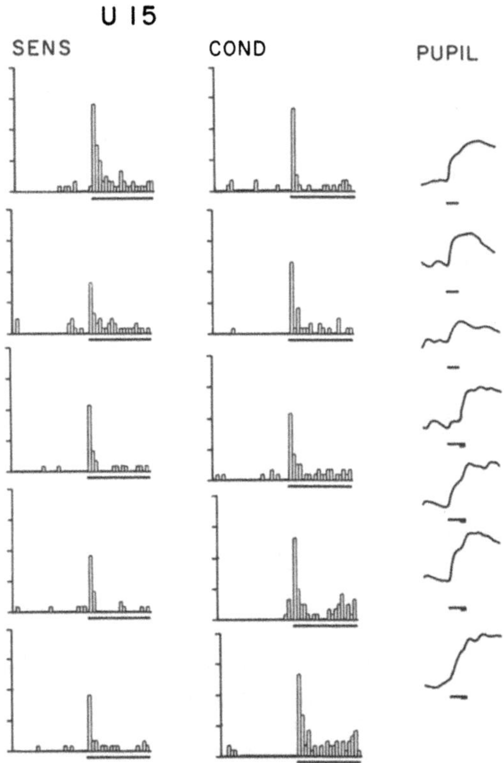

FIG. 10. Histograms and pupillary records for cell U-15 illustrating background discharges and discharges during the one-second acoustic stimulus (horizontal marker). Each histogram is the sum of two consecutive trials, each bar represents 50 msec. Data for the ten trials of sensitization and the first ten trials of conditioning are presented. Note the decrement during sensitization and the extremely rapid increment during conditioning. Calibration: 6 spikes per division; horizontal bar, 1 second. Sample pupillary records from top to bottom: sensitization trials 1, 5, 10 and conditioning trials 1, 3, 5, 7. In this and Fig. 11, 12, and 14, the horizontal line indicates the one-second presentation of the conditioned stimulus and the downward deflection represents the 375 msec presentation of the unconditioned stimulus.

from Group A, showing histograms for blocks of two trials for the ten trials of sensitization and the first ten trials of conditioning. There is a clear and rapid decrement in evoked activity during sensitization. Such rapid habituation has been reported often in the literature in both invertebrate and vertebrate preparations. The systematic and extremely rapid increment in response during the first ten trials of conditioning is noteworthy; a potentiated response, relative to the end of sensitization is present in the third histogram (trials 5–6). Pupillary records from selected trials are also given. The purpose of these records is simply to show that a pupillary conditioned response also developed rapidly; there has been no attempt to try to draw strict relationships between the cellular and behavioral plasticity in this experiment as the behavior is used mainly as a control.

The extremely rapid cellular learning for Group A is persistent within the time limits of this experiment. Figure 11 provides histograms of successive

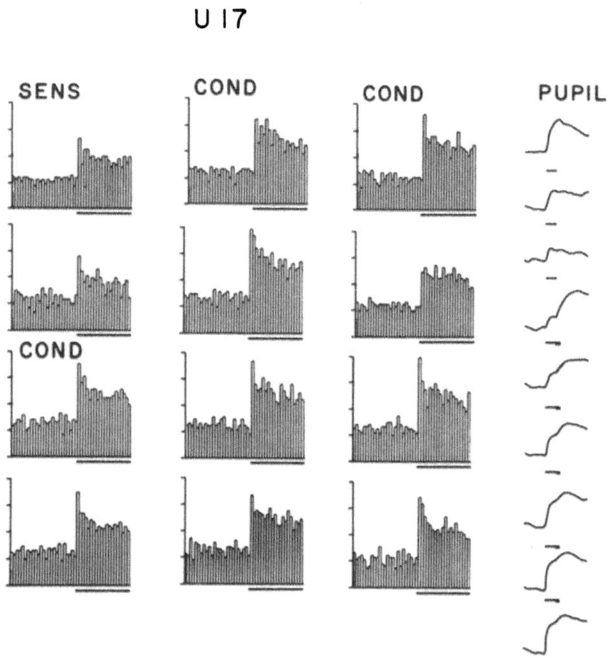

FIG. 11. Histograms and pupillary records for cell U-17. Each histogram is the sum of five consecutive trials; each bar represents 50 msec. Data for all sensitization and conditioning trials are presented. Note that the response to the conditioned stimulus has been potentiated within the first five trials of conditioning; this effect is persistent, block eight (trials 36–40) alone is not significantly greater than the sensitization response. Note also the absence of any systematic change in background activity. Calibration: 12 spikes per division. Sample pupillary records illustrates trials 1,7, and 10 during sensitization (top three records) and trials 1,5,10,20,30, and 45 during conditioning, from top to bottom. Note the decrement in pupillary response during sensitization and the subsequent development of the conditioned response during conditioning. Note also the constant size of the dilation to the shock during conditioning and the growth of the response to the CS relative to this unconditioned response.

blocks of five trials for another cell from Group A. The evoked response relative to sensitization is already potentiated by the end of the first five trials of classical conditioning. This enhancement lasts throughout the 50 trials during which contact with this neuron was maintained. As in the case of other cells that learned, the pupil also developed a rapid and lasting conditioned response.

Cells in Group C did not learn; this might be related to their increase in background activity. Figure 12 provides data for this type of neuron. An increase in the number of discharges during CS presentation is evident during conditioning, but this is balanced by an increase in background activity. The

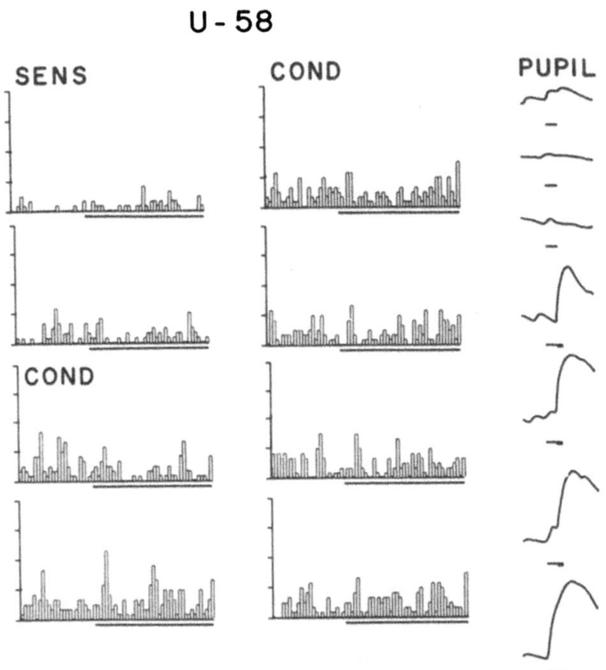

FIG. 12. Histograms and pupillary records for cell U-58. Each histogram is the sum of five consecutive trials; each bar represents 25 msec. Data for all sensitization and conditioning trials are shown. This cell failed to develop an increase in response to the CS greater than the increase in background activity. As in the case of other non-learning cells (Group C), there was no pronounced onset response to the conditioned stimulus at the beginning of training (compare with cells in Group A, Fig. 10). Calibration: 6 spikes per division, 1 second. Pupil records, top to bottom: sensitization trials 1,5,10 and conditioning trials 1,5,10, and 25. The failure of the cell to learn is not attributable to a possibly poor preparation because, as with all other cells in Group C, a pupillary dilation conditioned reflex was established (compare the first and fourth records during conditioning).

failure of this cell to learn (and other cells in Group C as well) is due to relative non-plasticity of the neurons rather than a possibly poor preparation; the adequacy of the preparation is independently indexed by the pupillary records, revealing the acquisition of a very large pupillary dilation conditioned reflex.

Discharge characteristics of all cells were analyzed for the period preceding conditioning in order to determine whether there is a physiological characteristic that predicts subsequent conditioning. Several parameters of background activity, recorded during a period proceding the initiation of sensitization, were calculated; e.g., mean spontaneous rate, standard deviation of the spontaneous rate, and the "alpha" and "beta" indices used by O'Brien and Fox (1969a,b) and O'Brien et al. (1973). None of these measures differentiated among or between the four groups of cells. Initial responsiveness to the conditioned and unconditioned stimuli was also examined, the values taken from the first five CS and US trials of sensitiza-

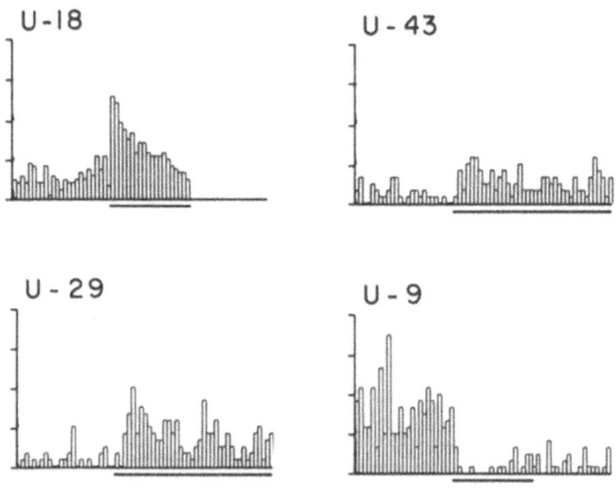

FIG. 13. Histograms illustrating types of cellular responses to the CS, representing discharges during the first five CS trials of the sensitization period. (Inhibitory responses were rare; an example, U-9, is included for the sake of completeness). Note the histograms of U-18, U-29, and U-43, each of which shows an excitatory response to the acoustic stimulus. The overall responses during the entire CS presentation are similar; z scores (discharges during the CS divided by the standard deviation of discharges prior to CS onset) are: U-18 = 0.780; U-29 = 1.098; U-43 = 0.775. In contrast, the z scores for the first 100 msec of CS presentation are: U-18 = 27.150; U-29 = 1.62; U-43 = 3.420. Whereas the peak evoked discharge for U-18 occurred during the first 100 msec, the peaks for the other cells occurred later than 100 msec. Cell U-18 is from Group A, those cells showing the greatest and most persistent learning; U-29 is from Group B showing less pronounced and less persistent learning; U-43 is from Group C, the non-learning group. Calibration: 6 spikes per division, one second.

tion, respectively. Degree of "bimodal convergence" (response to both the CS and US) was also determined. Again, there were no statistically significant differences between or among groups. Thus, under the circumstances of this experiment, which include an independent behavioral assessment of associative learning, neither "bimodal convergence" (e.g., Yoshii and Ogura, 1960) nor spontaneous rate (e.g., Kotlyar and Mayorov, 1971) differentiate learning from non-learning neurons.

Inspection of the histograms for each cell suggested that the *pattern* of response to the conditioned stimulus was different among the groups (Fig. 13). Specifically, it appeared that cells exhibiting a *large onset* response (Group A, U-18) were also those which conditioned rapidly and persistently, in contrast to cells which had an equal or larger overall response to the CS, but *without* a pronounced "onset" response (U-43, U-29). The data were reanalyzed on the basis of the first 100 msec of CS presentation. Indeed it was found that Group A had a significantly larger onset response, relative to background activity, than any of the other three groups, none of which differed from the other (Table 2).

Table 2. Onset Response (First 100 ,sec)

Group	*N*	*Onset Score*⁺	*Mann-Whitney U*		
			B	*C*	*D*
A	8	20.88	7**	9**	9*
B	9	1.05	—	35	20
C	10	1.90		—	39
D	7	3.79			—

+Mean z score for the first five CS trials of sensitization

$$\text{where } z = \frac{\bar{X}\text{ Evoked}}{\text{S.D. Background}}$$

*$p < .028$, two-tailed
**$p < .01$, two-tailed

Thus, overall responsiveness to the conditioned stimulus does not predict rapid and persistent cellular learning, whereas the presence of a large onset response *does* predict learning.

The importance of using a concurrent behavioral control to interpret negative data is illustrated in Fig. 14. The cell in question has a pronounced onset response, which as we have just seen, should predict learning. However, this cell failed to learn. The right side of this figure presents samples of pupillary data. During pairing of the CS and the US, unconditioned

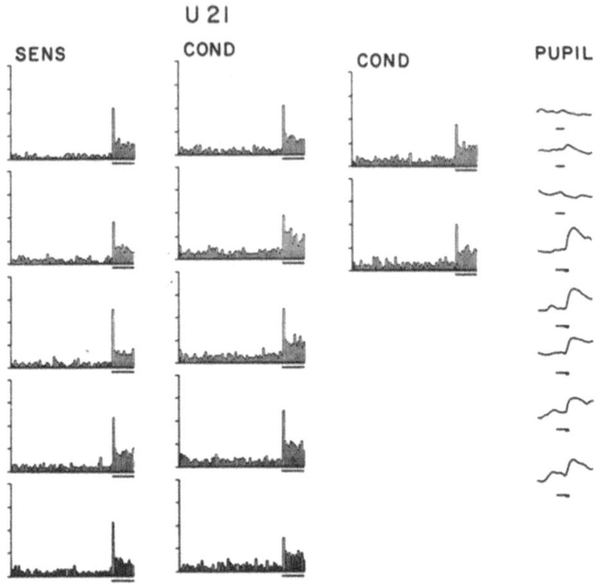

FIG. 14. Hostograms and pupillary records for cell U-21. Each histogram is the sum of five consecutive trials; each bar represents 83.3 msec. Data for all sensitization and conditioning trials are shown. Although this unit is characterized by a pronounced onset response (greatest response during the first 100 seconds.), there was no systematic change in response (i.e., increase) during conditioning, nor a decrement during sensitization (apparent habituation). Calibration: 12 spikes per division, one second. Sample pupillary records illustrate trials 1,3, and 10 during sensitization and trials 1,6,16,26, and 35 during conditioning. The pupil was minimally responsive during sensitization, and a conditioned pupillary dilation response did not develop, despite the presence of an unconditioned response.

responses were large, but a pupillary dilation conditioned response did not develop. Therefore, the preparation was substandard and hence the failure of the cell to learn cannot be interpreted as an instance of non-learning. If a behavioral control had not been used, the cell would have been classified as a non-learner and as it is characterized by a pronounced onset response, this feature would apparently not be confined to learning cells. With the behavioral control, the importance of an onset response of the cell to the conditioned stimulus remains as a valid predictor of rapid cellular learning.

CONCLUSIONS

Investigations of the neuronal bases of associative learning can profitably exploit the rapid development of conditioned arousal in the search for cellular processes underlying learning. Conditioned arousal, as indexed by development of a pupillary dilation conditioned response, provides an opportunity to record the discharges of single neurons throughout the course of classical conditioning training, thus providing comprehensive data from a single neuron concurrent with behavioral findings. Furthermore, the measurement of conditioned behavioral arousal using an autonomic index permits the use of neuromuscular paralysis which provides strict control of stimulus intensity and a highly stable preparation for electrophysiological recordings.

Under such conditions, neuronal learning develops in the system that processes the signal stimulus, the auditory system. Thus, a sensory system analyzes not only the physical parameters of stimuli, but also the psychological parameters, that is, the meaning or importance of a physically constant stimulus whose significance is changed by virtue of its use as a conditioned stimulus.

While the auditory cortex is sensitive to both parameters, its thalamic source of input is organized differently. At this level, the tonotopically organized ventral subdivision of the medial geniculate does not develop neural conditioned responses in contrast to the less specific magnocellular region which is plastic. The particular plasticity of the magnocellular medial geniculate has been replicated in two other laboratories. Research initiated by the late James Olds indicates that multiple-unit conditioned responses to acoustic stimulation develop in the medial but not ventral division of the medial geniculate nucleus in the rat (Birt et al., 1978).[7] The training situation involved an appetitive hybrid classical-instrumental conditioning paradigm. Miller (1979) reported similar findings for the rabbit trained in an instrumental avoidance situation. The replication of our initial report and extension to two other species and two other conditioning paradigms strongly supports the notion that cells within the magnocellular subdivision of the medial geniculate nucleus are especially plastic during learning.

It is also of interest that the organization of this nucleus is essentially the same across a very wide and diverse range of mammals. In addition to the rat, cat, and rabbit, these include the tree shrew (Oliver and Hall, 1975), the squirrel monkey (Jordan, 1973), the owl monkey (Fitzpatrick and Imig, 1978), and the oppossum (M. Robards, unpublished). The magnocellular medial geniculate nucleus may constitute an especially conditionable substrate of an evolutionarily conservative nature, i.e., one that was attained early in mammalian evolution and thereafter maintained.

Within the magnocellular region, over 70 percent of the cells do learn, as evidenced by systematic changes in evoked activity to a conditioned stimulus. Learning is not related to the ability of a neuron to respond to both the conditioned and unconditioned stimuli. Rather, the best learning

[7] Disterhoft and Stuart (1976) failed to find significant learning in the medial geniculate nucleus of the rat, but pooled data from the various subdivisions.

cells are characterized by a *pronounced onset response* to the acoustic conditioned stimulus *before* training is initiated. Thus, it is the *pattern* of response to a stimulus, not simply the occurrence of a response, that seems to be important for rapid and persistent cellular learning.

Hypotheses about the circuitry and the mechanisms of cellular associative learning now can be formulated. For example, the pronounced onset response suggests that rapid and persistent cellular learning occurs in neurons which have a rather direct and effective input pathway from the primary auditory system. But further discussion of such hypotheses would be premature until the locus-of-learning issue has been settled. The magnocellular area is likely to be a site of active learning processes because it receives the same input as the ventral region, which does not learn. However, a definitive answer depends upon more direct experiments, which are now in progress.

Closely related to this issue of cellular mechanism is the more general problem of the neuronal events that permit the establishment of neuronal and ultimately behavioral conditioned responses. Here, too, the level of arousal appears intimately related to learning, even to learning of conditioned arousal. Thus, learning is not efficient, perhaps not possible, during sleep (Simon and Emmons, 1955; Emmons and Simon, 1956). It now appears that sleep is amnestic (Guilleminault and Dement, 1977). At the other extreme, the level of central neural tonus, as indicated by the particular frequency of hippocampal theta activity, is predictive of the rate of learning of the classically conditioned nictitating membrane response of the rabbit (Berry and Thompson, 1978). Also, the level of neuronal firing in the reticular formation of the cat (another index of central tonus) is predictive of the rate of habituation of eye movements toward a sound source (Weinberger et al., 1969). Finally there is accumulating evidence that learning and memory are modulated by the degree of incremented arousal evoked by the training stimulus in several situations; the mechanism seems to involve the degree of release of peripheral catecholamines which provide feedback to the brain regarding the level of "peripheral arousal" (McGaugh et al., 1980).

These findings suggest that neuronal learning as reported here may be modulated by the level of background arousal or neural tonus. Such experiments should provide critical data about cellular mechanisms of learning. However, this issue is likely to be complicated. Certainly, arousal is neither equivalent to, nor necessarily correlated with, simply an increased probability of neuronal discharge throughout the nervous system, because, as we have seen, conditioned arousal has highly differentiated and characteristic effects upon different groups of neurons within the magnocellular medial geniculate nucleus. It may be, as postulated by Konorski, that cellular modification during learning is dependent upon the presence of facilitatory input from non-specific "arousal" systems together with input from classical sensory systems (Konorski, 1967). Detection of this critical specific input may be difficult if it is itself insufficient to produce cellular discharge. Nonetheless, it should be detectable with precise microcellular techniques. It is, in any event, evident that arousal continues to provide a challenge to those concerned both with central activity states and their relationship to acquired behavior.

ACKNOWLEDGEMENTS

Research reported here was supported by the following: BNS76-81924 from the National Science Foundation and AA00334 from the National Institute on Alcohol Abuse and Alcoholism to Norman M. Weinberger, NIMH Predoctoral Fellowship No. MH 05440-02 to John H. Ashe, NIMH Predoctoral Fellowship No. MH 05424 to David K. Ryugo, and NIMH Predoctoral Fellowship No. MH 51324 to T.D. Oleson.

I wish to acknowledge with pleasure the secretarial assistance of Elain Hackelman, and the technical assistance of Lola Moffitt, Simon Boughey, Bill Hopkins, and Brad Koontz.

REFERENCES

Aitkin, L.M., Medial geniculate body of the cat: Responses to tonal stimuli of neurons in medial division. *J. Neurophysiol.* 36, 275–283 (1973).

Aitkin, L.M., and Webster, W.R. Medial geniculate body of the cat: Organization and responses to tonal stimuli of neurons in ventral division. *J. Neurophysiol.* 35, 365–380 (1972).

Ashe, J.H., Cassady, J.M., and Weinberger, N.M. The relationship of the cochlear microphonic potential to the acquisition of a classically conditioned pupillary dilation response. *Behav. Biol.* 16, 45–62 (1976).

Ashe, J.H., and Cooper, C.L. Multifiber efferent activity in postganglionic sympathetic and parasympathetic nerves related to the latency of spontaneous and evoked pupillary dilation. *Exp. Neurol.* 59, 413–434 (1978).

Ashe, J.H., Cooper, C.L., and Weinberger, N.M. Role of the parasympathetic pupillomotor system in classically conditioned pupillary dilation of the cat. *Behav. Biol.* 23, 1–13 (1978a).

Ashe, J.H., Cooper, C.L., and Weinberger, N.M. Mesencephalic multiple-unit activity during acquisition of conditioned pupillary dilation. *Brain Res. Bull.* 3, 143–154 (1978b).

Ben-Ari, Y., and LaSalle, G.E.G. Plasticity at unitary level. II. Modifications during sensory-sensory association procedures. *Electroenceph. Clin. Neurophysiol.* 32, 667–679 (1972).

Berry, S.D., and Thompson, R.F. Prediction of learning rate from the hippocampal electroencephalogram. *Science* 200, 1298–1300 (1978).

Birt, D., Nienhuis, R., and Olds, M. Separation of associative from non-associative short latency changes in medial geniculate and inferior colliculus during differential conditioning and reversal in rats. *Soc. Neurosci. Abs.* 4, 255 (1978).

Black, A.H. Cardiac conditioning in curarized dogs. The relationship between heart rate and skeletal behaviour, in *Classical Conditioning: A Symposium*. W.F. Prokasy, ed. Appleton-Century-Crofts, New York (1965), pp. 20–47.

Bradshaw, J.L. Pupil size and problem solving. *Quart. J. Exp. Psychol.* 20, 116–122 (1968).

Bruner, A. Reinforcement strength in classical conditioning of leg flexion, freezing, and heart rate in cats. *Cond. Reflex* 4, 24–31 (1969).

Bures, J., and Buresova, O. Relationship between spontaneous and evoked unit activity in the inferior colliculus in rats. *J. Neurophysiol.* 28, 641–644 (1965).

Champion, R.A. *Learning and Activation*. John Wiley and Sons, New York (1969).

Cohen, D.H. The neural pathways and informational flow mediating a conditioned autonomic response, in *Limbic and Autonomic Nervous Systems Research*. L.V. DiCara, ed. Plenum Press, New York (1974).

Davidson, R.E., and Richardson, A.M. Classical conditioning of skeletal and autonomic responses in the lizard. *Physiol. Behav.* 5, 589–594 (1970).

Delius, J.D. Irrelevant behaviour, information processing, and arousal homeostasis. *Psychol. Forsch.* 33, 165–188 (1970).

Dell, P. Reticular homeostasis and critical reactivity, in *Progress in Brain Research*, Vol. 1. G. Moruzzi, A. Fessard, and H.H. Jasper, eds. Elsevier Publishing Company, Amsterdam (1963), pp. 82–103.

Dell, P., Bonvallet, M., and Hugelin, A. Mechanisms of reticular deactivation, in *The Nature of Sleep*. G.E.W. Wolstenhomme and C.M. O'Connor, eds. Churchill, London (1961), pp. 86–107.

deToledo, L., and Black, A.H. Heart rate: Changes during conditioned suppression in rats. *Science* 152, 1404–1406 (1966).

Disterhoft, J.F., and Stuart, D.K. Trial sequence of changed unit activity in auditory system of alert rat during conditioned response acquisition and extinction. *J. Neurophysiol.* 39, 266–281 (1976).

Emmons, W.H., and Simon, C.W. The non-recall of material presented during sleep. *Am. J. Psychol.* 69, 76–81 (1956).

Fitzpatrick, K.A., and Imig, T.J. Projections of auditory cortex upon the thalamus and midbrain in the owl monkey. *J. Comp. Neurol.* 177, 537–556 (1978).

Galambos, R., and Rubert, A. Action of middle ear muscles in normal cats. *J. Acoust. Soc. Am.* 31, 349–355 (1959).

Galeano, C. Electrophysiological aspects of brain activity during conditioning: A review. *Acta Neurol. Latinoamer.* 9, 395–413 (1963).

Geral, A.A., and Obrist, P.A. Classical conditioning of the pupillary dilation response of normal and curarized cats. *J. Comp. Physiol. Psychol.* 55, 486–491 (1962).

Gluck, H., and Rowland, V. Defensive conditioning of electrographic arousal with delayed and differentiated auditory stimuli. *Electroenceph. Clin. Neurophysiol.* 11, 485–496 (1959).

Gormezano, I., Schneiderman, N., Deaux, E., and Fuentes, I. Nictitating membrane: Classical conditioning and extinction in the albino rabbit. *Science* 138, 33–34 (1962).

Graybiel, A.M. Some fiber pathways related to the posterior thalamic region in the cat. *Brain Behav. Evol.* 6, 363–393 (1972).

Guilleminault, C., and Dement, W.C. Amnesia and disorders of excessive daytime sleepiness, in *Neurobiology of Sleep and Memory*. R.R. Drucker-Colin and J.L. McGaugh, eds. Academic Press, New York (1977), pp. 439–456.

Holdstock, T.L., and Schwartzbaum, J.S. Classical conditioning of heart rate and galvanic skin response in the rat. *Psychophysiology* 2, 25–38 (1965).

Imig, T.J., and Weinberger, N.M. Auditory system multi-unit activity and behavior in the rat. *Psychon. Sci.* 18, 164–165 (1970).

Irvine, D.R.F., and Webster, W.R. Studies of peripheral gating in the auditory system of cats. *Electroenceph. Clin. Neurophysiol.* 32, 545–556 (1972).

John, E.R. Higher nervous functions: Brain functions and learning. *Ann. Rev. Physiol.* 23, 451–484 (1961).

John, E.R., Leiman, A.L., and Sachs, E. An exploration of the functional relationship between electroencephalographic potentials and differential inhibition. *Ann. N.Y. Acad. Sci.* 92, 1160–1182 (1961).

John, E.G., and Rockel, A.J. The synaptic organization in the medial geniculate body of afferent fibres ascending from the inferior colliculus. *Z. Zellforsch.* 113, 44–66 (1971).

Jordan, H. The structure of the medial geniculate nucleus (MGN): A cyto- and myeloarchitectonic study in the squirrel monkey. *J. Comp. Neurol.* 148, 469–479 (1973).

Kahneman, D., and Beatty, J. Pupil diameter and load on memory. *Science* 154, 1583–1585 (1966).

Konorski, J. *Integrative Activity of the Brain: An Interdisciplinary Approach*. University of Chicago Press, Chicago (1967).

Kotlyar, B.I., and Mayorov, V.I. Activity of the visual cortex units in rabbits in the course of association of sound with rhythmic light. *Zh. Vyssh. Nerv. Deiat.* 21, 157–163 (1971) (Rus.).

Lindsley, D.B. The role of nonspecific reticulo-thalamo-cortical systems in emotion, in *Physiological Correlates of Emotion*. P. Black, ed. Academic Press, New York (1970), pp. 147–188.

Love, J.A., and Scott, J.W. Some response characteristics of cells of the magnocellular division of the medial geniculate body of the cat. *Can. J. Physiol. Pharmacol.* 47, 881–888 (1969).

Marsh, J.T., Worden, F.G., and Hicks, L. Some effects of room acoustics on evoked auditory potentials. *Science* 137, 280–282 (1962).

McGaugh, J.L., Martinez, J.L., Jr., Jensen, R.A., Messing, R.B., and Vasquez, B.J. Central and peripheral catecholamine function in learning and memory processes, in *Neural Mechanisms of Goal-Directed Behavior and Learning*. R.F. Thompson and U.B. Shvyrkov, eds. Academic Press, New York (1980), pp. 75–81.

Miller, J.D. Multiple unit activity in the rabbit thalamus and inferior colliculus during differential avoidance conditioning and reversal. Dissertation submitted in partial fulfillment of the requirements for the Ph.D., U. of Texas at Austin (1979).

Mirsky, A.F., and Pragay, E.B. EEG characteristics of impaired attention accompanying secobarbital and chlorpromazine administration in monkeys, in *Attention—Contemporary Theory and Analysis*. D.I. Mostofsky, ed. Appleton-Century-Crofts, New York (1970), pp. 403–415.

Moore, R.Y., and Goldberg, J.M. Ascending projections of the inferior colliculus in the cat. *J. Comp. Neurol.* 121, 109–136 (1963).

Moore, R.Y., and Goldberg, J.M. Projections of the inferior colliculus in the monkey. *Exp. Neurol.* 14, 429–438 (1966).

Morest, D.K. The neuronal architecture of the medial geniculate body of the cat. *J. Anat.* (Lond.) 98, 611–630 (1964).

Morest, D.K. The laminar structure of the medial geniculate body of the cat. *J. Anat.* (Lond.) 99, 143–160 (1965a).

Morest, D.K. The lateral tegmental system of the midbrain and the medial geniculate body: Study with Golgi and Nauta methods in cat. *J. Anat.* (Lond.) 99, 611–634 (1965b).

Morrel, F. Electrophysiological contributions to the neural basis of learning. *Physiol. Rev.* 41, 443–494 (1961).

Moruzzi, G. The sleep-waking cycle, in *Neurophysiology and Neurochemistry of Sleep and Wakefulness.* M. Jouvet and G. Moruzzi, eds. Springer-Verlag, Berlin (1972), pp. 1–165.

Nunnaly, J.C., Knott, P.D., Duchnowski, A., and Parker, R. Pupillary response as a general measure of activation. *Percept. Psychophys.* 2, 149–155 (1967).

O'Brien, J.H., and Fox, S.S. Single-cell activity in cat motor cortex. I. Modifications during classical conditioning procedures. *J. Neurophysiol.* 32, 276–284 (1969a).

O'Brien, J.H., and Fox, S.S. Single-cell activity in cat motor cortex. II. Functional characteristics of the cell related to conditioning changes. *J. Neurophysiol.* 32, 285–296 (1969b).

O'Brien, J.H., and Packham, S.C. Conditioned leg movement in the cat with massed trials, trace conditioning, and weak US intensity. *Cond. Reflex* 8, 116–124 (1973).

O'Brien, J.H., Packham, S.C., and Brunnhoelzl, W.W. Features of spike train related to learning. *J. Neurophysiol.* 36, 1051–1061 (1973).

Oleson, T.D., Ashe, J.H., and Weinberger, N.M. Modification of auditory and somatosensory system activity during pupillary conditioning in the paralyzed cat. *J. Neurophysiol.* 38, 1114–1139 (1975).

Oleson, T.D., Vododnick, D.S., and Weinberger, N.M. Pupillary inhibition of delay during Pavlovian conditioning in paralyzed cat. *Behav. Biol.* 8, 337–346 (1973).

Oleson, T.D., Westenberg, I.S., and Weinberger, N.M. Characteristics of the pupillary dilation response during Pavlovian conditioning in paralyzed cats. *Behav. Biol.* 7, 829–840 (1972).

Oliver, D.L., and Hall, W.C. Subdivisions of the medial geniculate body in the tree shrew (*Tapaia glis*). *Brain Res.* 86, 217–227 (1975).

Parrish, J. Classical discrimination conditioning of heart rate and bar-press suppression in the rat. *Psychon. Sci.* 9, 267–268 (1967).

Rowland, V. Steady potential phenomena of cortex, in *The Neurosciences: A Study Program.* G.C. Quarton, T. Melnechuk, and F.O. Schmitt, eds. The Rockefeller Press, New York (1967), pp. 482–496.

Ryugo, D.K., and Weinberger, N.M. Differential plasticity of morphologically distinct neuron populations in the medial geniculate body of the cat during classical conditioning. *Soc. Neurosci. Abs.* 2, 435 (1976).

Ryugo, D.K., and Weinberger, N.M. Differential plasticity of morphologically distinct neuron populations in the medial geniculate body of the cat during classical conditioning. *Behav. Biol.* 22, 275–301 (1978).

Schneiderman, N., Fuentes, I., and Gormezano, I. Acquisition and extinction of the classically conditioned eyelid response in the albino rabbit. *Science* 136, 650–652 (1962).

Sharpless, S., and Jasper, H. Habituation of the arousal reaction. *Brain 79*, 655–680 (1956).

Simon, C.W., and Emmons, W.H. Learning during sleep? *Psychol. Bull.* 52, 328–343 (1955).

Simpson, H.M., and Hale, S.M. Pupillary changes during a decision-making task. *Percept. Mot. Skills* 29, 495–498 (1969).

Smith, K. Conditioning as an artefact. *Psychol. Rev.* 61, 217–225 (1954).

Sokolov, E.N. Higher nervous functions: The orienting reflex. *Ann. Rev. Physiol.* 25, 545–580 (1963).

Sokolov, E.N. The neuronal mechanisms of the orienting reflex, in *Neuronal Mechanisms of the Orienting Reflex.* E.N. Sokolov and O.S. Vinogradova, eds. Lawrence Erlbaum Publishers, Hillsdale, New Jersey (1975), pp. 217–235.

Thomas, G.J. Neurophysiology of learning. *Ann. Rev. Psychol.* 13, 71–106 (1962).

Thompson, R.F., Patterson, M.M., and Teyler, T.J. The neurophysiology of learning. *Ann. Rev. Psychol.* 23, 73–104 (1972).

Van Twyver, H.B., and King, R.L. Classical conditioning of the galvanic skin response in immobilized cats. *Psychophysiology* 5, 530–535 (1969).

Weinberger, N.M., Velasco, M., and Lindsley, D.B. The relationship between cortical synchrony and behavioral inhibition. *Electroenceph. Clin. Neurophysiol.* 23, 297–305 (1967).

Weinberger, N.M., Nakayama, K., and Lindsley, D.B. Electrocortical recruiting responses during classical conditioning. *Electroenceph. Clin. Neurophysiol.* 24, 16–24 (1968).

Weinberger, N.M., Goodman, D.A., and Kitzes, L.M. Is behavioral habituation a function of peripheral auditory system blockade? *Comm. Behav. Biol.* 3, 111–116 (1969).

Weinberger, N.M., Oleson, T.D., and Haste, D. Inhibitory control of conditional pupillary dilation response in the paralyzed cat. *Behav. Biol.* 9, 307–316 (1973).

Weinberger, N.M., Oleson, T.D., and Ashe, J.H. Sensory system neural activity during habituation of the pupillary orienting reflex. *Behav. Biol.* 15, 283–301 (1975).

Wiener, J.M., Pfeiffer, R.R., and Backus, A.S.M. On the sound pressure transformation by the head and auditory meatus of the cat. *Acta Otolaryngol.* 61, 255–269 (1966).

Winer, J.A., Diamond, I.T., and Raczkowski, D. Subdivisions of the auditory cortex of the cat: The retrograde transport of horseradish peroxidase to the medial geniculate body and posterior thalamic nuclei. *J. Comp. Neurol.* 176, 387–418 (1977).

Woody, C.D., and Brozek, G. Gross potential from facial nucleus of cat as an index of neural activity in response to glabella tap. *J. Neurophysiol.* 32, 704–716 (1969).

Yehle, A., Dauth, G., and Schneiderman, N. Correlates of heart-rate classical conditioning in curarized rabbits. *J. Comp. Physiol. Psychol.* 64, 98–104 (1967).

Yoshii, N., and Ogura, H. Studies on the unit discharge of brainstem reticular formation in the cat. I. Changes of reticular unit discharge following conditioning procedure. *Med J. Osaka Univ.* 11, 1–17 (1960).

PART II

Learning and Memory

Copyright © 1982, Spectrum Publications, Inc.
The Neural Basis of Behavior

5

The Evolution Of Concepts Of Memory

Seymour S. Kety

Animate as opposed to inanimate matter has had the unique propensity to grow more complex and more adaptively responsive to environmental change over the hundreds of millions of years in which its existence on earth has been recorded. Its increasingly adaptive responsiveness is the crux of its endurance and evolution. Genetic mutation and natural selection have, since the time of Darwin, been seen as the dual mechanisms responsible for the increasing adaptation, explaining how a species develops and adapts to nature with augmenting efficiency. The process is slow and requires millions of years. Even the highly developed behavioral patterns and complex societies of insects are explicable in terms of natural selection if account is taken of the brief generational and maturational time and the large number of individuals produced in each generation.

There is an equally important manner in which the individual member of a species adapts to nature with progressive efficiency, but in the brief span of an individual lifetime. That process we call learning and the crucial component of it is memory—the ability to store experience in a manner which makes possible its later retrieval and utilization in modifying future behavior to make it more effective and adaptive.

The scientific study of memory began only 100 years ago and was undertaken by neuropsychiatrists who were stimulated by the obvious disorders of memory in human beings. In his volume, *Diseases of Memory*, Ribot (1882) described the clinical and pathological features of memory disorders and their natural history. In his treatise, *Uber das Gedachtnis*, Ebbinghaus (1885) described the characteristics of normal human memory derived from his classical experiments. Korsakoff (1889), in "Etude Medico-Psychologique sur une Forme des Maladies de la Memoire," depicted in vivid detail the symptoms of the amnesia which has since borne his name. Thus, the scientific study of memory began with a consideration of the phenomenology of memory and its disorders.

The *localization of memory* has occupied the attention of scientists ever since it was realized that loss of memory could be associated with disease in particular regions of the brain. Lashley's "In Search of the Engram" (1950) described his many ingenious but unsuccessful attempts at localization. A general conclusion has seemed to be apparent; in the octopus, J.Z. Young identified a "memory lobe," but in vertebrates and particularly in mammals, memory appears to be widely distributed throughout the brain and spinal cord. Although the process does not occur exclusively in one place, certain areas are more important and even essential, and among these the temporal lobe and particularly the hippocampus are of special significance. Changes have also been seen in the electrical activity of certain structures which appear to be correlated with simple forms of learning. Perhaps the most interesting and most clearly pertinent of these has been the demonstration by Thompson and co-workers (1978) of the building up of a pattern of electrical activity in the hippocampus uniquely correlated in time and contour with the development of a conditioned response.

Even more challenging than *where* memory is located is the question of *how* it is mediated. That problem has been the stimulus of great activity recently and it is that problem which each of the three chapters in this section will address. Although Aristotle speculated on how memory was brought about, the modern period of hypothesis and research goes back about 100 years to Cajal and the neuron doctrine.

With the realization that the nervous system was a network of interconnected neurons, the points of connection naturally assumed great significance, and it was quickly recognized that these junctions were probably plastic rather than hard-wired. Various morphological hypotheses developed to account for the increased functional state at the synapse that was assumed to underlie memory. Some speculated that this would be by virtue of a tighter contact at the synapse, while others, like Sherrington (1887: 1117), postulated an increase in number or area of synapses:

> ...the nerve cell directs its pent-up energy towards amplifying its connections with its fellows, in response to the events which stir it up. Hence, it is capable of an education unknown to other tissues.

Regardless of how the synaptic change was imagined, however, a general thesis developed, that *repetitive use of a synapse somehow produces a lasting increase in its conductivity.*

In the light of new knowledge regarding the nature of the synapse, many more possibilities than tightening or multiplication present themselves to account for, or contribute to, an increased synaptic conductivity. The chemical nature of the synapse suggests these, among others: increased synthesis or release of transmitter, its greater persistence in the synaptic cleft, an enhanced ionic flux, increased area of synaptic contact, increased number or sensitivity of receptors, and enhancement of post-synaptic processes such as those involving second messengers.

Although short- and long-term memory were differentiated by the clinical studies of the last century, it was just thirty years ago that the two types of memory were hypothetically differentiated in terms of their electrical or chemical nature, respectively. Such hypotheses were stated independently by C.P. Duncan (1949), D.O. Hebb (1949), and by R.W. Gerard (1949: 170), who put it thus:

> All is not over when an impulse flashes across a synapse and onto its destination. It leaves behind ripples in the state of the system. The fate of a later impulse can thus be at least a little influenced by the past history of the neurons involved. . . . Reverberant circuits, in principle, could last indefinitely, but in practice their duration is doubtful. . . . Perhaps there is a short-lasting active memory, depending on circuits, and a more enduring static one.

Observations on the time-delays in the "consolidation" of memory which led them to this hypothesis have been extensively replicated and enlarged since that time, resulting in a general consensus that it is possible to interfere with the establishment of a memory for a short time after an experience by disrupting or suppressing the electrical activity of the brain through electrical convulsions or drugs that could interrupt reverberant circuits by blocking synaptic activity. After that time, however, the experience appears to be stored in a more permanent form, presumably by chemical or morphological changes, since it is now resistant to electrical disruption.

The roughly exponential decay of the memory of nonsense syllables demonstrated by Ebbinghaus suggested to some the dissociation of a complex chemical molecule and, for a brief period after the discovery of the genetic code, there were attempts to extend the concept of the storage of genetic information to that of experiential information in some form of macromolecular coding. This has now subsided with the recognition that memories could more plausibly be stored as persistent circuits in the vast neuronal network and the possible synaptic changes involved in an increase in conductivity could lie in the synthesis of enzymes, membranes, or receptors. Thus the macromolecules necessary for memory storage could be seen as facilitating the establishment of specific interconnections and patterns of increased conductivity, with the specificity of the memory lying there rather than in the macromolecules themselves. Almost forgotten are the early experiments of Dingman and Sporn (1961), who showed that inhibition of RNA synthesis could block memory consolidation, and the ingenious studies by Chamberlain and co-workers (1963) of an induced postural asymmetry in the rat's spinal cord. The asymmetry was produced by a unilateral cerebellar lesion and was indefinitely maintained within the spinal cord if the unbalanced input was permitted to go on for a period up to an hour. Drugs which appeared to stimulate or inhibit RNA synthesis were found to facilitate or retard this process.

There has been a large amount of research on RNA and protein synthesis and their effects on consolidation by Hyden, Agranoff, Barondes, Flexner, and Glassman, among others, all of which points to an involvement of protein synthesis in long-term memory formation (Jarvick, 1970). It is difficult to say more than that since it is not easy to select among the more imaginative and specific hypotheses of where and how the protein syntheses is involved on the basis of current evidence. The recent work of Victor Shashoua (this volume) has considered and controlled many of the variables which confound research on complex brains, and provides new evidence compatible with the association of particular proteins with learning as well as an indication of where, in the brain, they may be formed.

The work of Chamberlain, Halick, and Gerard in 1963 demonstrated that, for some types of learning, it was enough to stimulate repetitively for many minutes in order to establish a persistent alteration in synaptic behavior, and that alteration is indeed the essential feature of learning. There is no reason to stop there, however, or to ignore the many additional processes that may have evolved to modulate and to reinforce that primordial process. There are many higher forms of learning in which that elemental process (i.e., alteration of synaptic behavior) could be effectively enhanced, and made more adaptive and efficient, if the significance of an experience to the survival of the individual (or the species) exerted an effect upon that process to determine which experiences were consolidated and for how long (Kety, 1965).

I have elsewhere (1970, 1976) suggested the possibility that in such types of learning, some of the biological concomitants of affective state may act to favor the persistence of the neural patterns preceding them. More specifically, biogenic amines, modulators, and hormones released in such states may affect trophic processes occurring at recently activated synapses in order to promote selectively the persistence of those circuits that have led to reward or the relief of pain or discomfort.

Psychologists have long recognized the importance of affective state and of reward and punishment in facilitating and intensifying the memorization process. Biological theories of memory, however, have tended to ignore this and consequently lack the additional dimension it could add to their hypotheses. This may have been because, until recently, what was known about the biology of emotional states was unable to contribute to a hypothesis of memory at the biological level. Recent information on the manifold associations between affective state, neurohormones, and neurotransmitters has made it highly plausible that affect could influence memory at the chemical synapse.

An appropriate electrical model of this interaction was already available in the "memistor," developed by Widrow and Angell (1962) as the essential unit in an ingenious learning machine. Each memistor consists of a very thin strip of metal immersed in a solution of its salts. An independent input can bring about a persistent change in the conductivity of the metal strip by depositing or removing the metal from it, depending on the sign and the intensity of the "plating" current. Knowledge of the monoamine systems of the brain began to develop at the same time, by virtue of histofluorescence techniques. This made it possible to surmise that monoamine terminals in the cortex, activated in various emotional states, could serve as contingent inputs at more specific synapses, altering their conductivity through biochemcal rather than electrochemical means. It was suggested that the monoamine input was diffuse and nonspecific and, in this context, it is interesting that the majority of these endings have recently been shown to terminate without making specific contacts, but rather to release the neurotransmitter over a region (Descarries et al., 1975; Chan-Palay, 1977). It was also suggested that other chemical modulators associated with affect could operate in this way. For example, neurohormones released into the cerebrospinal fluid from non-synaptic terminals or from neurosecretory cells in the brain, or hormones in the blood stream passing across the choroid plexus, would thus be broadcast over fields of cortical synapses, where they might thereby effect persistent changes in synaptic conductivity that would be contingent upon the state of arousal, attention, reward, or displeasure accompanying and following particular experiences.

A substantial number of studies have examined this hypothesis in the last nine years; the results are compatible with an involvement of amines such as norepinephrine or serotonin, or peptides such as vasopressin or fragments of ACTH (Anlezark et al., 1973; van Ree et al., 1978; Dismukes and Rake, 1972; Kasamaku and Pettigrew, 1976; Gallagher et al., 1977; Libet and Tosaka, 1970; Randt et al., 1971). These compounds, and others not identified as yet, may play some role in consolidation through modification of synaptic protein synthesis or cyclic AMP metabolism to bring such trophic changes about. Recent clinical studies suggest that Korsakoff's amnesia is associated with a cerebral deficiency of norepinephrine (McEntee and Mair, 1978) or that L-dopa may improve memory functions where it is disordered (Murphy et al., 1972). However, the results are by no means consistent and, dealing as such studies have with the complexity of the mammalian brain and behavior, all of the variables have not been controlled nor have alternative explanations been ruled out. There are some observations that stand out, however, and effectively support the idea of contingent monoaminergic inputs to particular synapses that can produce a persistent change in their function. Eric Kandel has provided such information most definitively and describes his findings in this volume.

Within this volume may be found contributions that represent the cutting edge of the field of memory research, elucidating both the electrophysiological and neurochemical processes that operate to convert significant individual experiences to neural changes that persist and modify subsequent behavior.

REFERENCES

Anlezark, G.M., Crow, T.J., and Greenway, A.P. Impaired learning and decreased cortical norepinephrine after bilateral locus coeruleus lesions. *Science* 181, 682–684 (1973).

Chamberlain, T.J., Halick, P., and Gerard, R.W. Fixation of experience in the rat spinal cord. *J. Neurophysiol.* 26, 662–673 (1963).

Chan-Palay, V. *Cerebellar Dentate Nucleus.* Springer-Verlag, Berlin (1977).

Descarries, L., Beaudet, A., and Watkins, K.C. Serotonin nerve terminals in adult rat neocortex. *Brain Res.* 100, 563–588 (1975).

Dingman, W., and Sporn, M.B. The incorporation of 8-azaguanine into rat brain RNA and its effect on maze learning by the rat: An inquiry into the biochemical basis of memory. *J. Psychiat. Res.* 1, 1–11 (1961).

Dismukes, R.K., and Rake, A.V. Involvement of biogenic amines in memory formation. *Psychopharmacologia* 23, 17–25 (1972).

Duncan, C.P. The retroactive effect of electroshock on learning. *J. Comp. Physiol. Psychol.* 42, 32–44 (1949).

Ebbinghaus, H. *Uber das Gedachtnis.* Duncker, Leipzig (1885).

Gallagher, M., Kapp, B.S., Musty, R.E., and Driscoll, P.A. Memory formation: evidence for a specific neurochemical system in the amygdala. *Science* 198, 423–425 (1977).

Gerard, R.W. Physiology and psychiatry. *Am. J. Psychiat.* 106, 161–173 (1949).

Hebb, D.O. *The Organization of Behavior*, John Wiley & Sons, New York (1949).

Jarvick, M.E. Effects of chemical and physical treatments on learning and memory. *Ann. Rev. Psychol.* 62, 125–132 (1970).

Kasamatsu, T., and Pettigrew, J.D. Depletion of brain catecholamines: failure of ocular dominance shift after monocular occlusion in kittens. *Science* 194, 206–209 (1976).

Kety, S.S. The incorporation of experience into the central nervous system, in *Deafferentation Experimentale et Clinique.* J. de Ajuriaguerra, ed. Georg et Cie, Geneva (1965), pp. 251–256.

Kety, S.S. The biogenic amines in the central nervous system: Their possible roles in arousal, emotion and learning, in *The Neurosciences: Second Study Program.* F.O. Schmitt, ed. Rockefeller University Press, New York (1970), pp. 324–336.

Kety, S.S. Biological concomitants of effective states and their possible role in memory processes, in *Neural Mechanisms of Learning and Memory*. M.R. Rosenzweig and E.L. Bennett, eds. MIT Press, Cambridge (1976), pp.321–336.

Korsakoff, S.S. Etude medico-psychologique sur une forme des maladies de la memoire. *Revue Philosophique* 5, 501–530 (1889).

Lashley, K.S. In search of the engram. *Symp. Soc. Exper. Biol.*, 4, 454–482 (1950).

Libet, B., and Tosaka, T. Dopamine as a synaptic transmitter and modulator in sympathetic ganglia: a different mode of synaptic action. *Proc. Natl. Acad. Sci. USA* 67, 667–673 (1970).

McEntee, W.J., and Mair, R.G. Memory impairment in Korsakoff's psychosis: a correlation with brain noradrenergic activity. *Science* 202, 905–907 (1978).

Murphy, D.L., Henry, G.M., and Weingartner, H. Catecholamines and memory: enhanced verbal learning during L-dopa administration. *Psychopharmacologia* 27, 319–326 (1972).

Randt, C.T., Quartermain, D., Goldstein, M. and Anagnoste, B. Norepinephrine biosynthesis inhibition: effects on memory in mice. *Science* 172, 498–499 (1971).

Ribot, T.A. *The Diseases of Memory*. Appleton Co., New York (1882).

Sherrington, C.S. Chapter in Foster's *Neurophysiology*. (1887), p. 1117.

Thompson, R.F., Berger, T.W., Berry, S.D., and Hoehler, F.K. The search for the engram II. Presented at the 50th Anniversary Symposium, Dept. of Psychology, U. of Texas at Austin (1978).

van Ree, J.M., Bohus, B., Versteeg, D.H.G., and de Wied, D. Neurohypophyseal principles and memory processes. *Biochem. Pharmacol.* 27, 1793–1800 (1978).

Widrow, B., and Angell, J.B. Reliable trainable networks for computing and control. *Aerospace Engineering* 21, 78–123 (1962).

Copyright © 1982, Spectrum Publications, Inc.
The Neural Basis of Behavior

6

Some Capacities for Structural Growth and Functional Change in the Neuronal Circuitries of the Adult Hippocampus

Gary Lynch
Kevin Lee

INTRODUCTION

It has become increasingly clear that the various circuits of the hippocampal formation are capable of dramatic structural reorganization and extremely long-lasting changes in their operating characteristics. Axons and dendrites in this structure will on occasion generate large numbers of new connections while brief periods of repetitive electrical stimulation cause semi-permanent increases in synaptic strength. Structural and physiological plasticites of these types are of interest because they offer possible explanations for the extreme flexibility which is the hallmark of behavior in the "higher" vertebrates. However, attempts to test for such relationships between neuronal and behavioral change are impeded by an almost complete lack of information about the cellular machinery responsible for the former as well as the physiological events which accompany the latter. The present review is concerned with these issues and specifically with the cellular substrates of neuronal plasticity. We shall first describe the "sprouting" response of intact fibers in the partially deafferented hippocampus and use these findings to discuss various hypotheses about the factors which initiate and regulate axonal growth in the adult central nervous system. Following this, we will turn to the remarkable long-term potentiation of synaptic response found in several hippocampal pathways following repetitive stimulation. The emphasis of this section will be on the types of biochemical and structural mechanisms which might be responsible for rapidly appearing, stable changes in synaptic physiology.

SPROUTING OF NEW TERMINALS AND SYNAPSES IN THE PARTIALLY DEAFFERENTED HIPPOCAMPUS

Partial denervation of muscle or skin causes the remaining intact axons to the muscle to grow ("sprout") new collateral branches which then largely replace the degenerating contacts (see Edds, 1953 for a review). A process analogous to this occurs in hippocampus (Lynch et al., 1972) and other brain structures (Raisman, 1969; Lund and Lund, 1971; Moore, 1974) following destruction of one or more of their primary afferents. The hippocampus because of its comparatively simple and rigidly laminated organization has proven particularly useful for analyses of the temporal parameters and developmental sequence of the sprouting effect. The dentate gyrus is composed of a layer of densely packed granule cells whose dendrites fan out to form a molecular layer some 250–300 μm in depth. The proximal 25–30 percent of this layer is occupied by fibers and synapses originating in the pyramidal cell fields of the ipsilateral and contralateral hippocampi (the ipsilateral projection is called the "associational" system while that coming from the contralateral side comprises the "commissural" system). The remaining distal segments of the dendritic field (the middle and outer molecular layers) receive a massive input from the ipsilateral entorhinal cortex (perforant path) (see Lynch and Cotman, 1975 for a review). Following lesions of the entorhinal cortex in the adult rat, the commissural and associational projections extend collateral branches into a 50 μm strip immediately above their normal termination sites (Lynch et al., 1973). Thus, sprouting by the remaining intact projections does occur, but for some reason these fibers fail to gain access to the more distal aspects of the deafferented dendritic field. Studies using a variety of neuroanatomical techniques have shown that the commissural projections begin their sprouting response at about five to six days after the lesion (Lynch et al., 1977; Lee et al., 1977), after which time they rapidly form synapses on the newly invaded territory (Lee et al., 1977; Matthews et al., 1976). Unfortunately, estimates of the rate of reinnervation and the ultrastructural details of this process are made difficult by tissue shrinkage and related pathologies which occur in the

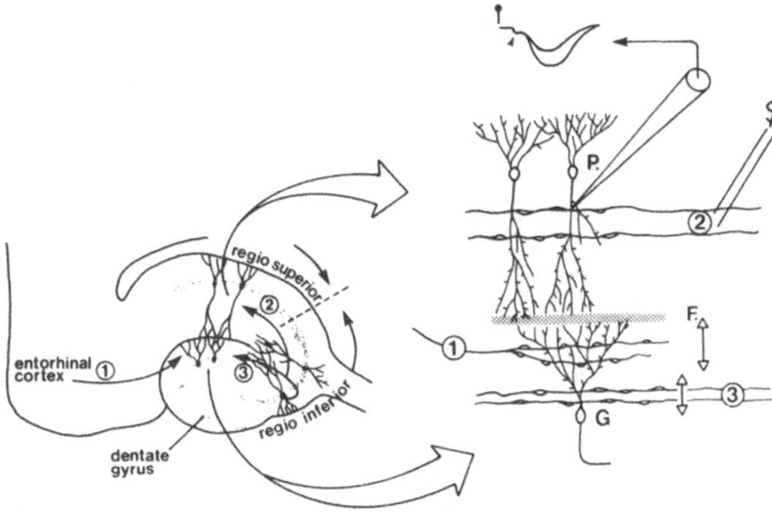

FIG. 1. Schematic representation of certain interconnections within the hippocampal formation. Pathway 1 (perforant path) arises from the entorhinal cortex and innervates the distal two-thirds of the dentate gyrus granule cell dendrites. Pathways 2 and 3 are of regio inferior pyramidal cell origin and project to the apical dendrites of regio superior pyramidal cells (pathway 2: Schaffer collaterals), and to the proximal one-third of the granule cell dendrites (pathway 3: associational system). Following high frequency stimulation of the Schaffer collateral pathway, the evoked potential recorded in the apical dendrites of regio superior pyramidal cells (arrow) is enhanced. This enhancement (long-term potentiation) is stable and has been shown to persist for days and in some cases for months. P: pyramidal cell; G: granule cell layer; F: hippocampal fissure.

denervated zone. For these reasons the temporal parameters of sprouting have seen re-examined using the afferents of the inner molecular layer. Specifically, the commissural inputs to this layer were removed by aspiration of the contralateral hippocampus and the response of the remaining associational system was studied using quantitative electron microscopy (McWilliams and Lynch, 1978; 1979). The advantage of this paradigm is that little or no shrinkage occurs in the denervated zone. Presumably this is the case because only a minority of the afferent input is eliminated and the lesion is placed at a considerable distance from the site sampled by electron microscopy. However, it should be emphasized that unlike the case following lesions of the entorhinal cortex, the sprouting associational fibers are located in the zone they reinnervate—hence there is no need for collateral branches to form, and the growth response probably consists of an addition of boutons to an existing population of fibers. These experiments again showed that the sprouting response began only after a delay of 5–6 days and

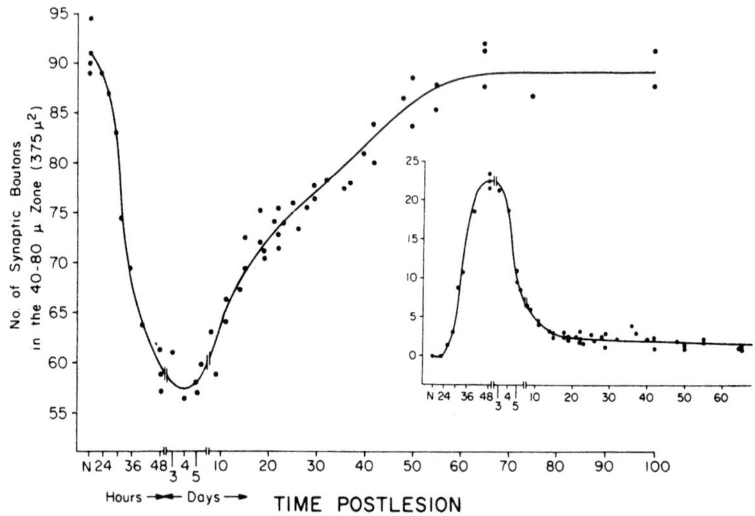

FIG. 2. Plots are shown of the numbers of intact and degenerating (inset) synaptic boutons in the inner molecular layer of the dentate gyrus following removal of the contralateral hippocampus (adapted from McWilliams and Lynch, 1978). The proliferation of new synaptic sites begins only after a postlesion delay of five days, and an approximately normal density of innervation is achieved by 60 days postlesion.

that once underway the growth reaction produced synapses in the denervated zone at a rate of 0.3 contacts/100 μm^2/24 hours. Beyond day 15 postlesion reinnervation proceeded more slowly and the population of synapses did not return to its normal values until 60 days after the lesion.

These experiments provide some important details about the sprouting response in the hippocampus:

1. Synaptogenesis begins only after a delay of several days;
2. Synaptic sites are generated at a rate which is only a fraction of that seen in the developing brain.
3. In the case of the commissural/associational sprouting after lesions of the entorhinal cortex the growth response penetrates only a limited percentage of the denervated territory.

Thus sprouting in the adult rat is delayed in its onset, restricted in its extent, and in terms of reinnervation follows a rather leisurely pace.

Understanding the sprouting response and hence the possible role of this form of growth in the normal operation of brain will require some insight into the reasons that sprouting response exhibits the characteristics just described. Research into these questions is in its earliest stages, but some interesting observations have been made regarding several of the parameters of sprouting. The rate of reinnervation is correlated with the rate at which degenerating endings are removed as first suggested by Raisman and Field (1973). However, detailed quantitative studies suggest that the relationship is not one to one but instead new contacts are added more quickly than old ones are removed (McWilliams and Lynch, 1979). This suggests that two factors may set the pace for reinnervation: 1) the removal of degeneration and hence possibly the "freeing-up" of appropriate postsynaptic sites (Raisman and Field, 1973), and 2) the generation of entirely new postsynaptic sites by the target dendrites.

The five-day lag between the lesion and the onset of sprouting remains a puzzle. One possibility is that this is the time period required by the brain to begin removing the degeneration products and thereby accrue "space" (or postsynaptic vacancies) for the intact fibers to grow into. However it is becoming increasingly clear that this is not likely to be the case. Electron microscopic studies have shown that the process of stripping the degenerating terminals from the dendrites and their removal from the dentate gyrus begins within hours of the lesion and that a substantial portion, perhaps the majority, of these endings are eliminated well in advance of any evidence of sprouting (McWilliams and Lynch, 1979). This leaves two very different categories of hypotheses which might be used to explain the delay in the onset of sprouting: 1) the five-day period may reflect the time needed to generate a signal to the intact fibers and/or to mobilize their growth responses; 2) some factor(s), other than degenerating endings, may be present in the neuropil which blocks the growth response during the five days after the lesion. It should be noted that these two models point to different versions of fiber growth in the adult brain. In the former the axons are relatively static and must be "called" into action after a lesion while the second hypothesis implies that growth is continually present but its manifestation after lesions is blocked by elements associated with deafferentation.

There are factors present in the denervated zones which seem appropriate to the blocking of the growth response. Within 24 hours of the lesion the astroglial population begins to hypertrophy in the region of deafferentation; this response subsides on the fifth day postlesion (Rose, et al., 1976) a change which is temporally correlated with a sudden reduction in the rate at which degeneration is removed (McWilliams and Lynch, 1979). Together these results suggest that the onset of sprouting is closely tied to a marked change in the behavior of the astroglia. It is thus possible that the astrocytic hypertrophy physically hinders the axonal growth process and as the former undergoes a sudden reduction the latter appears. Alternatively, the abrupt change in the astrocyted behavior could be associated with the production of a "trigger" for sprouting. In either event the above results point to an important role for the astroglia in the phenomenon of sprouting.

Research into the development of the hippocampus has also begun to provide important clues about the factors which regulate the sprouting response in the adult. It is evident that some population of commissural-associational fibers in the two-week-old rat generate a sprouting response (following entorhinal lesions) which is unaffected by the restrictions found in older rats. Thus commissural axons begin to invade the deafferented territory within hours of the lesion and are not restricted in their upward extension but instead within one to two days spread throughout the entire molecular layer (Gall and Lynch, 1978). These projections form synapses in the denervated zones at a rate which is well in excess of that found during normal development, and, interestingly enough, this sprouting response does not retard the innervation of the normal targets of the commissural-association fibers (Gall et al., 1979, in press). Sprouting in the neonatal brain occurs with minimal delay, is unrestricted in its extent, and occurs at

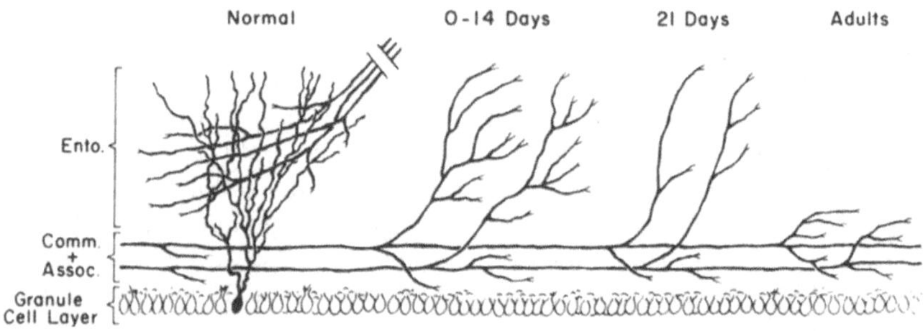

FIG. 3. Schematic illustration of the sprouting response of the commissural and associational afferents to the dentate gyrus in response to the removal of the perforant path at various postnatal ages. Following entorhinal cortex ablation in the early postnatal period, the remaining intact afferents send collaterals throughout the full extent of the denervated zone. By 21 days of age, however, this capacity for growth is markedly diminished in both density and extent. With lesion placement in adult animals, the axonal sprouting is restricted to the 50 μm of the deafferented territory adjacent to the normal region of commissural/ associational innervation.

an extremely rapid pace—it follows then that the severe restrictions present in the adult are not due to absolute limits on capacity of the axons to form collaterals or synapses but more likely are reflections of developmental changes in axons or additions to the neuropil. Recent experiments using a histological method selective for axons have further clarified the nature of the sprouting response as it is found in the immature brain. It appears that one group of axons exhibits an "adult" growth reaction to deafferentation at 14 days postnatal (dpn) in that it is delayed in its onset and quite restricted in its extent; if confirmed with other methods, these findings indicate that at two weeks postnatal some axons are capable of rapid explosive

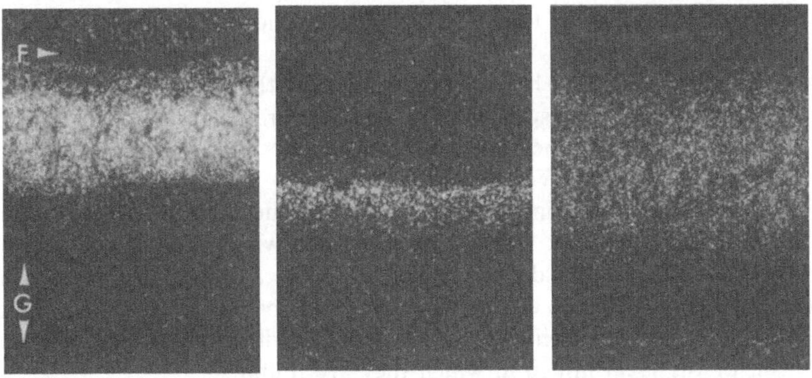

FIG. 4. The above dark-field micrographs of ^{3}H-leucine labeled axonal projections to the rat dentate gyrus molecular layer illustrate the normal lamination of afferents to this region and the changes of this laminar arrangement following partial deafferentation (G-granule cell layer, F-hippocampal fissure). In the left panel the perforant path input is labeled and can be seen to innervate the outer two-thirds of the molecular layer, while the commissural terminals (*center panel*) occupy the inner one-third of this zone. Following removal of the perforant path input in a 14-day-old rat, the commissural axons "sprout" to innervate the deafferented zone (*right panel*). Correlative electron microscopic studies have shown that this growth occurs without a concomitant loss of synaptic density in the normally-innervated inner molecular layer (Gall et al., 1979).

sprouting while others execute the more sluggish growth response seen in the adult (Gall and Lynch, unpublished). Possibly the 14 dpn dentate gyrus contains both mature and immature fibers, and this is the explanation of the two forms of sprouting seen at this age. If this is correct then the restrictions on sprouting seen in the adult may be due to some maturation-related changes in the afferent fibers of the hippocampus.

LONG-TERM POTENTIATION OF SYNAPTIC RESPONSES IN HIPPOCAMPUS

The hippocampus possesses a second capacity for change which in terms of its rapid onset and extreme duration appears analogous to behavioral plasticity. Brief trains of high frequency stimulation delivered to any of several pathways in hippocampus result in long-term potentiation ("LTP") of the synaptic responses generated by subsequent "single pulse" stimulation of that pathway (Bliss and Lomo, 1973). Unlike the more classical forms of synaptic facilitation (e.g., post-tetanic potentiation at the neuromuscular junction), LTP is induced with very brief trains (less than one second), and, more importantly, is extremely stable; it has been reported to persist for weeks or longer (Bliss and Gardner-Medwin, 1973; Douglas and Goddard, 1975).

A number of studies have sought to identify the locus of the cellular adjustments which are responsible for LTP. Several experiments have led to the conclusion that the repetitive stimulation does not alter the axons (Schwartzkroin and Wester, 1975; Andersen et al., 1977; Dunwiddie 1978) while studies using multiple inputs to the same cells (or dendritic fields) have shown that LTP is not correlated with generalized changes in the target cells (Dunwiddie and Lynch, 1978). By a process of exclusion then the effect appears to be due to some extremely persistent adjustment in the axon terminals, the spines of the target dendrites, the synapses between them, or the local milieu in which they are found.

Research has also been directed at the issue of what factors are responsible first for triggering LTP and second for maintaining it. With regard to the first question experiments using the *in vitro* slice method (Yamamoto, 1972) have shown that LTP is difficult to induce when the concentration of calcium in the bathing medium is reduced from 2.5 to 1.0–1.5 mM (with a corresponding increase in magnesium). Under these conditions transient potentiation is still found after the stimulation train, but the percentage of slices exhibiting LTP is reduced as is the magnitude of the effect when it is obtained (Dunwiddie and Lynch, 1979). This has led to the hypothesis that calcium accumulation in the terminals, and perhaps target dendrites as well, is responsible for triggering the long-term potentiation (Fig. 5).

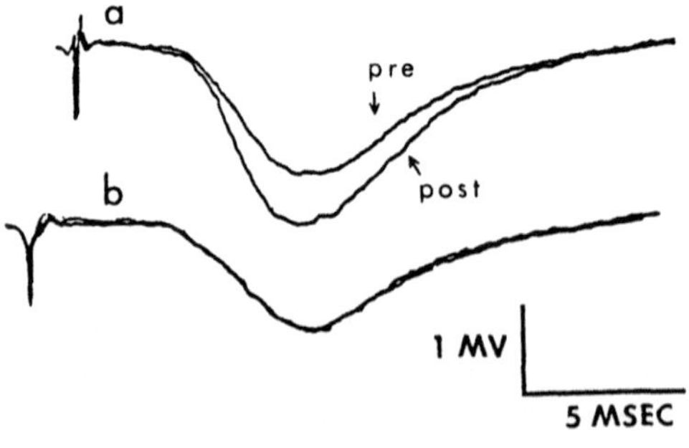

FIG. 5. Evoked potentials recorded from the stratum radiatum of CA1 in response to stimulation of the Schaffer collateral pathway. In a evoked potentials recorded before and after a burst of high frequency stimulation (100 per second for 1 second) are shown. The response is clearly enhanced following this type of stimulation. In b, superimposed traces are shown for responses taken prior to and following low frequency stimulation (0.2 per second for 2 minutes). In this case the size and shape of the evoked potentials was unchanged following stimulation.

Many of the intracellular effects of calcium are now known to be mediated by calcium-sensitive protein kinases, enzymes which phosphorylate a variety of substrate proteins. Recently it has been shown that the phosphorylation of certain synaptic proteins is stimulated by calcium, and, in particular, Hershkowitz (1978) has suggested that a protein (protein "B") of about 40,000 daltons is particularly sensitive to calcium concentration. Attempts to measure the effect of high frequency stimulation on protein phosphorylation, utilizing a post-hoc assay system (see Lynch et al., 1979 for a review), have shown that the induction of LTP is accompanied by a significant and selective change in the subsequent endogenous phosphorylation of a protein with a molecular weight of 40,000 daltons (Browning et al., 1979a). Phosphorylation of this protein was not inhibited by removal of magnesium from the incubation medium (Browning, unpublished data), a result that was also found by Hershkowitz for the protein "B."

As mentioned, calcium induces phosphorylation by the direct or indirect activation of protein kinases. In light of the above set of results, it was of interest to ascertain which of these enzymes was responsible for the phosphorylation of the 40K material. Cyclic-AMP, the c-AMP-dependent kinase, as well as the catalytic subunit of that enzyme, did not markedly phosphorylate the 40K protein, although, in agreement with others, these compounds did phosphorylate a number of synaptic proteins. However, phosphorylase b kinase (PBK), a kinase which is extremely sensitive to calcium and which is known to be present in the brain (Ozawa, 1973), phosphorylated the 40K protein and only this protein (see Browning et al., 1979b). Taken together, these results suggest the following hypothesis: with repetitive stimulation calcium accumulates in the terminal (and perhaps dendrites of the affected pathway), where it activates a PBK-like enzyme which in turn phosphorylates the 40K protein.

While these cellular events are correlated with the induction of LTP, their relationship to that effect are unclear. That is, the identity and functions of the 40K protein are unknown, and at present we have no evidence linking it to alterations in synaptic efficiency. If, indeed, phosphorylation does participate in the production of potentiation, it presumably does so as an intermediate step between the very brief train of stimulation pulses and the appearance of the persistent change which is the substratum of the functional change. Pertinent to this, recent experiments have shown that the disturbances in the endogenous phosphorylation of the 40K material produced by stimulation gradually decrease and, by 15–20 minutes after the high frequency stimulation, disappear (Browning, unpublished data).

The extreme stability of the long-term potentiation effect invites the speculation that it may be caused by a structural modification, and, as described in the first section of this review, the hippocampus certainly possesses abundant capacity for anatomical plasticity. Fifkova and Van Harreveld (Van Harreveld and Fifkova, 1975; Fifkova and Van Harreveld, 1977) have reported that repetitive stimulation of the entorhinal cortex causes a swelling of spines in the outer molecular layer of the dentate gyrus. However, they did not employ concommitant neurophysiological recording in their studies, and it is possible that the effects were related to physiological changes other than LTP (e.g., seizures, long-lasting depression). More recently, it was found that the induction of LTP in slices or *in vivo* was accompanied by increase in the number of synaptic contacts on dendritic shafts (Lee et al., 1979). This effect, while modest in terms of the total number of synapses, did represent a significant increment in the shaft contact population. The number of spine, multiple, and perforated synapses was unaffected by repetitive stimulation. However, more recent studies using acute anesthesized rats detected changes in the within-animal distribution of three measures of the dendritic spines. Specifically, the post-synaptic density (psd) length, neck width, and area of dendritic spines all displayed significantly diminished coefficients of variation in the potentiated animals. Thus, while the mean size of each of these measures was unaltered, there was an apparent shift in their distribution, presumably resulting from a modification of the spine. One possible explanation of these data is that the dendritic spines are undergoing a change in shape which renders their profiles more homogeneous in an analysis of random section. (For example, if the head of a spine were to change from an ovoid to a more spherical configuration, the mean spine size could remain constant with the variation amongst the encountered profiles decreased).

It seems then that repetitive stimulation of the Schaffer-commissural fibers produces changes of very different types in the shaft and spine synapses, and the question arises as to the relationship between these and long-term potentiation. This complex question is made difficult by a lack of information regarding the number of axons and synapses which are actually "driven" in the region sampled by the recording electrode tip. Thus, if a small percentage of the total population of fibers was involved, then the magnitude of the morphological change which would be expected would be relatively small when considered against the background of "non-stimulated" synapses, spines, etc. There is also uncertainty regarding the relative potency of shaft versus spine synapses. It is certainly possible that the former are particularly effective, since they influence dendritic physiology without an interposed spine which probably forms a high impedance coupling element. It is not inconceivable then that the addition of a few shafts contacts to the stimulated fibers might significantly enhance the size of the EPSP's generated in the shafts and somata of their target pyramidal cells. A further complication to the interpretation of the data is added by the possibility that the majority of shaft contacts are formed with specialized target cells. We have routinely noted that shaft synapses are found in large numbers on dendritic processes which have few if any neighboring spines and in certain ultrastructural features appear different from the pyramidal cell dendrites. It is thus possible that most, if not all, shaft contacts in CA1 are found on a specialized class of cells (i.e., the occasional interneurons which have dendrites in this region). While intracellular studies of LTP are few in number (Schwartzkroin and Wester, 1975; Andersen et al., 1977), it appears that the effect is readily observed in the pyramidal cell population, and therefore represents a change in the dendrites of these cells. Thus, we must be alert to the possibility that the increase in shaft synapses produced by repetitive stimulation is not occurring on the neurons which exhibit LTP, and if so, is not a likely candidate for the substratum of the effect.

The observed change in distribution of the spine synapse measures, on the other hand, is a modification which is probably expressed across a large population of synapses. While no major changes in the means of the spine area, psd length, or neck width were observed, an alteration of the shape of these elements is suggested by the significant decreases in within animal variance which were seen. Shape change could enhance synaptic transmission by modifying the apposition site of terminal and spine (i.e., the postsynaptic density) or by improving the coupling between the receptor sites and the dendritic shaft.

In any event, these experiments indicate that repetitive stimulation produces structural modification in the target region of the activated axons and therefore strengthens the possibility that morphological alteration is at the basis of long-term potentiation. This is clearly an area in which further and more detailed ultrastructural analyses are required.

In summary, brief trains of high frequency stimulation produce long-term potentiation and both biochemical and structural alterations. Links between these latter effects and the physiological change (as well as to each other) have yet to be established, but causal relationships are certainly not implausible. By way of a working hypothesis we suggest that calcium accumulates in the constituents of the synaptic connections during repetitive stimulation and triggers a phosphorylation reaction which in turn alters the relationship of the terminal to its target—this alteration results in ultrastructural changes in both shaft and spine synapses.

SUMMARY AND COMMENT

These studies suggest that during the second and third weeks of postnatal life, axons in the rat hippocampus lose their ability to undergo explosive sprouting, and that growth beyond these ages a) requires a period of mobilization, and b) is hindered by various elements in the neuropil. Nonetheless, the mature hippocampus does exhibit substantial axonal and dendritic growth responses following removal of input. The question that must now be faced is whether these growth responses or the cellular machinery that is responsible for them are used by neuronal circuitries in circumstances which do not involve deafferentation. It does appear that brief trains of high frequency stimulation induce subtle changes in the ultrastructure of the regions innervated by the "driven" axons. While we are far from having a satisfactory picture of the anatomical effects which accompany long-term potentiation, the data so far collected indicate that structural alterations can be induced in intact adult circuitries. It may prove to be the case, then, that phenomena like sprouting and long-term potentiation are produced by similar cellular machinery operating in dissimilar circumstances. It is hoped that investigation into questions such as the significance of the phosphorylation changes which accompany LTP and the reasons for the five-day lag in the onset of sprouting will identify specific biochemical processes and thus provide insight into this question.

REFERENCES

Andersen, P., Sundberg, S., Sveen, O., and Wigstrom, H. Specific long-lasting potentiation of synaptic transmission in hippocampal slices. *Nature* 266, 736–737 (1977).

Bliss, T., and Lomo, T. Long-lasting potentiation of synaptic transmission in the dentate area of the anaesthetized rabbit following stimulation of the perforant path. *J. Physiol.* 232, 331–356 (1973).

Bliss, T., and Gardner-Medwin, A. Long-lasting potentiation of synaptic transmission in the dentate area of the unanaesthetized rabbit following stimulation of the perforant path. *J. Physiol.* 232, 357–374 (1973).

Browning, M., Bennett, W., and Lynch, G. Phosphorylase kinase phosphorylates a membrane protein influenced by repetitive synaptic activation. *Nature* 278, 273–275 (1979a).

Browning, M., Dunwiddie, T., Bennett, W., Gispen, W., and Lynch, G. Synaptic phosphoproteins: specific changes after repetitive stimulation of the hippocampal slice. *Science* 203, 60–62 (1979b).

Douglas, R., and Goddard, D. Long-term potentiation of the perforant path-granule cell synapse in the rat hippocampus. *Brain Res.* 86, 205–215 (1975).

Dunwiddie, T., and Lynch, G. Long-term potentiation and depression of synaptic responses in the hippocampus: localization and frequency dependency. *J. Physiol.* 276, 353–361 (1978).

Dunwiddie, T., and Lynch, G. The relationship between extracellular calcium concentration and the induction of hippocampal long-term potentiation. *Brain Res.* 169, 103–110 (1979).

Dunwiddie, T., Madison, V., and Lynch, G. Synaptic transmission is required for initiation of long-term potentiation. *Brain Res.* 150, 413–417 (1978).

Edds, M.V. Jr. Collateral nerve regeneration. *Quart. Rev. Biol.* 28, 260–276 (1953).

Fifkova, E., and Van Harreveld, A. Long-lasting morphological changes in dendritic spines of dentate granular cells following stimulation of the entorhinal area. *J. Neurocytol.* 6, 211–230 (1977).

Gall, C., and Lynch, G. Rapid axon sprouting in the neonatal rat hippocampus. *Brain Res.* 153, 357–362 (1978).

Gall, C., and Lynch, G. Regulation of fiber growth and synaptogenesis in the developing hippocampus. *Dev. Biol.* (in press).

Gall, C., McWilliams, R., and Lynch, G. The effect of collateral sprouting on the density of innervation of normal target sites: Implication for theories on the regulation of the size of developing synaptic domains. *Brain Res.* 175, 37–47 (1979).

Gall, C., McWilliams, R., and Lynch, G. Accelerated rates of synaptogenesis by "sprouting" afferents in the neonatal hippocampus. *J. Comp. Neurol.* (in press).

Hershkowitz, M. Influence of calcium on phosphorylation of a synaptosomal protein. *Biochim. Biophys. Acta* 542, 274–283 (1978).

Lee, K., Oliver, M., Schottler, F., Creager, R., and Lynch, G. Ultrastructural effects of repetitive synaptic stimulation in the hippocampal slice preparation: A preliminary report. *Exp. Neurol* . 65, 478–480 (1979).

Lee, K., Stanford, E., Cotman, C.W., and Lynch, G. Ultrastructural evidence for bouton proliferation in the partially deafferented dentate gyrus of the adult rat. *Exp. Brain Res.* 29, 475–485 (1977).

Lund, R., and Lund, J. Synaptic adjustment after deafferentation of the superior colliculus of the rat. *Science* 171, 804–806 (1971).

Lynch, G., Browning, M., and Bennett, W. Biochemical and physiological studies of long-term synaptic plasticity. *Fed. Proc.* 38, 2117–2132 (1979).

Lynch, G., and Cotman, C.W. The hippocampus as a model for studying anatomical plasticity in the adult brain, in *The Hippocampus, Vol. 1*. R. Isaacson and K. Pribram, eds. Plenum Publishing Co., New York (1975), pp. 123–155.

Lynch, G., Gall, C., and Cotman, C.W. Temporal parameters of axon "sprouting" in the brain of the adult rat. *Exp. Neurol.* 54, 179–183 (1977).

Lynch, G., Matthews, D., Mosko, S., Parks, T., and Cotman, C.W. Induced acetylcholinesterase-rich layer in dentate gyrus following entorhinal lesions. *Brain Res.* 42, 311–318 (1972).

Lynch, G., Stanfield, B., and Cotman, C. Development differences in post-lesion axonal growth in the hippocampus. *Brain Res.* 59, 155–168 (1973).

Matthews, D.A., Cotman, C.W., and Lynch, G. An electron microscopic study of lesion-induced synaptogenesis in the dentate gyrus of the adult rat. II. Reappearance of morphologically normal synaptic contacts. *Brain Res.* 115, 23–41 (1976).

McWilliams, J.R., and Lynch, G. Terminal proliferation and synaptogenesis following partial deafferentation. *J. Comp. Neurol.* 180, 581–615 (1978).

McWilliams, R., and Lynch, G. Terminal proliferation in the partially deafferented dentate gyrus: Time course for the appearance and removal of degeneration and the replacement of lost terminals. *J. Comp. Neurol.* 187, 191–198 (1979).

Moore, R.Y., Bjorklund, A., and Stenevi, U. Growth and plasticity of adrenergic neurons, in *The Neurosciences Third Study Program*. F.O. Schmitt and F.G. Worden, eds. MIT Press, Cambridge, Massachusetts (1974), pp. 961–977.

Ozawa, E. Activation of phosphorylation kinase from brain by small amounts of calcium ion. *J. Neurochem.* 20, 1487–1488 (1973).

Raisman, G. Neuronal plasticity in the spinal nuclei of the adult rat. ***Brain Res.*** 14, 25–48 (1969).

Raisman, G., and Field, P. A quantitative investigation of the development of collateral reinnervation after partial deafferentation of the septal nuclei. ***Brain Res.*** 50, 241–264 (1973).

Rose, G., Cotman, C.W., and Lynch, G. Hypertrophy and redistribution of astrocytes in the deafferented hippocampus. ***Brain Res. Bul.*** 1, 87–92 (1976).

Schwartzkroin, P., and Wester, K. Long-lasting facilitation of a synaptic potential following tetanization in the *in vitro* hippocampal slice. ***Brain Res.*** 89, 107–119 (1975).

Steward, O., and Loesche, G. Quantitative autoradiographic analysis of the time course of proliferation of contralateral entorhinal afferents in the dentate gyrus denervated by ipsilateral entorhinal lesions. ***Brain Res.*** 125, 11–21 (1977).

Van Harrevald, A., and Fifkova, E. Swelling of dendritic spines in the fascia dentate after stimulation of the perforant fibers as a mechanism of post-tetanic potentiation. *Exp. Neurol.* 49, 736–749 (1975).

Copyright © 1982, Spectrum Publications, Inc.
The Neural Basis of Behavior

7

Habituation, Sensitization and Associative Learning in *Aplysia*

E.T. Walters
T.J. Carew
E.R. Kandel

INTRODUCTION

A central problem in the study of behavior is how various forms of learning are interrelated. Are they governed by separate mechanisms or by variations on a common mechanism? A particularly important question concerns the relationship between simple nonassociative learning and more complex associative forms. A comparison of the mechanisms underlying these different types of learning requires an experimentally advantageous animal in which both nonassociative and associative learning can be studied on the cellular level. Because of the relative simplicity of its nervous system, the marine snail *Aplysia* has been useful for cellular studies of the mechanisms of nonassociative learning. We have found recently that this animal is also capable of associative learning. This capability permits us to compare these two classes of learning.

Over the last few years various aspects of *Aplysia's* behavioral repertory have been worked out on the cellular level (Kupfermann and Kandel, 1969; Kupfermann et a;., 1971, 1974; Mayeri et al., 1974; Carew and Kandel, 1977; Weiss et al., 1978; Hening et al., 1979; Rayport and Kandel, 1979). Here we consider only two defensive behaviors: the gill-withdrawal reflex and escape locomotion. We have used the gill-withdrawal reflex to examine the mechanisms of nonassociative learning, and escape locomotion to examine, on a behavioral level, the relation of nonassociative to associative learning. We will first review work on two forms of nonassociative learning: habituation and sensitization of the gill-withdrawal reflex (Fig. 1).

HABITUATION OF GILL-WITHDRAWAL

Habituation is probably the most ubiquitous behavioral modification found in animals. It refers to a decrease in behavioral response that occurs when an initially novel stimulus is repeatedly presented. Although remarkably simple, habituation is important in everyday life. Through habituation, animals including humans learn to ignore stimuli that have lost novelty or meaning; it thereby frees their attention for stimuli that are rewarding or significant for survival. Habituation is one of the earliest learning processes to emerge in humans and is commonly used in infants to study the development of intellectual processes such as attention, perception, and memory (Leaton and Tighe, 1976).

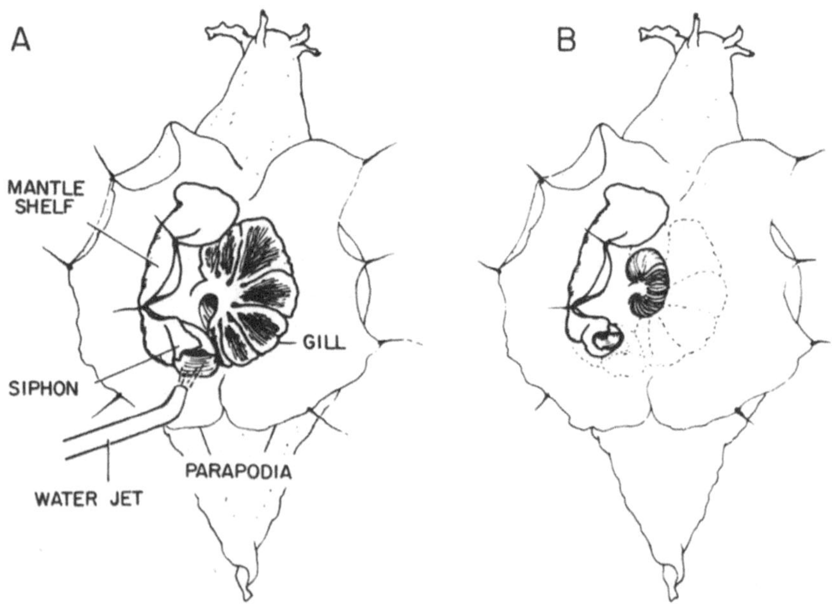

FIG. 1. Defensive withdrawal reflex of the siphon and gill in *Aplysia.* Dorsal view of an intact animal. The parapodia and mantle shelf have been retracted to allow direct observation of the gill. *A.* Relaxed position. *B.* Defensive-withdrawal reflex in response to a weak tactile stimulus to the siphon (a seawater jet). The relaxed position of the gill is indicated by the dotted lines.

An interesting feature of habituation in both *Aplysia* and humans is that it has both short- and long-term forms. The short-term form of habituation of gill-withdrawal in *Aplysia* is produced by a single training session of 10 mechanical stimuli delivered to the siphon (Fig. 1). Recovery is complete within a few hours, and partial recovery can occur within 15 minutes (Pinsker et al., 1970). Recovery is equivalent to forgetting a learned response. Thus, the time it takes for the response to recover indicates the duration of the memory. With repeated training sessions of 10 trials each, the memory for habituation can be prolonged so as to last days and even weeks (Fig. 2), and the reflex becomes almost completely depressed (Carew et al., 1972).

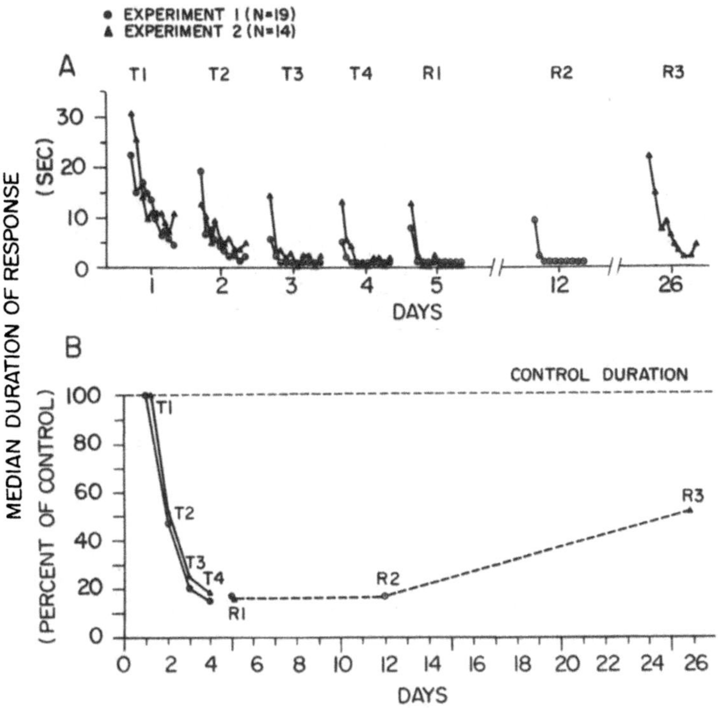

FIG. 2. *A*. Long-term habituation of siphon withdrawal in *Aplysia*. Habituation during four daily sessions of training (T1 to T4), and retention for 1 day (R1), 1 week (R2), and 3 weeks (R3) after training. Each session consisted of 10 trials with an interstimulus interval of 30 seconds. Data from two experiments are compared. In experiment 1, retention was tested 1 day (R1) and 1 week (R2) after training. In experiment 2, retention was tested 1 day (R1) and 3 weeks (R3) after training. Each point is the median response in a single trial. *B*. Time course of habituation based on data illustrated in *A*. The score for each daily session is the median of the sum of responses on trials 1 to 10 for each animal. Control duration (100 percent) is the response time during the first day of training. From Carew et al., 1972.

By examining various sites within the neural circuit of the gill-withdrawal reflex (Fig. 3) during habituation, Castellucci, Kupfermann, Pinsker, and Kandel (1970) found that the mechanism underlying short-term habituation

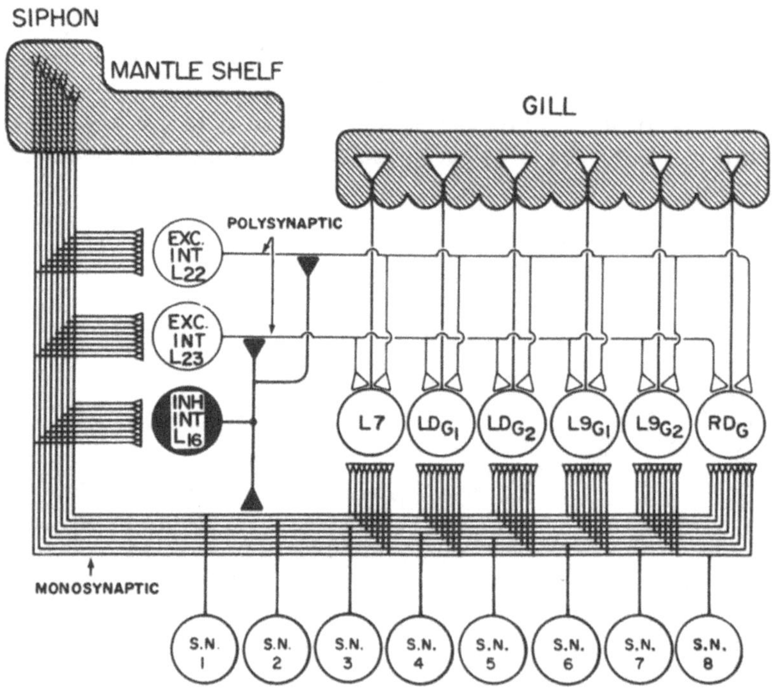

FIG. 3. Simplified wiring diagram of the defensive gill-withdrawal reflex. The siphon skin is innervated by approximately 24 mechanorecepter sensory neurons. The diagram illustrates that a tactile stimulus to any point on the siphon skin excites approximately 8 sensory neurons (S.N.). The sensory neurons make monosynaptic connections to 6 identified gill motor neurons and to at least 1 inhibitory interneuron (L16) and 2 excitatory interneurons (L22 and L23). From Kandel et al., 1976.

was a depression in excitatory synaptic transmission. This depression was localized to the synapses made by the sensory neurons on their central target cells, the motor neurons and interneurons. Using a quantal analysis, Castellucci and Kandel (1974) further localized the synaptic depression to the presynaptic terminals of the sensory neurons. The depression resulted from a progressive decrease in the amount of transmitter released from these terminals by each action potential.

What is responsible for the decrease in the amount of transmitter released? Transmitter is released from the presynaptic terminals in multimolecular packets or quanta. The number of quanta released is largely determined by the concentration of free calcium in the presynaptic terminal. The depolarizing action of the action potential leads to an influx of Ca^{++}, which is then thought to allow transmitter vesicles to bind to discharge sites—a critical step for exocytotic release. Klein and Kandel (1978) found that the Ca^{++} current produced by each action potential was not fixed but could vary. Repeated activation of the sensory neurons leads to a decrease (inactivation) of the Ca^{++} current, and thus a decrease in transmitter release.

We mentioned previously that repeated training sessions can completely depress the behavior. Does long-term habituation training produce an even more profound synaptic depression than that produced by short-term habituation? Can repeated training produce a complete and persistent inactivation of a previously functioning synapse?

With these questions in mind, Castellucci, Carew, and Kandel (1978) next explored the mechanisms whereby the long-term effect is generated. They found that in untrained animals most sensory cells (93 percent) make functional connections to the motor neurons. By contrast, in animals given long-term habituation training, 70 percent of these connections had been inactivated, so that most sensory cells no longer made functional synaptic connections to the gill motor neurons. This synaptic inactivation persisted for one week and was only partially restored at three weeks (Fig. 4). Thus, whereas short-term habituation involves a transient decrease in synaptic efficacy, long-term habituation leads to a more prolonged and profound change: a functional inactivation of previously existing connections. These data provide direct evidence that instances of long-term memory can be mediated by a persistent change in synaptic efficacy. Furthermore, these results make clear that short- and long-term habituation share a common neural locus: the synapses that the sensory neurons make onto the motor neurons and interneurons. Moreover, short- and long-term habituation involve aspects of the same cellular mechanism: depression of excitatory transmission. We now need to do a quantal analysis on long-term depressed synapses to see whether the synaptic depression is pre- or postsynaptic. If long-term depression, like short-term depression, proves to be presynaptic, this would support the hypothesis that a single trace can underlie both short- and long-term memory.

SENSITIZATION OF GILL-WITHDRAWAL

Sensitization, an opposite form of learning to habituation, is a process whereby an animal learns to increase its responsiveness to stimuli as a result of the presentation of a strong or noxious stimulus. Thus, whereas during habituation an animal learns to ignore a particular stimulus because its con-

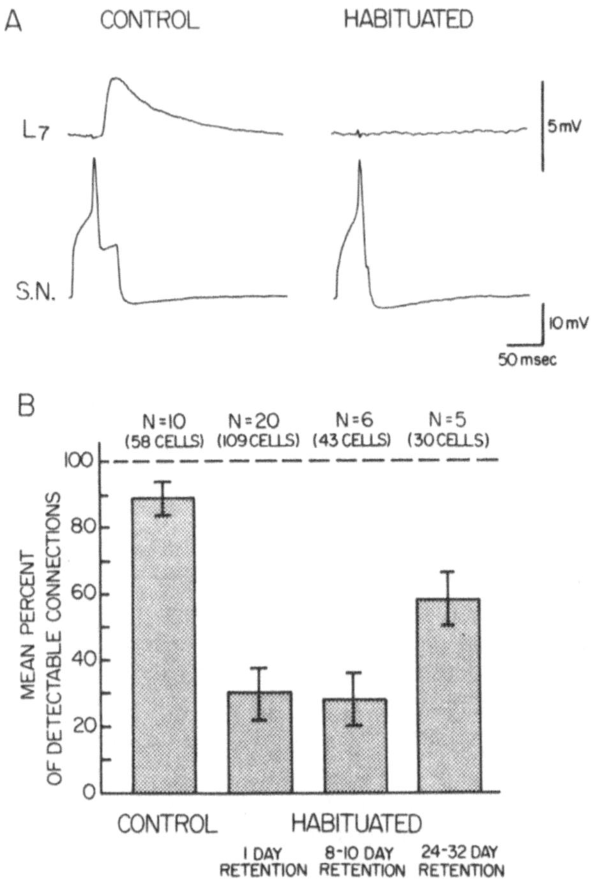

FIG. 4. Long term habituation. *A*. Comparison of synaptic connection between a sensory neuron (S.N.) and the motor neuron L7 in control (untrained) animals and in animals given long-term habituation training. The synaptic connection in trained animals is undetectable. *B*. The mean percent of detectable connections in control and habituated animals tested 1 day, 1 week, and 1 month after long-term habituation training. Error bars indicate standard error of the mean (SEM). From Castellucci et al. (1978).

sequences are innocuous or trivial, during sensitization an animal learns to attend to stimuli because they may be accompanied by painful or dangerous consequences (Fig. 5).

On the cellular level, sensitization of gill-withdrawal produced by shocking the neck involves an enhancement of synaptic transmission at the same locus which is involved in habitation (Castelluci and Kandel, 1976). In this case, however, transmitter release is *enhanced* because Ca^{++} influx is increased (Klein and Kandel, 1978). Thus, sensitization involves a presynaptic facilitation whereby terminals from pathways mediating sensitization modulate the calcium current in the sensory neuron terminals. The same synaptic locus can thereby be modulated in opposite ways by opposing forms of learning: it can be depressed by habituation and it can be facilitated by sensitization (Fig. 6). These cellular results support findings in mammals that habituation and sensitization are independent and opposing forms of learning (Spencer et al., 1966).

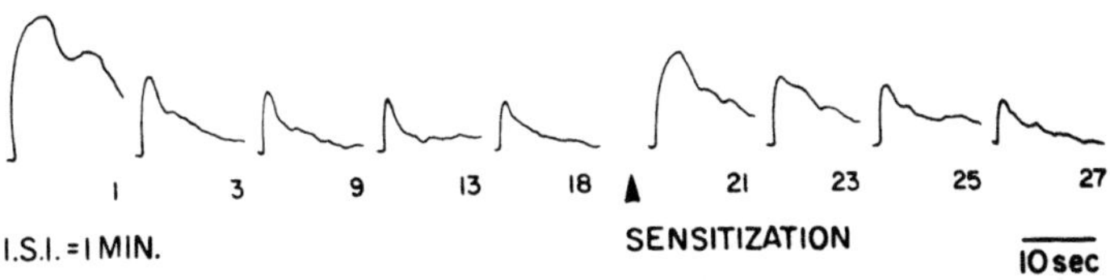

FIG. 5. Short-term sensitization of the gill-withdrawal reflex in *Aplysia*. Photocell recordings of gill-withdrawal showing sensitization following habituation of the reflex. Habituating tactile stimuli were presented to the siphon at 1 minute interstimulus intervals (I.S.I.). After 20 presentations a noxious sensitizing stimulus was applied to the neck. This produced a facilitation of the reflex lasting several minutes. From Pinsker et al. (1970).

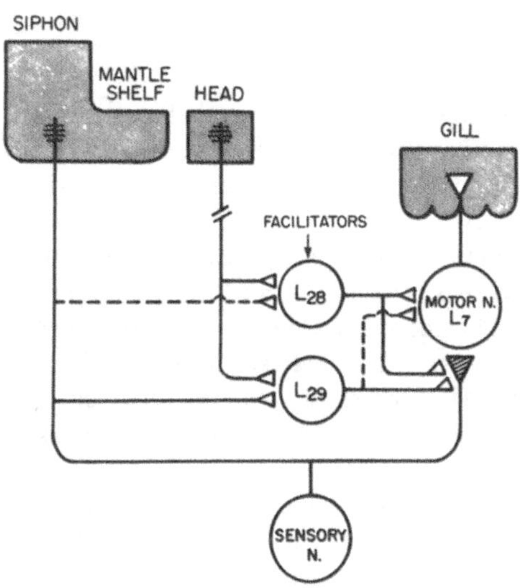

FIG. 6. Locus of plastic changes underlying habituation and sensitization of the gill-withdrawal reflex. For schematic purposes only one sensory neuron (S.N.), one motor neuron (L7), and two identified interneurons (L28 and L29) are shown. The terminal (*shaded*) of the sensory neuron onto the motor neuron is the common plastic locus for both the synaptic depression underlying habituation and presynaptic facilitation underlying sensitization. The pathway from the head that mediates sensitization activates a group of interneurons (facilitators), two of which (L28 and L29) are indicated here. These interneurons produce presynaptic facilitation of transmission between the sensory neuron and L17. Solid lines indicate direct monosynaptic connections. Dashed lines indicate polysynaptic connections. From Hawkins (1981).

The diagram in Fig. 7 summarizes these results and provides a somewhat speculative model of the mechanisms underlying sensitization and habituation. In the resting state, the depolarization produced by each action poten-

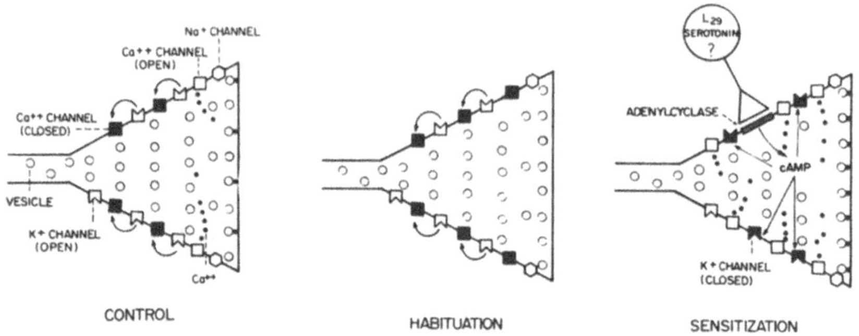

FIG. 7. Model of short-term habituation and sensitization. In the control state an action potential in the sensory neuron terminal membrane opens a number of Ca^{++} channels (*squares*) in parallel with Na^{+} channels (*hexagons*). Sensitization is produced by interneurons including L28 and L29 which are thought to be serotonergic. Serotonin activates an adenyl cyclase in the terminals, which stimulates cAMP synthesis. cAMP then broadens the spike by decreasing the activation of K^{+} channels, leading to a greater Ca^{++} influx, greater binding of vesicles to release sites, and increased probability of release. During habituation repeated action potentials decrease the number of open Ca^{++} channels, in the limit shutting them down completely. The resulting depression in Ca^{++} influx would inactivate the synapse.

tial opens up a number of Ca^{++} channels. Ca^{++} flows in and allows the vesicles to bind to the membrane, a prerequisite for release. Sensitization appears to be mediated by serotonergic cells which act on a serotonin-sensitive adenylate cyclase to increase the level of cAMP in the sensory cell terminals. The cAMP is thought to enhance transmitter release by decreasing the opposing K^{+} current so as to increase the duration of the action potential and thereby the size of the Ca^{++} current (Klein and Kandel, 1980). Attempts are now being made to carry this analysis to the molecular level by examining whether cAMP decreases the K^{+} current by phosphorylating the K^{+} ion channels (Paris, Kandel, and Schwartz, work in progress).

Thus far we have considered only nonassociative forms of learning. A further step in complexity is associative learning and in particular, classical conditioning. Classical conditioning resembles sensitization in that activity in one pathway can modify the activity of another pathway. These two forms of learning differ mainly in the requirement that, in classical conditioning, activity in the two pathways must have a specific temporal relationship. Because of the similarities between sensitization and classical conditioning, several authors have suggested that they have mechanisms in common (Kimmel, 1964; Kandel, 1967; Wells, 1968; Razran, 1971). We have thus far not been able to obtain clear evidence for classical conditioning in the gill-withdrawal reflex. To explore the relationship between non-associative and associative learning we have turned to a more complex behavior—escape locomotive, a behavior that shows both sensitization and classical conditioning.

SENSITIZATION OF ESCAPE LOCOMOTION

Locomotor responses in *Aplysia* offer several advantages for examining more complex forms of learning. First, pedal locomotion in *Aplysia* consists of discrete, regular steps which are unusually large (Fig. 8; see also Parker, 1917). These features are useful for monitoring the behavioral and neural changes accompanying the modulation of locomotion by learning, as well as for investigating the neural mechanisms underlying the locomotor sequence. Using quantitative videotape techniques we have obtained a detailed behavioral characterization of the normal locomotor sequence and thus can evaluate the changes produced by learning (Hening et al., 1979).

Second, individual motor neurons as well as distinct classes of motor neurons subserving locomotion have been identified in the pedal ganglia (Hening et al., 1979). By recording from these motor neurons, Hening et al. (1979) found that the locomotor program is generated centrally, and is manifest even in the isolated circumesophageal ganglia (see also Jahan-Parwar and Fredman, 1978a, b). An advantage of using a central program as the index for learning is that the learned changes should also be readily apparent in the isolated nervous system, a preparation that is very convenient experimentally.

Like gill-withdrawal, escape locomotion can be sensitized by noxious electrical stimuli applied to the head, a point remote from the site used to test the behavior. Sensitization of escape locomotion can be tested by triggering escape with a weak shock to the tail. Figure 9 shows that after even a single sensitization training trial (head shock), trained animals tend to walk more than untrained controls in the subsequent test session. This tendency is maintained through nine trials, at which point there is significant facilitation of locomotion in trained animals compared to untrained animals. Similarities between the sensitization of gill-withdrawal and escape locomotion suggest that each may be an expression of the same general process, perhaps a form of defensive arousal.

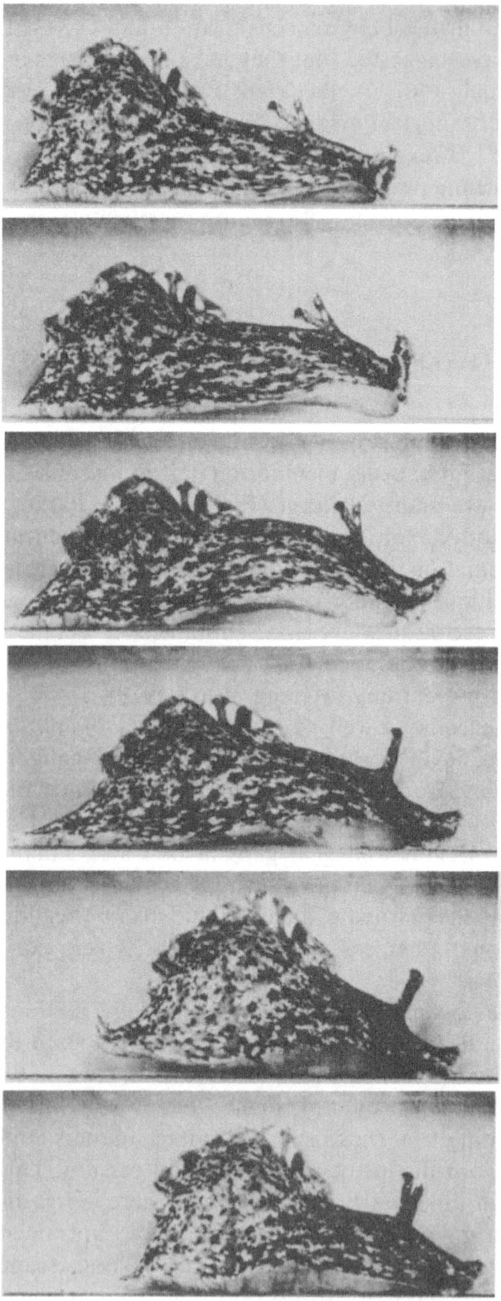

FIG. 8. One complete step in the *Aplysia* locomotor sequence. The step begins in the top frame with elevation and extension of the head. As the locomotor wave travels backwards the body arches (*middle frames*). The step ends with retraction of the tail, a discrete and easily observed movement. In these experiments each step is counted at the moment of tail retraction.

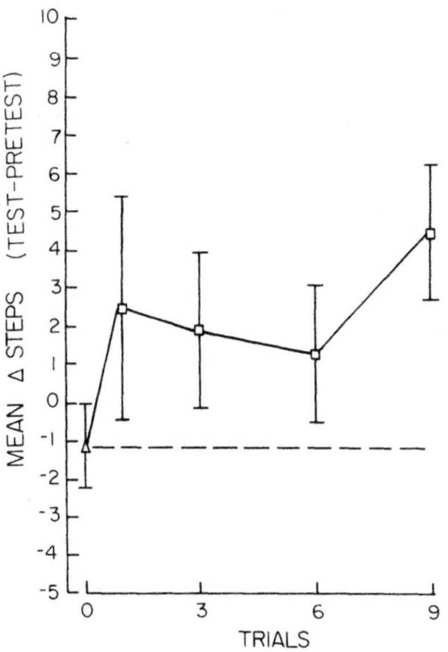

FIG. 9. Sensitization of pedal locomotion. Data are plotted as the mean difference in the number of steps taken in the PRETEST before training and the TEST after training. A training trial consisted of a strong electric shock to the head. Three trials were given per day, separated by 3 hours. Different groups of animals were given 1, 3, 6, or 9 trials. The control group received no head shocks and was tested 3 days after its pretest. The test stimulus was a weak shock to the tail. In order to compare these results to results presented later (Fig. 15), an additional stimulus, a crude shrimp extract, was present during the TEST. This chemosensory stimulus produces no unconditioned facilitation of locomotion.

ASSOCIATIVE LEARNING

To investigate the relationship between sensitization and classical conditioning, we have used a classical aversive conditioning paradigm (Pavlov, 1927). This paradigm has allowed us to produce classical conditioning using the same noxious training stimulus (head shock) and the same test pathway (escape locomotion to tail shock) that we used to produce sensitization. The only difference between sensitization training and classical conditioning is the presence of a specifically paired conditioned stimulus in the latter procedure.

In classical aversive conditioning, one stimulus, the conditioned stimulus (CS), is repeatedly paired with an aversive unconditioned stimulus (US). In vertebrates this training commonly gives rise to a set of conditioned responses which can be expressed in two different ways. First, after conditioning the CS sometimes develops the ability to elicit overt motor responses. Second, the CS sometimes acquires the ability to modulate a variety of test behaviors not necessarily involved in the original conditioning procedures (Estes and Skinner, 1941; Brown et al., 1951). We have examined the conditioned modulatory effects of the CS, both for technical convenience and because these are of considerable theoretical interest (Rescorla and Solomon, 1967). For example, the finding in vertebrates that the CS can modulate other behaviors indicates that learning produces widespread effects, *any* of which can serve as indicators of learning, and none of which represents the actual learning process itself (Rescorla, 1978). Despite the extensive use of this approach in vertebrate studies, it has not been directly explored in invertebrates.

Conditioning Procedures

The experimental procedures we used are summarized in Fig. 10. All experiments began with the PRETEST on Day 1 to assess baseline locomotor

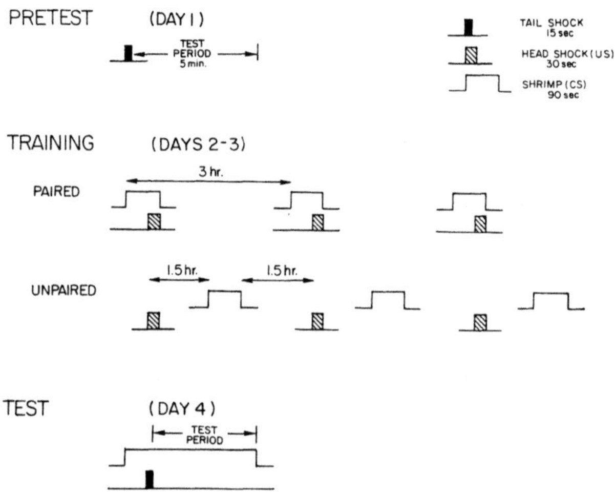

FIG. 10. Classical conditioning procedures. The test stimulus was a weak shock to the tail. The US was a strong head shock. The CS was a small volume of crude shrimp extract applied over the oral tentacles. The CS was applied after the animal's pan was separated from the home tank (and from chemosensory contact with the other animals). This procedure was identical for all groups. From Walters et al., 1979.

responsiveness before training. The test stimulus was a weak electric shock applied to the tail. The latency of the first step and the number of steps taken within a five minute period following the shock were recorded using criteria illustrated in Fig. 8.

Animals were matched on the basis of their PRETEST scores and assigned to one of three training groups. The "untrained" group received no further treatment. The "unpaired" group was trained with the conditioned stimulus (CS = shrimp extract) and the unconditioned stimulus (US = shock to head) explicitly unpaired. The "paired" group was trained with specific temporal pairing of the CS and US (Fig. 10). Three training trials per day were given for two days. The animals in the paired group first received the CS applied over the anterior tentacles and then, 60 seconds later, the US was applied to the head. The unpaired group was trained with the same CS and US as the paired animals, but received the CS 90 minutes after the US on each trial. Eighteen hours after the last training trial, all animals were tested. In the TEST session each animal received the CS for 60 seconds and then, with the CS still present, the same test stimulus used in the PRETEST (weak tail shock) was delivered. These training and testing procedures demonstrated a form of conditioning characterized by (1) temporal specificity, (2) a requirement of CS presence for the learning to be expressed, and (3) rapid acquisition.

Temporal Specificity

The critical feature of associative learning is temporal specificity. In both classical and instrumental learning, the subject displays a change in behavior due to specific temporal relationships between events. A common interpretation is that one event (the CS in classical conditioning and the operant response in instrumental conditioning) comes to predict the occurrence of the other (the US or reinforcement), allowing the subject to respond accordingly (Rescorla, 1967). One question that we have examined is whether training with a pattern of temporally paired CS and US presentations produces a different outcome than training with a pattern of explicitly unpaired presentations (Walters et al., 1979). In the TEST session after training (Fig. 11), the animals in the paired group walked significantly more than those in either control group (Fig. 11A). The same data presented as the difference in escape locomotion before and after training (Fig. 11B) clearly show that not only is the paired group different in the amount of escape locomotion exhibited in the TEST session, but it is also different in the direction of the effect: both control groups show a decrease in locomotion in the TEST session whereas the paired group shows a significant increase.

In addition, training with either the US alone, or with the CS alone, failed to produce the conditioned facilitatory effect of the CS on escape responses (Walters et al., 1979). These findings indicate that the ability of the CS to enhance escape locomotion is dependent upon the specific temporal relationship between CS and US during conditioning.

The CS Must Be Present for Conditioning to be Expressed

Associative learning is often characterized by marked stimulus specificity (Miller, 1967). The presence of the CS is necessary for expression of the conditioned effect: it is not elicited by other stimuli, except by closely related ones. As a first step in investigating stimulus specificity, we examined whether the CS was required during the TEST session (Walters et al., 1979). If paired training had merely produced a general increase in responsiveness, one would predict that the test stimulus alone, in the absence of the CS, might elicit the conditioned effect.

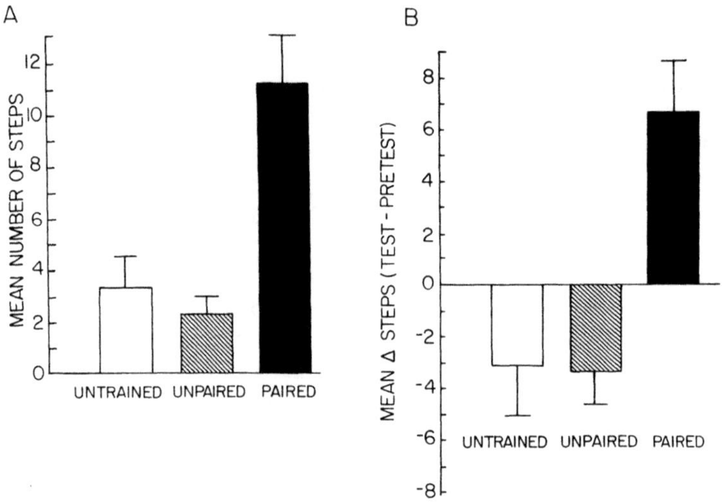

FIG. 11. Classical conditioning in *Aplysia*. *A*. Responses in the TEST session. Each score is the mean (±SEM) number of steps taken within 5 minutes of the test stimulus. Paired animals (N= 18) walked significantly more than untrained (N= 12) or unpaired (N= 18) animals. *B*. Differences between TEST and PRETEST scores (from the same experiment as A). The paired animals walked significantly more in the TEST than in the PRETEST. The decrease in locomotion in the untrained group is not statistically significant, whereas the decrease in the unpaired group is significant. Such decreases are often seen in untrained and unpaired groups while increases have never been seen in these controls. From Walters et al., 1979.

To examine this possibility we first trained animals with the standard paired and unpaired protocols (Fig. 10). Each group was then tested twice, first in the absence of the CS, and then, three hours later, in the presence of the CS. In the absence of the CS both groups showed a decrease in escape locomotion in comparison to the PRETEST scores (Fig. 12). However, in the presence of the CS the paired group exhibited significantly more escape locomotion to the test stimulus than did the unpaired group and, in addition, significantly more locomotion than it had shown to the same test stimulus in the absence of the CS (Fig. 12). This indicates that the CS is re-

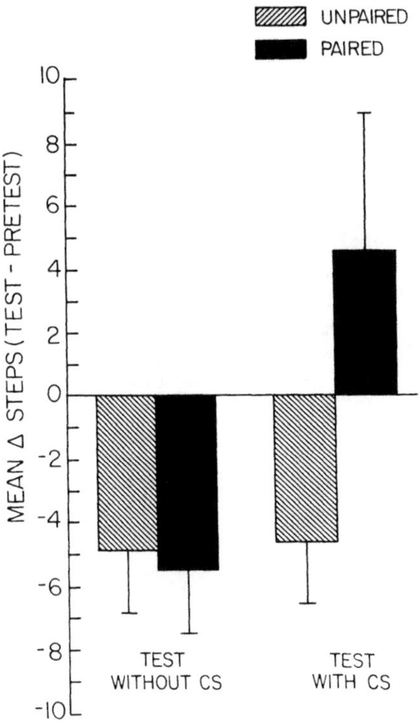

FIG. 12. CS requirement for expression of conditioning. Mean differences (±SEM) between TEST and PRETEST scores in the absence and (three hours later) in the presence of the CS. The paired animals (N = 8) walked significantly more in the presence of the CS than they had in the absence of the CS. In addition, in the presence of the CS the paired animals walked significantly more than the unpaired animals (N = 8). From Walters et al., 1979.

quired for the conditioned effect to be expressed and suggests that the conditioning does not merely produce a nonspecific increase in responsiveness.

Aplysia Shows Rapid Acquisition of Aversive Conditioning

We examined the acquisition of the learned response by training different groups of animals with different numbers of trial (from 0 to 12 trials). Each group was tested the morning after its last training trial. Fig. 13 shows the results of paired and unpaired training.

The major effect of training was a profound increase in the amount of escape locomotion elicited in the paired animals. This effect reached its maximum at six trials and was maintained through 12 training trials. The unpaired animals showed the opposite trend, a progressive decrease in the amount of escape locomotion elicited with increasing numbers of training trials.

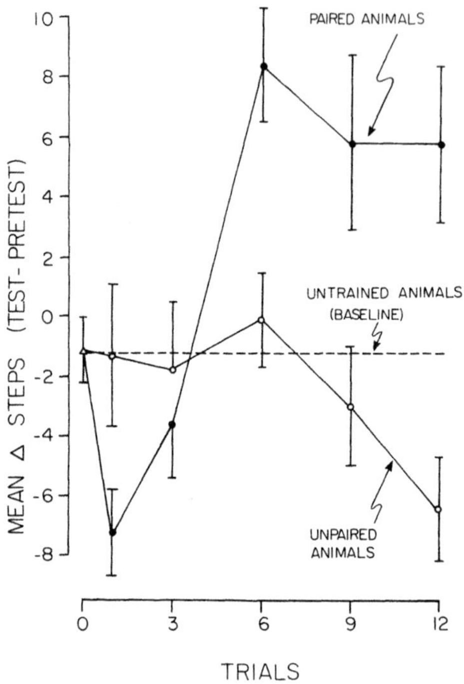

FIG. 13. Acquisition. Different groups (13 to 18 animals per group) were given 0, 1, 3, 6, 9, or 12 trials (three trials per day) and tested 18 hours after the last trial. Each point is the mean difference (±SEM) in walking between the TEST and the PRETEST (see Fig. 10). The dashed baseline corresponds to untrained (0 trials) performance. Paired animals walked significantly more than unpaired and untrained animals at 6, 9, and 12 trials. Paired animals also walked significantly *less* than unpaired animals after only one trial. We are currently examining this effect.

CONCLUSIONS

The recent elucidation of the cellular mechanisms of two forms of nonassociative learning in *Aplysia* and the possibility of carrying this analysis to the molecular level have encouraged our attempt to analyze associative learning. Moreover, by focusing on a system (escape locomotion) which manifests both sensitization and classical conditioning, we hope to be able to determine the interrelationships between these forms of learning. In addition, since several forms of associative learning have recently been described in other gastropod mollusks (Mpitsos and Davis, 1973; Mpitsos and Collins, 1975; Gelperin, 1975; Crow and Alkon, 1978), it may soon be possible to compare different forms of associative learning in related species.

Although a full understanding of these interrelationships will require a cellular analysis, the behavioral studies themselves have proven important in setting limits on the nature of the associative changes and in indicating interactions between associative and nonassociative effects. The associative learning expressed in escape locomotion does not simply result from the direct conditioning of a locomotor response by CS-US pairing, since no locomotion is elicited by the CS when it is presented alone after conditioning. The conditioned effect must therefore involve one of two alternative mechanisms: 1) conditioning of another motor response, such as head withdrawal or a postural response, which itself facilitates locomotor responses to tail shock, or 2) conditioning of a motivational or arousal state which facilitates escape responses. On the basis of our behavioral data, we cannot distinguish fully between these possibilities. However, the learning does not appear to be due to the conditioning of a motor response that facilitates locomotion because, in the testing which follows conditioning, neither head withdrawal nor postural changes distinguish paired from unpaired animals. The learning is more consistent with the conditioning of a motivational state (defensive arousal), which manifests itself in the modulation of responses not directly elicited by the CS.

The Conditioned Motivational State Hypothesis

The finding that aversive conditioning in *Aplysia* can occur without the conditioning of an overt response to the CS is interesting for two reasons. First, this finding is consistent with many interpretations of vertebrate aversive conditioning of a central state (Mowrer, 1960; Rescorla and Solomon, 1967; Konorski, 1967; Estes, 1941; Hammond, 1970). In vertebrates, the conditioned state has been called alternatively "conditioned fear" (Mowrer, 1960; Rescorla and Solomon, 1967), "conditioned emotional state" (Hammond, 1970), or "conditioned motivational state" (Mackintosh, 1974).

Second, in vertebrates conditioned internal states have been found to have motivationally consistent effects: the conditioned "fear" produced by the CS (after paired training) enhances defensive responses and inhibits appetitive responses (Rescorla and Solomon, 1967; Scobie, 1972). One implication for *Aplysia* of the conditioned motivational state hypothesis is that a range of behaviors will be modulated by the CS following conditioning, and that these modulations will be appropriate to a state of defensive arousal ("fear"). Defensive responses such as head withdrawal, inking, and escape locomotion should be facilitated; appetitive responses such as feeding and mating should be inhibited; and general homeostatic systems, such as those controlling cardiac activity, should be adjusted in whichever direction is most compatible with the defensive state.

These implications suggest a speculative, but testable, model of aversive classical conditioning in *Aplysia* (Fig. 14) that has four features. One, a defensive arousal system which can modulate various effector systems. Two, a US that has a relatively effective connection to the defensive arousal system. This inference is supported by the finding that, when presented nonassociatively, the US (head shock) produces appropriate modulatory ef-

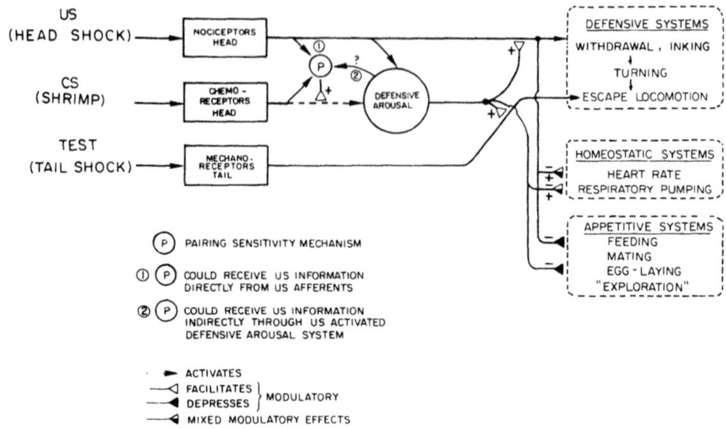

FIG. 14. Schema for the conditioned motivational state hypothesis as applied to *Aplysia*.

fects, enhancing both escape locomotion and head withdrawal, and suppressing feeding (Walters et al., 1978; Kupfermann and Pinsker, 1968). Three, a CS pathway that makes functionally ineffective connections to the defensive arousal system. This is suggested by the fact that repeated stimulation with the CS alone does not result in facilitation by the CS of escape locomotion. Four, the connections from the CS pathway to the defensive arousal system are strengthened when activity in the CS pathway is repeatedly paired with activity in the US pathway (and/or activity of the defensive arousal system). Thus, following conditioning the CS becomes effective in activating the defensive arousal system, and this results in the modulation of test responses such as escape locomotion triggered by tail shock.

Interrelationships of Sensitization and Classical Conditioning

Escape locomotion triggered by tail stimulation can be enhanced both by nonassociative training (sensitization) and by associative training (classical conditioning) using the same training and test pathways. This interesting finding allows a direct comparison of these two forms of learning. For example, sensitization develops early, does not change markedly with successive trials, and produces only moderate facilitation of escape locomotion (Fig. 9). By contrast, the classically conditioned facilitation of escape develops later, reaches its peak rapidly, and produces powerful facilitation of escape locomotion (Fig. 13; see also Walters et al., 1979).

Thus, similar long-term behavioral effects can be produced in two different ways: 1) by providing the animal with a cue stimulus which can predict the US, and 2) by simply repeating the US. Although superficially similar, these behavioral effects are actually quite different. In classical conditioning, the enhanced responsiveness appears to be specific both to the temporal pairing of the CS and the shock during training and to the presence of the CS during testing. The paired animal does not appear to be defensively aroused except when the CS is present. By contrast, in long-term sensitization, there is a continuous, nonspecific state of enhanced responsiveness; the sensitized animal appears to be chronically aroused. One might say that whereas aversive classical conditioning produces a specific "fear," long-term sensitization training produces a nonspecific, chronic "anxiety."

Complex Features of Classical Conditioning in Aplysia

As shown in Fig. 15, after nine training trials animals trained with head shock alone (sensitization training) show significantly more escape than

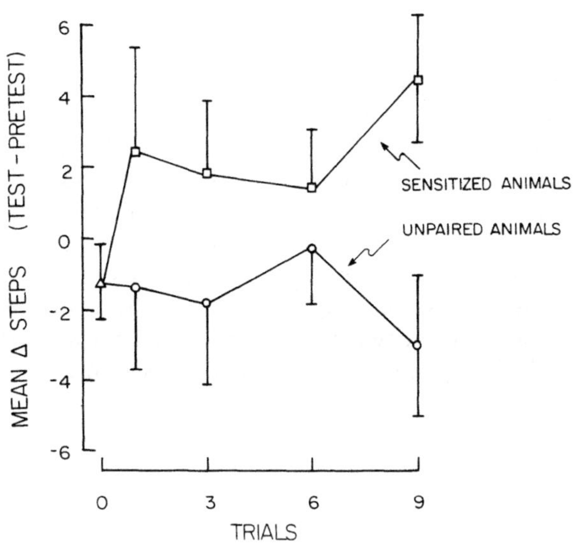

FIG. 15. Comparison of acquisition curves for groups given specifically unpaired training and group given sensitization (US alone) training. After nine trials unpaired animals showed significantly *less* escape than sensitized animals in the TEST session, indicating that specifically unpaired training also produced a form of associative learning.

animals trained with explicitly *unpaired* presentations of the shrimp CS and head shock US. This difference indicates that the unpaired animals, as well as the paired animals, show associative learning. The learning in the unpaired animals is expressed as a modulation opposite to the produced by paired training. Applying the general definition suggested by Rescorla (1969), this unpaired effect would appear to be an instance of conditioned inhibition, a form of associative learning not previously described in the invertebrates. A common interpretation of conditioned inhibition is that the explicitly unpaired animal learns that the CS predicts the *absence* of the US. The CS comes to have opposite meanings (a "danger" signal or a "safety" signal) for animals exposed to opposite contingencies between the CS and US.

Further experiments (for example, summation and retardation tests; see Rescorla, 1969) need to be carried out before we can evaluate the similarity of this unpaired effect in *Aplysia* to the conditioned inhibition described for vertebrates. However, this finding shows that associative learning in *Aplysia* has interesting, complex features which may allow us to extend to invertebrates the principles of learning derived from vertebrate studies.

Towards a Cellular Analysis of Associative Learning

Although *Aplysia* may provide behavioral insights into associative learning, its greatest attraction clearly lies in its advantages for cellular analyses. We have therefore been encouraged by our recent findings that (1) the aversive conditioning persists after restraining the animal and exposing its central nervous system for intracellular study, and (2) that neural correlates of conditioning can be observed in identified pedal motor neurons (Walters et al., in preparation). It may therefore prove possible to bring to bear on associative learning the same analytic tools which have proved so useful in the analysis of nonassociative learning. This would allow a comparison on the cellular level of the mechanisms underlying these two classes of learning.

ACKNOWLEDGEMENTS

This work was supported by National Institutes of Health Predoctoral Fellowship to E.T.W. (5T32MH15740), Career Development Award to T.-J.C. (5K02MH0081), Career Scientist Award to E.R.K. (5K05MH18558), and by grants from the National Institutes of Health (NS12744 and GM23540), and the McKnight Foundation.

REFERENCES

Brown, J.S., Kalish, H.I., and Farber, I.E. Conditioned fear as revealed by magnitude of startle response to an auditory stimulus. *J. Exp. Psychol.* 41, 317–328 (1951).

Carew, T.J., and Kandel, E.R. Inking in *Aplysia californica.* I. Neural circuit of an all-or-none behavioral response. *J. Neurophysiol.* 40, 692–707 (1977).

Carew, T.J., Pinsker, H.M., and Kandel, E.R. Long-term habituation of a defensive withdrawal reflex in *Aplysia. Science* 175, 451–454 (1972).

Castellucci, V.F., Carew, T.J., and Kandel, E.R. Cellular analysis of long-term habituation of the gill-withdrawal reflex of *Aplysia californica. Science* 202, 1306–1308 (1978).

Castellucci, V., and Kandel, E.R. A quantal analysis of the synaptic depression underlying habituation of the gill-withdrawal reflex in *Aplysia. Proc. Natl. Acad. Sci. USA* 71, 5004–5008 (1974).

Castellucci, V., and Kandel, E.R. Presynaptic facilitation as a mechanism for behavioral sensitization in *Aplysia. Science* 194, 1176–1181 (1976).

Castellucci, V., Pinsker, H., Kupfermann, I., and Kandel E.R. Neuronal mechanisms of habituation and dishabituation of the gill-withdrawal reflex in *Aplysia. Science* 167, 1745–1748 (1970).

Crow, T.J., and Alkon, D.L. Retention of an associative behavioral change in *Hermissenda. Science* 201, 1239–1241 (1978).

Estes, W.K., and Skinner, B.F. Some quantitative properties of anxiety. *J. Exp. Psychol.* 29, 390–400 (1941).

Gelperin, A. Rapid food-aversion learning by a terresterial mollusk. *Science* 189, 567–570 (1975).

Hammond, L.J. Conditioned emotional states, in *Physiological Correlates of Emotion.* P. Black, ed. Academic Press, New York (1970), pp. 245–259.

Hawkins, R.D. Interneurons involved in mediation and modulation of the gill-withdrawal reflex in *Aplysia.* III. Identified facilitating neurons increase the Ca^{++} current in sensory neurons. *J. Neurophysiol.* 45, 327–339 (1981).

Hening, W.A., Walters, E.T., Carew, T.J., and Kandel, E.R. Motorneuronal control of locomotion in *Aplysia. Brain Res.* 179, 231–253 (1979).

Jahan-Parwar, B., and Fredman, S.M. Control of pedal and parapodial movements in *Aplysia.* II. Cerebral ganglion neurons. *J. Neurophysiol.* 41, 609–620 (1978).

Jahan-Parwar, B., and Fredman, S.M. Pedal locomotion in *Aplysia.* I. Sensory and motor fields of pedal nerves. *Comp. Biochem. Physiol.* 60A, 459–465 (1978b).

Kandel, E.R. Cellular studies of Learning, in *The Neurosciences: A Study Program.* G.C. Quarton, T. Melnechuk, and F.O. Schmitt, eds. Rockefeller U. Press, New York (1967), pp. 666–689.

Kandel, E.R., Brunelli, M., Byrne, J., and Castellucci, V. A common presynaptic locus for the synaptic changes underlying short-term habituation and sensitization of the gill-withdrawal reflex in *Aplysia*, in *Cold Spring Harbor Laboratory Symposium on Quantitative Biology*, Vol. XL. Cold Spring Harbor (1976), pp. 465–482.

Kimmel, H.D. Theoretical note: A further analysis of GSR conditioning: A reply to Stewart, Stern, Winokur, and Fredman. *Psychol. Rev.* 71, 160–166 (1964).

Klein, M., and Kandel, E.R. Presynaptic modulation of voltage-dependent Ca^{2+} current: Mechanism for behavioral sensitization in *Aplysia californica. Proc. Natl. Acad. Sci. USA* 75, 3512–3516 (1978).

Klein, M., and Kandel, E.R Mechanism of calcium current modulation underlying presynaptic facilitation and behavioral sensitization in *Aplysia. Proc. Natl. Acad. Sci. USA* 77, 6912–6916 (1980).

Konorski, J. *Integrative Activity of the Brain.* U. Chicago Press, Chicago (1967).

Kupfermann, I., Carew, T.J., and Kandel, E.R. Local, reflex and central commands controlling gill and siphon movements in *Aplysia. J. Neurophysiol.* 37, 996–1019 (1974).

Kupfermann, I., and Kandel, E.R. Neuronal controls of a behavioral response mediated by the abdominal ganglion of *Aplysia. Science* 164, 847–850 (1969).

Kupfermann, I., and Pinsker, H. A behavioral modification of the feeding reflex in *Aplysia californica.Comm. Behav. Biol. (A)* 2,13–17 (1968).

Kupfermann, I., Pinsker, H., Castellucci, V., and Kandel, E.R. Central and peripheral control of gill movements in *Aplysia. Science* 174, 1252–1256 (1971).

Leaton, R.N., and Tighe, T.J. Comparisons between habituation research at the developmental and animal-neurophysiological levels, in *Habituation: Perspectives From Child Development, Animal Behavior, and Neurophysiology*. T.J. Tighe and R.N. Leaton, eds. Lawrence Erlbaum Associates, Hillsdale, New Jersey (1976), pp. 321–340.

Mackintosh, N.J. *The Psychology of Animal Learning*. Academic Press, London (1974), pp. 81–85.

Mayeri, E., Koester, J., Kupfermann, I., Liebeswar, G., and Kandel, E.R. Neural control of circulation in *Aplysia:* I. Motorneurons, *J. Neurophysiol.* 37, 458–475 (1974).

Miller, N.E. Certain facts of learning relevant to the search for its physical basis, in *The Neurosciences: A Study Program.* G.C. Quarton, T.Melnechuk, and F.O. Schmitt, eds. Rockefeller U. Press, New York (1967), pp. 643–652.

Mowrer, O.H. *Learning Theory and Behavior.* Wiley, New York (1960).

Mpitsos, G.J., and Collins, S.D. Learning: Rapid aversive conditioning in the gastropod mollusk *Pleurobranchaea. Science* 188, 954–957 (1975).

Mpitsos, G.J., and Davis, W.J. Learning: Classical and avoidance conditioning in the mollusk *Pleurobranchaea. Science* 180, 317– 320 (1973).

Parker, G.H. The pedal locomotion of the sea hare *Aplysia. J. Exp. Zool.* 24, 139–145 (1917).

Pavlov, I.P. *Conditioned Reflexes: An Investigation of the Physiological Activity of the Cerebral Cortex.* Translated and Edited by G.V. Anrep. Oxford U. Press, London (1927).

Pinsker, H., Kupfermann, I., Castellucci, V., and Kandel, E.R. Habituation and dishabituation of the gill-withdrawal reflex in *Aplysia. Science* 167, 1740–1742 (1970).

Rayport, S., and Kandel, E.R. Identified cells R2 and P1 control mucus release in *Aplysia:* A model system for studying the development of behavior on the cellular level. *Soc. Neurosci. Abs.* 5, 259 (1979).

Razran, G. *Mind in Evolution: An East-West Synthesis of Learned Behavior and Cognition.* Houghton Mifflin Company, Boston (1971).

Rescorla, R.A. Pavlovian conditioning and its proper control procedures. *Psychol. Rev.* 74, 71–80 (1967).

Rescorla, R.A. Pavlovian conditioned inhibition. *Psychol. Bull.* 72,77–94 (1969).

Rescorla, R.A. Some implications of a cognitive perspective on Pavlovian conditioning, in *Cognitive Processes in Animal Behavior.* S.H. Hulse, H. Fowler, and W.K. Honig, eds. Lawrence Erlbaum Associates, New Jersey (1978) pp. 15–50.

Rescorla, R.A., and Solomon, R.L. Two process learning theory: Relationships between Pavlovian conditioning and instrumental learning. *Psychol. Rev.* 74, 151–182 (1967).

Scobie, S.R. Interaction of an aversive Pavlovian conditional stimulus with aversively and appetitively motivated operants in rats. *J. Comp. Physiol. Psychol.* 79, 171–188 (1972).

Spencer, W.A., Thompson, R.F., and Neilson, D.R. Decrement of ventral root electrotonus and intracellularly recorded PSPs produced by iterated cutaneous afferent volleys. *J. Neurophysiol.* 29, 253–274 (1966).

Walters, E.T., Carew, T.J., and Kandel, E.R. Conflict and response selection in the locomotor system of *Aplysia. Soc. Neurosci. Abs.* 4, 209 (1978).

Walters, E.T., Carew, T.J., and Kandel, E.R. Classical conditioning in *Aplysia californica. Proc. Natl. Acad. Sci. USA* 76, 6675–6679 (1979).

Weiss, K.R., Cohen, J.L., and Kupfermann, I. Modulatory control of buccal musculature by a serotonergic neuron (Metacerebral Cell) in *Aplysia. J. Neurophysiol.* 41, 181–203 (1978).

Wells, M. *Lower Animals.* McGraw-Hill, New York (1968), pp. 154–165.

Copyright © 1982, Spectrum Publications, Inc.
The Neural Basis of Behavior

8

Biochemical Changes In The CNS During Learning

Victor E. Shashoua

Three types of information storage and retrieval processes can be identified in living organisms. These are the genetic, the immunological, and what may be called the "experiential" systems. In the genetic and the immune system, DNA and the immunoglobulins, respectively, have been identified as macromolecules that have crucial functions. In the experiential system, however, we have yet to determine which specific molecules are involved in information processing and retrieval. We clearly know that the experiential system exists. The problem is to bridge the gap between behavior and biochemistry.

The brain, as a tissue, has a very high rate of metabolism; about 20 times that of a muscle at rest and approximately five times that of an active muscle (Lowry et al., 1964). If we search among its biochemical components for molecules that might participate in the storage of information, we find that everything except the DNA is in a dynamic state. The average half-life of proteins is anywhere between 6 and 14 days (Lajtha and Toth, 1966). RNA turnover can vary from one-half hour to about 24 hours (Appel, 1967; Shashoua, 1964). Lipids and carbohydrates are also in a rapid state of flux (Bazan et al., 1977). Essentially, there seems to be nothing present within the nervous system that has a lifetime comparable to that required for experiential memory; only the structure and connectivity patterns of the nervous system have distinctive features with sufficient stability for use in memory processes. The notion that the pattern of connectivity can change with experience is one of the oldest hypotheses about memory formation. Tanzi (1893) was first to suggest this, soon after Ramon Y Cajal showed that the neuron is the basic unit of the nervous system.

THE DESIGN OF EXPERIMENTAL APPROACHES

Several investigations indicating that ongoing brain protein and RNA synthesis are essential for the establishment of a long-term memory (Flexner et al., 1963; Agranoff, et al., 1967; Barondes and Cohen, 1967; Jarvik, 1972) have supported the concept that there are at least two critical phases in the formation of a new memory (Flexner et al., 1963). The first is "short-term" memory, which is resistant to inhibitors of protein synthesis, and the second is "long-term" memory, which is sensitive to protein synthesis inhibitors such as puromycin and cycloheximide.

Although protein synthesis is required for long-term memory formation, it is not clear how the absence of such synthesis might prevent the recording of a specific behavioral experience. In attempting to solve this problem, it may be helpful to consider what kind of mechanism could be responsible for coupling the dynamic nature of the biochemistry of the nervous system to the formation of specific changes in connectivity patterns. Figure 1 shows a hypothetical scheme by which such a link might be established (Shashoua, 1972). In this scheme, environmental information as detected by the heat, light, chemical, and mechanical sensory receptors of an organism is converted by a series of four transduction steps into a long-term metabolic "demand signal," which is specific to the type of information being processed in certain neural circuits available for a given input. The demand signal, through three additional transduction steps, initiates the synthesis of proteins that subsequently modify membranes in the activated neural circuits. Each of the transduction steps in Fig. 1 consists of multicomponent and multistep events which represent phases during the continuous processing of input into a suitable form for biochemical storage.

In the first step, information from the sensory receptors is transduced into the characteristic digital electrical spike train language of neurophysiology, i.e., in an "electrical-time" mode. The storage capacity in this mode is somewhat limited since the same sensory receptors that produce a given quantum of input must almost immediately be reutilized in order to generate the next segment of information. The constraint requires a second transduction process in which the time aspects of the input are changed to produce an "electrical-space" model. Such a postulate is supported by neurophysiological experiments indicating that digital spike trains are converted into analog signals at specific cellular elements (Grundfest, 1969; Werner and Mountcastle, 1965). Thus, this information may be considered to be a distribution of "space charges" in a three-dimensional network over many neural elements in different brain areas. Clearly, many complex factors will have to operate to link new with old preexisting information at this juncture (John, 1972). Also, experiments in which electroconvulsive shock

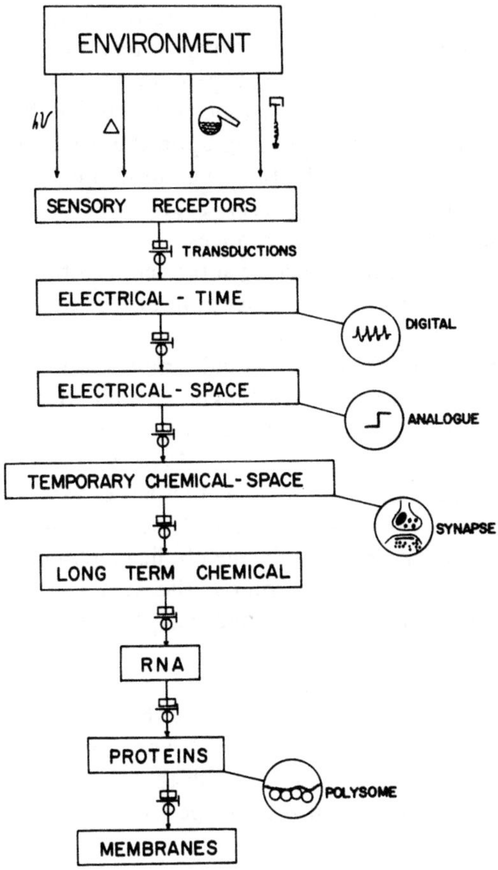

FIG. 1. Diagram of transduction processes in the nervous system. Symbols between environment and sensory receptors, from left to right: light inputs, heat inputs, chemical inputs, mechanical inputs. Each transduction process characterizes a stage of the information processing mechanism of the nervous system. These are considered to have specific time constants and to be the result of a multicomponent event representing the transit status of information.

(ECS) treatment within 10 seconds after training causes amnesia in rats (Chorover and Schiller, 1965) might be considered as evidence for the presence of such space charges. Thus, the memory trace in an electrical-space mode can be disrupted electrically. More recent experiments that suggest that ECS can disrupt memory at later times after training have been interpreted as secondary effects of the electrical events (McGaugh, 1966).

In the third transduction step, the electrical space-mode is converted into a "temporary chemical-space" signal. By this means, the information, residing as electrical charged sites and reflecting only the new aspects of the input, is used to generate a chemical signal at the same loci where the electrical charges were originally present. This storage mode no longer contains any electrical elements. Such changes are also temporary and may occur at synaptic sites to produce some sort of coupling between pre- and postsynaptic sites. Many types of chemical processes could be responsible for these chemical changes, such as formation of leaky synaptic membranes, changes in transmitter levels, production of small peptide molecules, development of temporary ionic gradients, etc. The time constant for this "temporary chemical-space" mode will vary depending upon the principle neurotransmitter used. It represents essentially the short-term memory phase of the process where information is preserved until the brain metabolic machinery can produce the permanent changes.

In the fourth transduction step, the events occurring at the cell membrane are communicated to the cell nucleus through the generation of "long-term chemical" signal (Rose, 1971; Shashoua, 1971). One substance that might participate in this process is cyclic AMP, which would bring about the phosphorylation of specific membrane proteins (Machlus et al., 1974; Browning et al., 1979). This hypothesis, described in a different chapter by Lynch and Lee, is implied by many studies in brain (Shashoua, 1970) and other tissues (Langan, 1968), which demonstrate that RNA synthesis is enhanced after cAMP production. Thus, phosphorylated proteins at targeted membrane sites could represent a holding pattern until the metabolic machinery, through the last two transduction steps, can promote the synthesis of proteins for transport to the membrane loci which had been targeted for change during acquisition of the behavior.

This type of analysis, in which behavior is coupled with biochemistry, reduces the problem to a search for a biochemical process that might be used in memory processing to alter neural membranes. Such a process might be a brain-specific process or it might be a process in all cells that is used in a special way in the nervous system. It could require brain-specific proteins in addition to non-brain-specific components.

One consequence of this type of analysis is that the molecules themselves do not have to have informational specificity. This specificity is provided by the neurocircuitry; the biochemical events provide only the means for a modification of this circuitry.

BEHAVIORAL EXPERIMENT

In our laboratory, goldfish were selected as the experimental animals for use in a search for specific proteins or biochemical processes that might be linked to behavior. A simple behavioral task was devised that would provide a maximum challenge to the nervous system of the goldfish (Shashoua, 1970). The animals were trained to swim with floats sutured at their ventral midlines at a position 1 mm caudal to the base of their pectoral fins. Figure 2 shows the diagram of the procedures. Each goldfish (weight, 7gm),

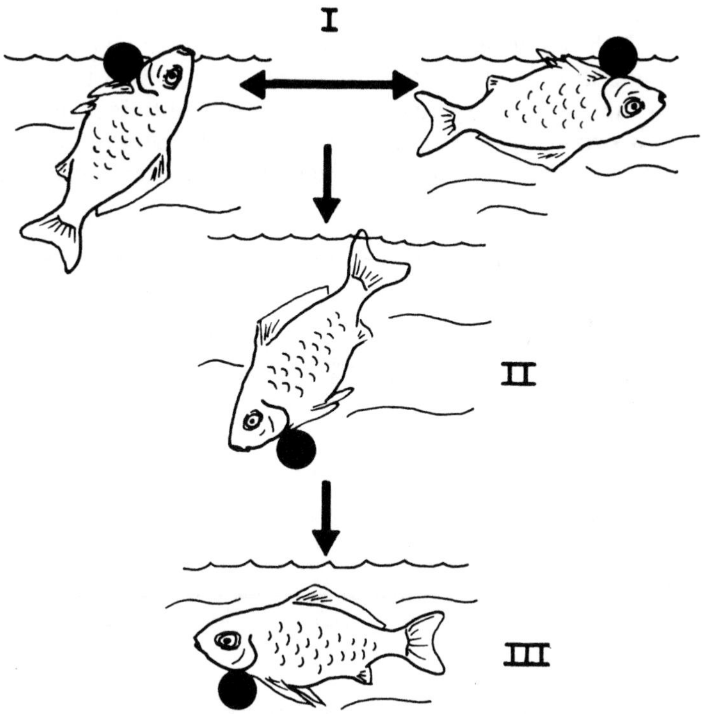

FIG. 2. The sequence of adaptation of a goldfish in the float-training task. Stage I—initial phase, each fish (7 g weight) has a 1 cm cylindrical styrofoam float (0.7 cm long). Stage II—intermediate phase, achieved after one hour. Stage III—final phase after four hours.

initially suspended by the float in an upside down position, adapts to the float through a series of reproducible stages until it can swim upright in a horizontal posture. This somewhat unconventional task challenges the nervous system in such a way as to involve motor, vestibular, cerebellar, and lateral line systems. An animal readjusts practically all of its motor movements in order to swim upright and it is presumed that such radical changes in swimming behavior should result in large biochemical changes in the nervous system. The training procedure lasts four to five hours. Periodically, each animal is observed for 30 seconds and its performance is evaluated according to a fixed set of criteria (Shashoua, 1976a) with 0 percent, 50 percent, and 100 percent performance scores representing swimming in an upside down, 45° angle, and a horizontal posture, respectively. More than 10,000 animals have been trained by this method. Test scores of groups of seven animals are used to generate the type of training curves for Trial I, shown in Fig. 3. When the animals were tested with the same floats 3 days later (Trial II), the goldfish were able to swim in a horizontal posture within 5 to 10 minutes after the floats were attached. This suggests that there is a retention of the previous experience (see Fig. 3). Well-trained animals can recall the new swimming skill for at least 11 days. This behavioral paradigm was used as a model system for investigations of biochemical changes.

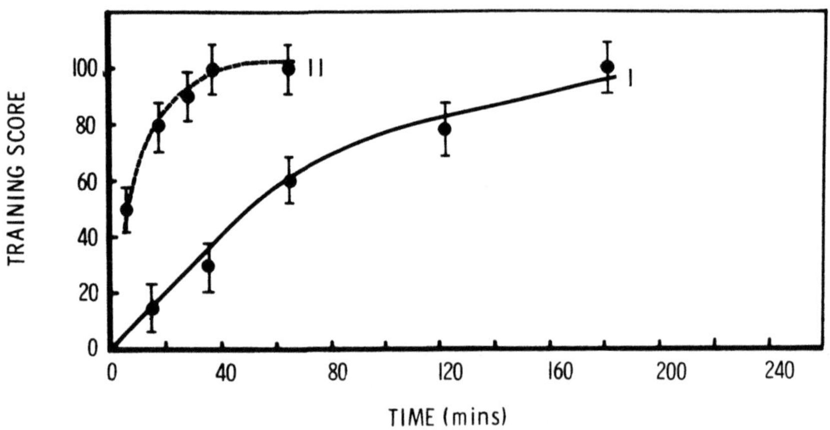

FIG.3. Learning (Trial I, day 1) and retention (Trial II, day 4) curves for the goldfish. Seven animals were trained on day 1, and the floats were removed. In Trial II on day 4, the same animals were tested with the same floats as on day 1.

BIOCHEMICAL EXPERIMENTS

Figure 4 outlines the type of biochemical experiments carried out. Generally, a group of seven animals was trained for four hours and then the floats were removed; one hour later the trained group of seven animals was labeled with radioactive [^{3}H]valine, while a group of seven untrained controls, in a separate tank, received injections of [^{14}C]valine. One hour after receiving the injections, the animals were anesthetized by cooling and the brains of the two groups were pooled together and homogenized in isotonic sucrose (Shashoua, 1976b). The homogenate was separated by centrifugation into nuclear, cytoplasmic, synaptosomal, myelin, and mitochondrial fractions. Each of these fractions contain newly synthesized proteins, the ^{3}H and ^{14}C products being derived from the trained animals and untrained controls, respectively. These products were separated on SDS-polyacrylamide gels by electrophoresis to give the type of patterns shown in Fig. 5.

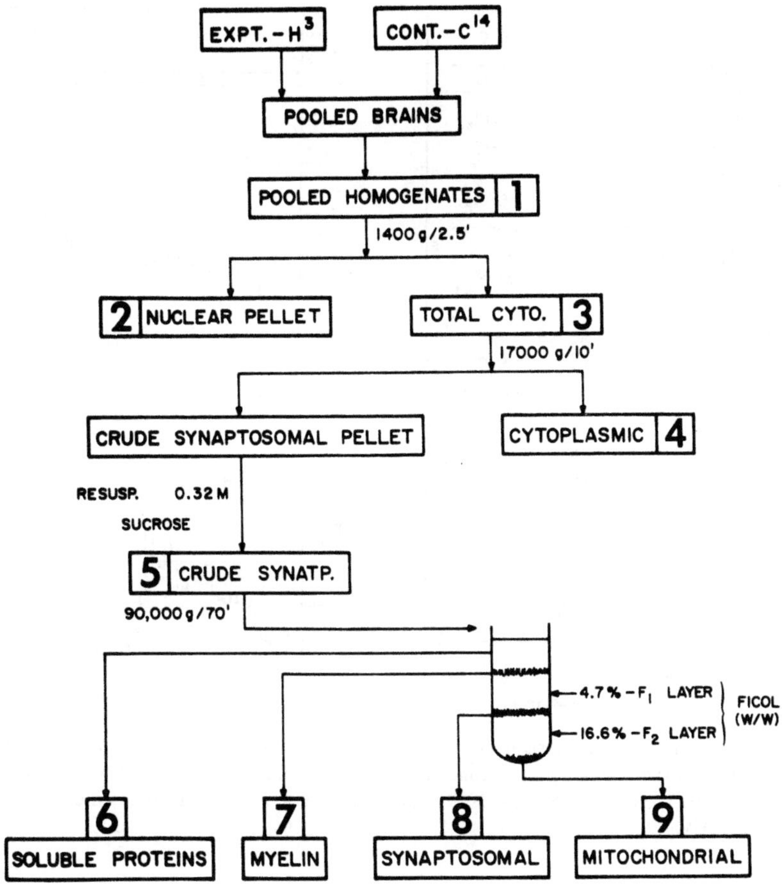

FIG. 4. Double labeling and subcellular fractionation procedure. After training seven goldfish received intracerebral injections of labeled valine [^{3}H]; an equal number of controls, in a separate tank, were labeled with valine [^{14}C]. The animals were labeled for one hour, then anesthetized in ice for 10 minutes. The brains of the two groups were pooled and homogenized in 0.32 M sucrose and fractionated by centrifugation methods.

In this double labeling procedure, any protein that is common to both the trained and control groups should have a constant ^{3}H to ^{14}C ratio. But any protein, whose synthesis is accelerated as a direct result of the training, should show a higher double labeling ratio. By this technique we found that there are three proteins, α, β, and γ, that are labeled to a greater extent in the trained than in the control animals (Shashoua, 1976b). The results are reproducible. Table 1 shows some of the data that demonstrate consistent

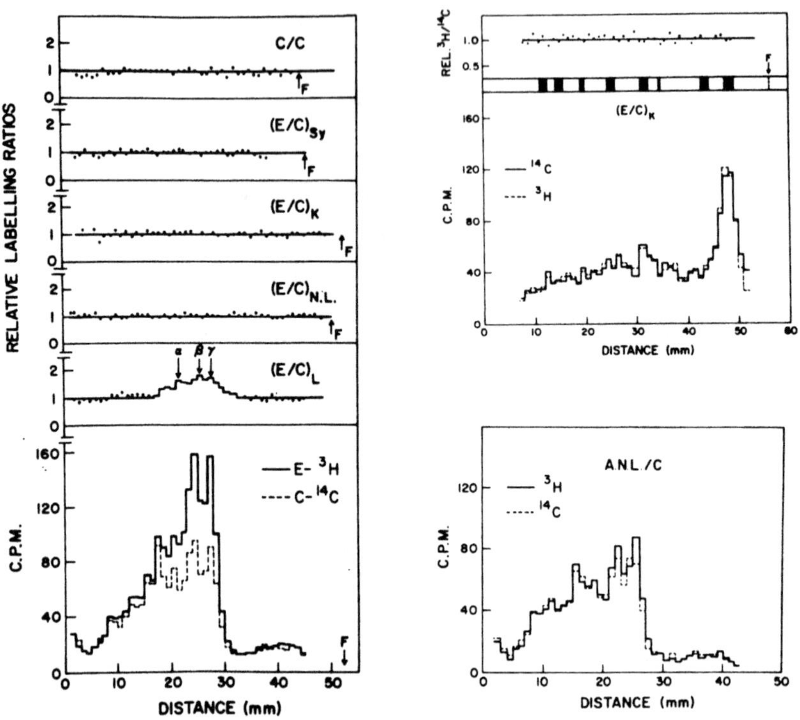

FIG. 5. Gel electrophoresis data for labeled goldfish brain proteins. C/C, control versus control; E/C, experimental versus control; Sy, synaptosomal cytoplasmic fraction; K, kidney cytoplasmic fraction. L, N.L., A.N.L. denote learning, non-learning, and active non-learning, respectively.

increases in α, β, and γ at three molecular weight regions (37,000, 32,000, and 26,000). The average increases in the ratios for these proteins were 46 percent, 59 percent, and 72 percent, respectively. The changes were confined to the brain cytoplasmic fractions. No protein changes were obtained for the synaptosomal, brain nuclear, or the kidney cytoplasmic fractions of the trained goldfish.

CONTROL EXPERIMENTS

The occurrence of changes in the pattern of labeling of specific protein molecules in goldfish brain after training does not necessarily indicate that these proteins are correlated with the learning aspects of behavior. Such changes might be a result of physiological stimulation of the animals or the

Table 1. Double-Labeling Data for Valine Incorporation

No.	*Type*	*Increase at bands %*		
1	Learners vs. untrained controls	60	80	100
2	Learners vs. untrained controls	60	78	100
3	Learners vs. untrained controls	41	47	91
4	Learners vs. untrained controls	37	44	43
5	Learners vs. untrained controls	22	26	31
6	Learners vs. untrained controls	35	30	40
7	Learners vs. untrained controls	15	20	30
8	Learners vs. untrained controls	17	25	18
	Control Experiments			
9	Passive non-learners vs. C		No changes	
10	Active non-learners vs. C		No changes	
11	Active non-learners vs. C		No changes	
12	Learner-forgetters vs. C		No changes	
13	Learner-forgetters vs. C		No changes	

Results are for gel electrophoresis data for incorporation of ^{3}H-valine versus ^{14}C-valine. In Experiments 7 and 8, the trained goldfish received ^{14}C-valine. All other trained groups received ^{3}H-valine. Each experiment compares seven experimental with seven control goldfish. Learner-forgetter animals are older goldfish (12 gm weight). All others are younger animals 5–7 gm weight.

stress or some other feature of the experiment. These possibilities were examined by conducting several types of behavioral control experiments. It was found that during most training sessions, some of the goldfish in each group of seven did not learn to swim upright after the floats were attached. Such goldfish could be separated into two groups according to their behavior: (1) passive non-learners, and (2) active non-learners. The passive non-learners, after the attachment of the floats, remained completely inactive in an upside down position during the four-hour training period. Such animals, when subjected to the double-labeling procedure, showed no protein changes. Thus, it is essential for the animal to do something for a change in the labeling to occur.

The second category of non-learners were the active non-learners. Here the animals were extremely active as soon as the floats were first attached, but their performance scores at the initiation of their training did not change significantly throughout the four-hour training period. For example. some animals would start with a 50 percent training score and continue to perform steadily at this rate throughout the experiment. Experiments 10 and 11 in Table 1 and Fig. 5 (ANL/C) show the type of results obtained in which the goldfish started with 29 percent and ended with 33 percent training scores or began with 46 percent and ended with 45 percent. These data suggest that learning is required in order to obtain protein changes. The active non-learners became physically exhausted by the vigorous swimming for up to a total of six hours without showing any changes in the pattern of protein synthesis. Thus physiological stimulation cannot be considered a primary factor for causing the enhanced labeling of the α, β, and γ proteins.

The possibility that stress during training was responsible for protein changes was also examined. Goldfish (one year old or less) were found to readily learn the float-training task and to recall the experience when tested at three or even 11 days later. Older goldfish (12 to 15 grams weight) learned the task at about the same rate as the young ones, but they could not recall the experience when tested three days later. Thus, the younger goldfish appear to have both short-term memory and long-term memory; that is, they can readily learn the task and recall the behavior three days later. The older animals, however, appear to have a short-term memory only, since they behave like naive animals when tested three days later. It is important to note that the float sizes chosen for the training procedures were the maximum that the animals could handle. Double-labeling studies showed that the younger animals had increased labeling in the α, β, and γ regions, whereas the older animals showed no such protein changes. If stress was a determinant of the protein changes, then both the young and older animals would be expected to show changes. Presumably, the effects of stress would be at a maximum during the acquisition phase of the behavior. The fact that no protein changes were obtained for the older goldfish, which could learn the task readily but not recall it, suggests that stress is not a major cause of the changes observed. However, one could perhaps argue that some other developmental factor, such as the size and age of the animal, might also be important in the sensitivity of an animal to stress, but this would not explain why the older animals could not retain the behavior. These results suggested that the α, β, and γ proteins might have some relationship to the acquisition process of a new behavior so that further studies of their properties seemed important.

ISOLATION AND PURIFICATION OF THE β PROTEIN FRACTION

Preparative gel electrophoretic methods were used to separate the α, β, and γ proteins from the total cytoplasmic proteins of goldfish brain. Generally, each preparation required the use of 300 goldfish brains. These were homogenized and purified (Shashoua, 1977a) to give the cytoplasmic fraction. Figure 6 shows the type of elution pattern obtained from one experiment in which [^{3}H]valine was used to label the trained group and the [^{14}C]valine for the controls. Measurements of the ratio of ^{3}H/^{14}C for each

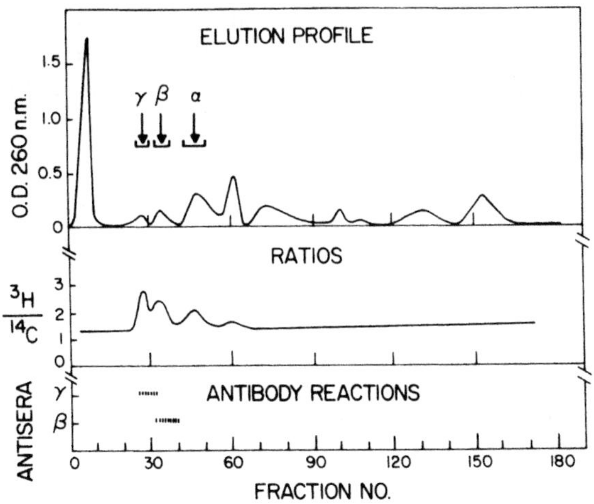

FIG.6. Data from preparative gel electrophoresis experiments. Upper graph shows O.D. 260 nm measurement of proteins on each fraction; middle graph shows the $^3H/^{14}C$ ratios of the proteins labeled with ^3H valine for the trained and ^{14}C valine for control untrained goldfish; lower graph shows the results of tests of each fraction with antisera to the *β* and *γ* proteins.

fraction were used to identify the positions of the *α*, *β*, and *γ* peaks. That all proteins at the *β* peak were identical was subsequently confirmed by immunological methods with antisera to *β*. The *β* protein was selected for further studies, and about 800 μg was isolated and used for detailed characterization experiments. The criteria for purity of the *β* protein were as follows:

(1) The protein migrated as a single staining band on two types of SDS-polyacrylamide (Neville, 1971) electrophoretic gels (see Fig. 7). The molecular weight of this product is about 32,000.

(2) No traces of impurities were detectable by radioactivity measurements or staining of proteins at all other regions of the gels.

(3) Analyses of the NH_2-terminal end groups by the method of Weiner et al. (1972) showed the presence of a single amino acid serine, for the *β* protein, indicating that the product contains a single polypeptide chain. Of course, it is possible that N-acylated chains might also be present, and these would not be detectable by end-group determinations.

(4) Analysis of the protein by isoelectric focusing further confirmed the degree of purity. As shown in Table 2, samples of the *β* protein in the absence of SDS contained a single major protein band at pH 7.4 and traces of a second product at pH 7.8. In the presence of SDS, analysis of *β* protein indicates some microheterogeneity. A single

major band with two intermediate and three trace products are obtained. These data are similar to results for other purified proteins such as aldolase A (Susor et al., 1969) where microheterogeneity is clearly indicated even with the crystalline form.

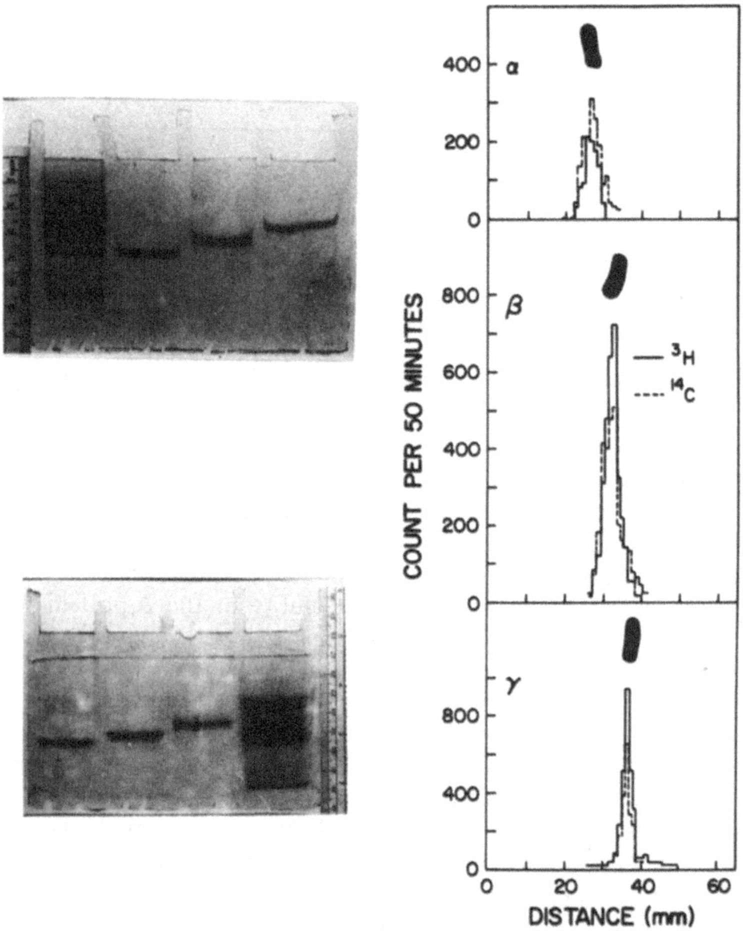

FIG. 7. Electrophorectic gel patterns of the purified of α, β, and γ proteins. A and B are photographs of SDS-polyacrylamide slab gels for the pH 6.9 Tris buffer and the borate pH 8.64–9.18 buffer systems, respectively. From left to right: A shows the total cytoplasmic proteins, γ, β, and α; B shows γ, β, α, and total cytoplasmic proteins. B has an upper stacking gel followed by the running gel system. C gives the pattern of labeling of a 1 cm wide strip from the A gel at the positions of α, β, and γ, respectively. The ^3H and ^{14}C counts represent the incorporation of valine for the trained and control goldfish, respectively. No counts were detected at position outside the indicated peaks.

Table 2. Isoelectric Focusing Data β Protein

Solvent	*Isoelectric Point*		
	Major	*Minor*	*Trace*
Urea buffer (no SDS)	7.4		7.2
Urea + SDS	7.6	7.7	7.4
		7.5	7.2

β protein samples separating as single bands on SDS-polyacrylamide gels were purified and run on isoelectric focusing gels according to the method of O'Farrell (1975) and Danno (1977).

(5) The β protein was capable of inducing the formation of specific antisera in rabbits. These appeared to be monospecific in that they gave single precipitin bands when tested against the purified β antigen or the total brain cytoplasmic fraction on Ouchterlony gels (Ouchterlony. 1967). This suggests that the antisera are directed against only one component in the goldfish brain cytoplasmic fraction.

(6) Table 3 shows a preliminary amino acid analysis of the β protein. The results indicate that the product is an acidic protein with aspartic and glutamic residues predominating and also a large serine content (Shashoua, 1977c).

Table 3. Amino Acid Analysis of the β Protein

Amino Acid	*Mole %*	*Amino Acid*	*Mole %*	*Amino Acid*	*Mole %*
Asp	9.0	Ala	8.0	Phe	2.9
Thr	5.6	Val	5.0	His	2.4
Ser	12.6	Met	1.0	Lys	4.6
Glu	13.6	Ileu	3.3	Arg	3.9
Pro	4.9	Leu	6.2		
Gly	15.8	Tyr	1.3		

Note: Tryptophane was not analyzed.

DISTRIBUTION OF THE PROTEIN IN SUBCELLULAR FRACTIONS OF GOLDFISH BRAIN

The β antiserum was used to study the distribution of the β protein in subcellular fractions of goldfish brain. The β protein was found to be a normal component of goldfish brain; that is, present in brains of untrained as well as trained goldfish. Similarly, immunological experiments with the γ protein showed that this also is a normal brain component. The fact that γ and β are normally present in the brain suggests that training simply increases the rate at which they are labeled. Presumably, exposure to the behavioral experience increases the turnover or demand for these proteins.

Studies of subcellular brain fractions with the antisera to the β and γ proteins showed that these proteins are largely confined to the cytoplasmic fraction. No precipitin bands were detectable in the nuclear, myelin, or membrane fractions (Shashoua, 1977a). Studies of specificity indicated that the antisera to β and γ did not cross-react with cytoplasmic proteins derived from mouse, rat, chick, or toad brain. The β antiserum did, however, show some cross-reactivity with cytoplasmic proteins from catfish brain, but it was not immunologically identical to it.

NEUROANATOMICAL LOCALIZATION OF THE β PROTEIN

The immunohistofluorescence techniques of Coons (1968) and Hartman (1973) were used to map the distribution of the β antigen in goldfish brain. Serial sections, 10 μM thick, were fixed in a mixture of $CHCl_3$ and MeOH (2:1 by volume) or with lysine-periodate (McLean and Nakane, 1974), and then stained with antisera to the β protein raised in the rabbits. After thorough washing to remove non-specific binding, the sections were stained with a second antibody raised in the goat against rabbit IgG. The goat antiserum to IgG, covalently linked with fluorescein molecules, binds to the β antibody within the tissue sections, so that its distribution can be visualized by fluorescence microscopy. Figure 8 shows the type of results obtained. In-

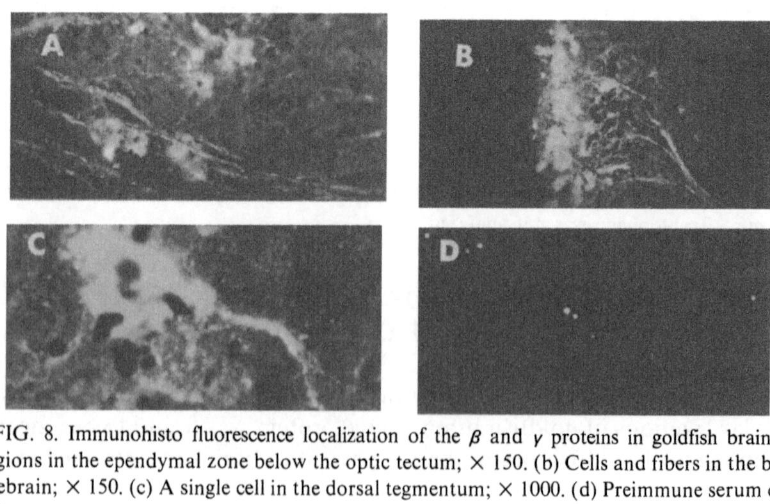

FIG. 8. Immunohisto fluorescence localization of the β and γ proteins in goldfish brain. (a) Regions in the ependymal zone below the optic tectum; × 150. (b) Cells and fibers in the basal forebrain; × 150. (c) A single cell in the dorsal tegmentum; × 1000. (d) Preimmune serum control.

dividual cells as well as fibrous elements were well stained, but only the cytoplasm of cells containing β protein was fluorescent. No nuclei were stained (Shashoua, 1977b). This is in agreement with the double labeling and the subcellular distribution studies which showed that the β and γ proteins were not present in the nuclear fraction. Figure 9 shows the neurohistochemical map of the distribution of β-containing cells in goldfish brain (Benowitz and Shashoua, 1977). The β protein was found to be localized in a group of cells in periventricular regions of goldfish brain, i.e., the ependymal zone. In this region of the optic tectum, the ependymal zone becomes substantial, comprising about 1/4 of the thickness of the tissue. The ependymal zone contains embryonic tissue even in the adult animal, so that some cell division can always be detected there. Most of the cells in the ependymal zone are considered to be glia (Vigh-Taichman and Vigh, 1970), so that the β protein may be a glial factor. Similar investigations indicate that γ

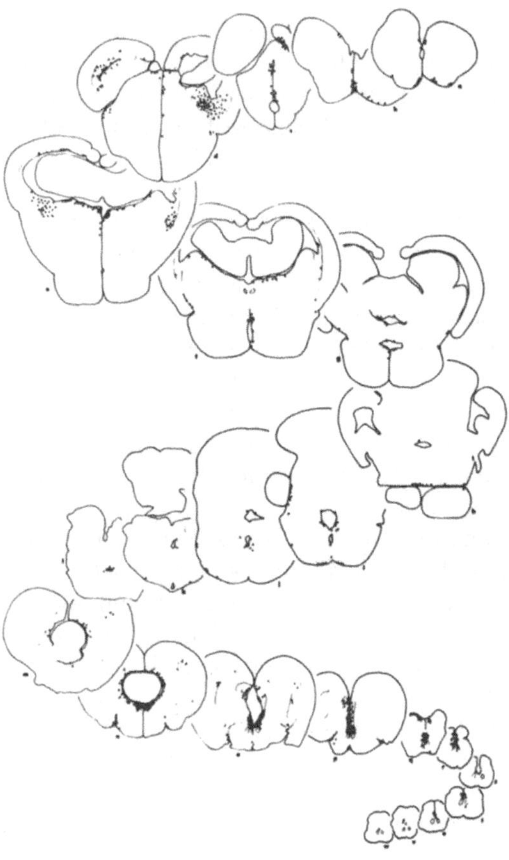

FIG. 9. Localization of β protein cells in goldfish brain. Serial cross-sections are drawn at 400 μm intervals. Triangles show the locations of individual β ependymal cells.

protein cells are also present in the ependymal zone. The identification of the glial or neuronal nature of the cells requires immunohistochemical electron microscopy. Because of the localization of the β and γ proteins, we have proposed the name "ependymin β and γ" for the proteins.

AMNESTIC EFFECTS OF THE ANTISERA TO THE β AND γ EPENDYMINS

There are several ways in which a protein such as ependymin β can be correlated with the acquisition of a new pattern of behavior. One possibility is that the specific system of β-containing cells is activated by the training. In this case, ependymin β would merely be a marker for specific neural circuits that are activated by the training, and, implicitly, would have no direct functional role in behavior acquisition. Alternatively, ependymin β could directly participate in some aspect of the plasticity process. As a test for this hypothesis, we investigated the effects of antisera on the retention of the training using methods similar to those used by other workers in studies of S-100 protein (Hyden and Lange, 1970), the ganglioside GMl (Karpiak et al., 1976), and synaptic plasma membrane proteins (Kobiler et al., 1976). The animals were trained with floats on day 1, then three hours after completion of training, were injected intracerebrally into the 4th ventrical with antisera to both the β and γ ependymins. Control animals were injected with normal rabbit serum or preimmune serum. The experiments were run blind. After three days, the floats were reattached, and the rate of reacquisition of the task was tested. Such experiments showed that the animals that received the antisera were amnestic, whereas control animals had complete recall of the behavior (Shashoua and Moore, 1978). Table 4 summarizes the data obtained in experiments of this type. The observations were highly reproducible; over 500 animals have been tested by this procedure. The data were also statistically significant. The animals that received the antisera could not recall the behavior.

There are several possible explanations for these results. For example, the antisera might produce some delayed toxicity reaction. As a control for this, we tested the effects of β and γ antisera by injecting them at 0.5 hour and 24 hours before training. As shown in Experiments 6 and 7 in Table 4, such treatments had no influence on the rate of learning or on recall, so toxicity does not appear to be a factor. Another possibility is that any antiserum to any brain protein injected into the CNS might produce amnestic effects. As a control for this, we tested the effects of an antiserum to a specific neural surface membrane protein, NS6 (Chaffee and Schachner, 1978). This antiserum can more easily find its antigenic target than the antisera to β and γ,

Table 4. Effect of Antisera on Behavior

Expt. No.	Antisera	Time (Hrs.)	Experimentals		Controls		T-test
			No. of Animals	Average % Retention Score	No. of Animals	Average % Retention Score	P-value
1	β	+8	28	36 ± 19	21	94 ± 7	<.0025
2	β	+8, +20	21	25 ± 11	21	94 ± 7	<0.0005
3	$\beta + \gamma$	+8, +20	98	49 ± 21	97	92 ± 16	0.0005
4	$\beta + \gamma$	+48	15	28 ± 33	14	81 ± 27	<0.1>0.05
5	$\beta + \gamma$	+72	13	70 ± 32	12	77 ± 37	<.35>1.3
				Controls			
6	$\beta + \gamma$	−0.5	21	90 ± 13	21	92 ± 6	<0.45>.4
7	$\beta + \gamma$	−24	21	94 ± 11	21	120 ± 35	<.2>.15
8	NS—6	+8	20	89 ± 39	20	88 ± 38	<.48>.45
9	$\beta + \gamma$ (antigen adsorbed)	+8, 20	12	82 ± 32	11	71 ± 24	<.2>.15

Experimental goldfish received injections into the brain fourth ventricle of antisera to either β or $\beta + \gamma$ ependymins. Controls received preimmune sera at the times specified prior or after the initiation of the five-hour training periods.

which must get into the cells in order to react with components in the cytoplasm. Antiserum to NS6 produced no amnestic effects, so that one cannot assume that every antibody to a brain specific protein produces amnesia. As an additional control, the antisera to β and γ were absorbed with the pure β and γ antigens, and then used in the training experiments. Again, (Experiment 9, Table 4) there were no amnestic effects, so no other components present in antiserum, other than the specific IgG molecules which react with β and γ, are important in producing the amnestic effects.

In another control experiment, we studied the time-course of action of the antisera. If ependymins β and γ are specifically correlated with the acquisition of behavior, there should be a certain time period within which antisera to these proteins can produce amnestic effects. The antisera were therefore injected at various times after training (see Experiments 3, 4, and 5 in Table 4). The antisera caused amnestic effects when injected between three hours and 24 hours after the completion of training. When injected 48 hours after training, they caused amnesia in about 50 percent of the animals, whereas when injected 72 hours after training, no amnestic effects were detectable. Clearly, antisera to the ependymins appear to be effective during the consolidation process, but not during the acquisition phase of the behavior. This suggests that the proteins might participate in some aspect of the formation of the long-term memory.

EVIDENCE FOR SECRETION OF THE β AND γ EPENDYMIN INTO THE CSF

One question that is raised by the above observations is how a high-molecular-weight antibody molecule directed against a cytoplasmic protein can find its target within the cells. Perhaps there is a specific mechanism for the uptake of IgG molecules within the nervous system. An alternative possibility is that the proteins are secreted into the extracellular fluid to produce effects elsewhere. This hypothesis was tested by three types of experiments.

In the first experiment, the cerebrospinal fluid from 20 goldfish was isolated and tested for immunological specificity. The antisera to ependymins β and γ produced strong precipitin bands against CSF by the Ouchterlony methods (Shashoua, 1979). This suggests that β and γ are present in the brain extracellular fluid. In the second type of experiment, the extracellular fluid from 100 brains was isolated and tested for the presence of β and γ by gel electrophoresis. Figure 10 shows a densitometer trace of the electrophoretic migration patterns of the proteins of the extracellular fluid as compared to those of the brain cytoplasmic fraction. The results clearly indicate that the major components in extracellular fluid are the proteins

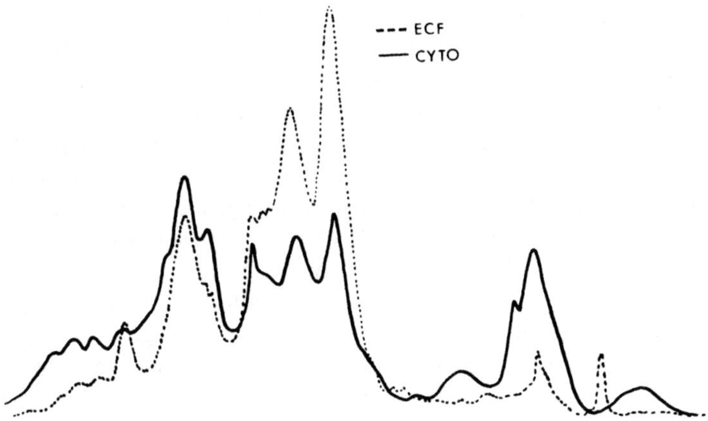

FIG. 10. Densitometer traces of electrophoretic migration patterns of ECF (extracellular fluid) and cytoplasmic goldfish brain proteins. The samples (50 μg each) were separated on 10 percent SDS-polyacrylamide gels and stained with Coomassie blue.

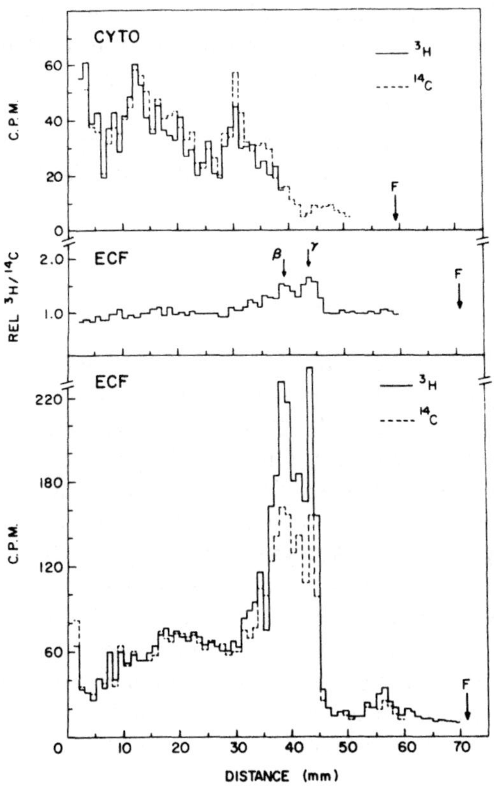

FIG. 11. Labeling patterns of the cytoplasmic and ECF brain proteins from trained and untrained control goldfish. The trained animals were labeled with [^{3}H]valine and untrained controls with [^{14}C]valine. Labeling time was one hour. The electrophorectic migration patterns on 10 percent SDS-polyacrylamide gels are for the cytoplasmic fraction after removal of the ECF. Note the more efficient removal of ECF in this experiment and the higher labeling at β and γ after the training.

migrating at the position of β and γ. In the third type of experiment, the brain proteins of trained and untrained goldfish were examined by the double labeling procedure in order to determine the rate at which β and γ are labeled and secreted into the extracellular fluid. Figure 11 shows the results of such an experiment. The animals were trained for five hours, prior to being injected with [^{3}H]valine; controls in a separate tank were injected with [^{14}C]valine. After one hour, the brains of the two groups were combined and gently extracted for 30 minutes at 0°C with isotonic sucrose to remove the adhering extracellular fluid. This fluid was then removed and the brains were homogenized in isotonic sucrose for isolation of the cytoplasmic protein fraction. The proteins were separated by SDS-gel electrophoresis and the labeling pattern of each fraction was determined. The results showed that intense labeling occurred at the β and γ regions of the gels used for the extracellular fluid fraction. There was a 50 percent increase in β and γ from the trained group compared to β and γ from the control group. In fact, in some experiments (see Fig. 11), the extraction procedure almost completely removed all labeled products at the β and γ region of the gels. This suggests that ependymins β and γ are rapidly labeled and secreted into the extracellular fluid and that the training merely enhances the rate at which they are synthesized and, hence, labeled. Thus, it is possible that the proteins function at sites away from their locus of synthesis; they may also have some type of neuroregulatory or nerve-growth function. In an attempt to explore this question, the ependymins were compared with NGF. The products, however, did not cross-react immunologically (Benowitz and Shashoua, 1979).

GLYCOPROTEIN NATURE OF EPENDYMIN β

The fact that the β and γ ependymins are secreted into the extracellular fluid raises the possibility that they may be glycoproteins. Figure 12 shows densitometer traces of the staining of extracellular fluid proteins separated on SDS electrophoretic gels. When the gels were stained by the periodic acid - Schiff (PAS) reaction (Clarke, 1964), strong staining occurred at the position of β and γ where maximum uptake by Coomassie blue also occurs. This suggests that β and γ are glycoproteins. Analysis of hydrolyzates by gas chromatography (Reinhold, 1972) confirmed this observation. J. Coddington found that β ependymin contains about 5 percent carbohydrate with substantial levels of mannose, N-acetyl glucosamine, and N-acetylneuraminic acid (Table 5). Such a chemical composition and the fact that β is a secreted protein suggests that this glycoprotein could participate in a variety of neuroregulatory, surface recognition, or developmental functions.

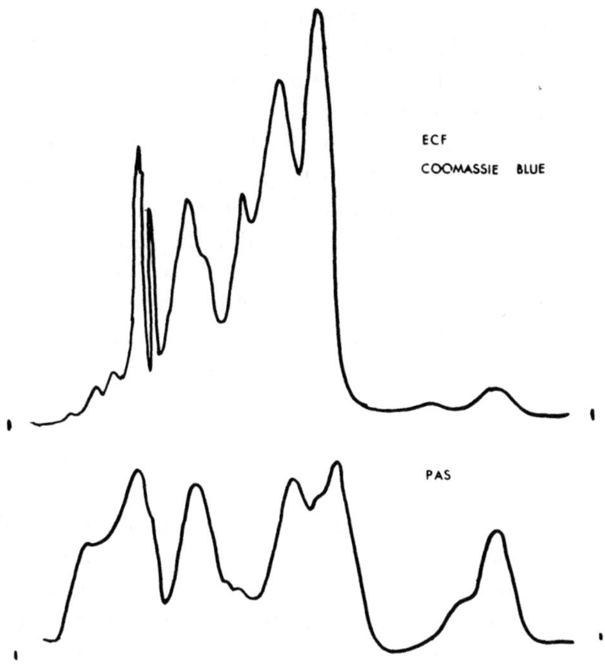

FIG. 12. Staining pattern of ECF proteins electrophoretically separated on 10 percent SDS-polyacrylamide. Coomassie blue data show densitometer tracings of proteins; PAS (periodic acid shifts base) show the patterns of carbohydrate staining.

Table 5. Ependymin β — Carbohydrate Analysis

	Weight %
Fucose	0.14
Xylose	0.16
Mannose	0.60
Galactose	1.21
Glucose	1.66
N-acetylglucosamine	1.93
N-acetyl-neuraminic acid	0.83
Total Carbohydrate	5.6

DISCUSSION

The above experimental results suggest that three proteins that occur in the goldfish brain are rapidly labeled after learning. Two of these proteins, ependymins β and γ, seem to be associated with cells within the brain ependymal zone. In the goldfish, this periventricular grey region extends all along the neuraxis and consists largely of glial cells. The β and γ ependymins appear to be secreted into the extracellular and cerebrospinal fluids. The proteins are normal components of the cerebrospinal fluid of untrained animals and their turnover rates in the fluid increase with the acquisition of a new behavior. They appear to participate in the consolidation step of long-term memory formation, since injections of antisera to β and γ into the brain after, but not before, training can inhibit the recall of the acquired experience. That the antisera are effective only within a specific window of time after training suggests that ependymins β and γ are required during a crucial phase of memory formation. They appear to have no role in short-term memory or the acquisition of a behavior.

The fact that the ependymins are highly concentrated in the extracellular fluid of untrained goldfish rules out the possibility that they are linked to a specific behavioral experience or to a training-specific function. It seems more likely that they might have a "maintenance" function in the consolidation process. One important aspect of their activity is indicated by the observation that, in some animals, injections of antisera to the β and γ ependymins, at times up to 48 hours after training, are capable of producing amnesia. This suggests that their function is continued for a long time after training so that any mechanisms that require fast conformation changes in membranes or immediate phosphorylation phenomena cannot be the primary consequence of activity of the ependymins, although such phenomena might be important in the activation of binding sites for the proteins. Two processes that have the appropriate time characteristics are differentiation and growth. If these processes were to occur after acquisition of new experience, then, in a sense, the consequences of training would be comparable to a micro event in the development of the nervous system. Such an hypothesis is represented in Fig. 13. Essentially, environmental inputs would transform certain pre-existing neural circuits into primed circuits. The primed circuits would then become "targeted" for change through a process which results in the "unmasking" of receptors for the ependymins. These activated receptors can then interact with ependymin β and γ to initiate a process for fixing information into a permanent state. Such a process could, perhaps, be comparable to the binding of a lectin to surface receptors. The transformed circuits might require ependymins with the correct newly synthesized glycopeptide fragment for their conversion to targeted circuits. The CSF is postulated as the route for the transport of the ependymins β and γ to their newly activated receptors. In this hypothesis, the ependymins are considered to be factors which might initiate the growth of new synapses or new dendritic spines, or convert silent synapses to active ones, or change the profile of firing of active axonal terminals. Clearly, we have no direct evidence for these possibilities. There are, nevertheless, certain aspects of the postulates which can be supported by current knowledge about the CNS.

The idea that these are pre-existing circuits which could subserve a given type of behavior is quite similar to the large body of neurophysiological and anatomical evidence that demonstrate the existence of pre-programmed behaviors such as reproductive behavior in *Aplysia* (Arch, 1976) and the mechanism of processing in the visual (Hubel and Weisel, 1965) and the somatosensory systems (Mountcastle, 1975). It is possible that certain types of pre-existing circuits are present in the CNS for use in learning a given type of behavior. When activated, such circuits could then require a factor to initiate a process for their modification. Once a system is altered it becomes part of the dynamic structure of the CNS, and its composition becomes subject to the same turnover rates of all other neural circuits. No molecules need to be permanent in this hypothesis; only the altered circuits remain stable. Clearly, there are many aspects to such a concept. We need to know how phosphorylation changes (Ueda and Greengard, 1977) and how hormonal factors (de Weid, 1974) and general biogenic amine activation events (Kety, 1970) can participate in the process. We also need to know how

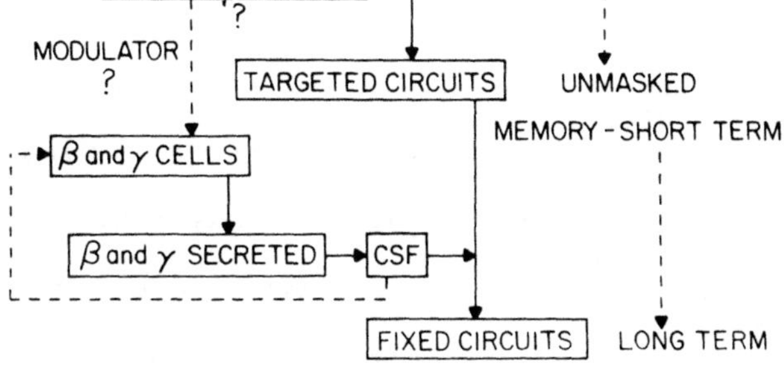

FIG. 13. A hypothetical mechanism for the role of β and γ ependymins in the CNS. Pre-existing neural circuits with specific receptors for β and γ become unmasked during the process of learning to change into "targeted" circuits. These are considered to be analogous to the short-term memory phase. β and γ ependymins arriving via the CSF can then interact with the targeted circuits to initiate a process which ultimately results in fixed circuits. These represent the long-term memory phase.

the receptors for β and γ ependymins, if they exist, can be stimulated. We do not yet know if there is any merit to this type of analysis of the problem, or if the ependymins have any direct role; however, the questions raised are testable and well within the realm of known biochemical processes that could participate in the phenomenon.

ACKNOWLEDGEMENT

This research was supported by the McKnight Foundation and the National Institute of Neurological and Communicative Disorders and Stroke (Grant No. NS 09407).

REFERENCES

Agranoff, B.W., Davis, R.E., and Brink, J.J. Memory fixation in the goldfish. *Proc. Nat. Acad. Sci. USA* 54, 788–793 (1967).

Appel, S.H. Turnover of brain messenger RNA. *Nature* 213, 1253–1254 (1967).

Arch, S. Neuroendocrine regulation of egg-laying in *Aplysia californica. Am. Zool.* 16, 167–175 (1976).

Barondes, S.H., and Cohen, H.D. Comparative effects of cycloheximide and puromycin on cerebral protein synthesis and consolidation of memory in mice. *Brain Res.* 4, 44–51 (1967).

Bazan, N.G., Brenner, R.R., and Giusto, N.M., eds. *Advances in Experimental Medicine and Biology*, Vol. 83. Plenum Press, New York (1977).

Benowitz, L.I., and Shashoua, V.E. Localizaton of brain protein metabolically associated with behavioral plasticity in the goldfish. *Brain Res.* 136, 227–242 (1977).

Benowitz, L.I., and Shashoua, V.E. Rapidly labeled and secreted proteins of the chick brain. *J. Neurochem.* 32, 797–809 (1979).

Browning, M., Dunwiddie, T., Bennett, W., Gispen, W., and Lynch, G. Synaptic phosphoproteins: Specific changes after repetitive stimulation of the hippocampus. *Science* 203, 60–62 (1979).

Chaffee, J., and Schachner, M. NS6, a new cell-surface antigen of brain, kidney, and spermatozoa. *Develop. Biol.* 62, 173–184 (1978).

Chorover, S.L., and Schiller, P.H. Short-term retrograde amnesia in rats. *J. Comp. Physiol. Psychol.* 59, 43–48 (1965).

Clarke, J.T. Simplified "disc" (polyacrylamide gel) electrophoresis. *Ann. N. Y. Acad. Sci.* 121, 428–436 (1964).

Coons, A.H. Fluorescent antibody methods, in *General Cytological Methods*. J.F. Danielle, ed. Academic Press, New York (1968), pp. 399–422.

Danno, G. Isoelectric focusing of proteins separated by SDS-polyacrylamide gel electrophoresis. *Anal. Biochem.* 83, 189–193 (1977).

de Weid, D. Pituitary-adrenal system hormones and behavior, in *The Neurosciences Third Study Program*. F.O. Schmitt and F.G. Worden, eds. M.I.T. Press, Cambridge, Massachusetts (1974), pp. 653–666.

Flexner, J.B., Flexner, L.B., and Stellar, E. Memory and cerebral protein synthesis in mice as effected by graded amounts of puromycin. *Science* 141, 57–59 (1963).

Grundfest, H. Synaptic and ephaptic transmission, in *Structure and Function of Nervous Tissue*, Vol. 2. G.H. Bourne, ed. Academic Press, New York (1969), pp. 463–491.

Hartman, B.K. Application of improved methodology to the localization of the peripheral and central noradrenergic nervous system. *J. Histochem. Cytochem.* 21, 312–332 (1973).

Hubel, D.H., and Wiesel, T.N. Receptive fields and functional architecture in non-striate visual areas of the rat. *J. Neurophysiol.* 27, 229–289 (1965).

Hyden, H., and Lange, P. Correlation of the S-100 brain protein with behavior. *Exp. Cell. Res.* 62, 125–132 (1970).

Jarvik, M.E. Effects of chemical and physical treatments on learning and memory. *Ann. Rev. Psychol.* 23, 457–486 (1972).

John, E.R. Switchboard versus statistical theories of learning and memory. *Science* 177, 850–864 (1972).

Karpiak, S.E., Serokosz, M., and Rapport, M.M. Effects of antisera to S-100 protein and to synaptic membrane fraction on maze performance and EEG. *Brain Res.* 102, 313–321 (1976).

Kety, S.S. The biogenic amines in the central nervous system: Their possible roles in arousal, emotion, and learning, in *The Neurosciences: Second Study Program.* F.O. Schmitt, ed. Rockefeller U. Press, New York (1970), pp. 324–336.

Kobiler, D., Fuchs, S., and Samuel, D. The effect of anti-synaptosomal plasma membrane antibodies on memory. *Brain Res.* 115, 129–139 (1976).

Lajtha, A., and Toth, J. Instability of cerebral proteins. *J. Biochem. Biophys. Res. Commun.* 23, 249–299 (1966).

Langan, T.A. Histone phosphorylation: Stimulation by adenosine 3',5'-monophosphate. *Science* 162, 579–580 (1968).

Lowry, O.H., Passoneau, J.V., Hasselberger, F.X., and Schulz, D.W. Effect of ischemia on known substrate and cofactors of the glycolytic pathway in brain. *J. Biol. Chem.* 239, 18–30 (1964).

Machlus, B.J., Wilson, J.E., and Glassman, E. Brain phosphoproteins: The effect of short experiences on the phosphorylation of nuclear proteins of the rat brain. *Behav. Biol.* 10, 43–62 (1974).

McGaugh, J.L. Time-dependent processes in memory storage. *Science* 153, 1351–1358 (1966).

McLean, I.W., and Nakane, P.K. Periodate-lysine-paraformaldehyde fixative: A new fixative for immunoelectron microscopy. *J. Histochem. Cytochem.* 22, 1077–1083 (1974).

Mountcastle, V.B. The view from within: Pathways to the study of perception. *Johns Hopkins Med. J.* 136, 109–131 (1975).

Neville, D.M. Molecular weight determination of protein-dodecyl sulfate complexes by gel electrophoresis in a discontinuous buffer system. *J. Biol. Chem.* 246, 6328–6334 (1971).

O'Farrel, P.H. High resolution two-dimensional electrophoresis of proteins. *J. Biol. Chem.* 250, 4007–4021 (1975).

Ouchterlony, O. Immunodiffusion and immunoelectrophoresis, in *Handbook of Experimental Immunology.* D.M. Weir, ed. Davis, Philadelphia, (1967), pp. 655–672.

Reinhold, V.N. Gas-liquid chromatographic analysis of constituent carbohydrates in glycoproteins, in *Methods of Enzymology*, Vol. 25. C.H.W. Hirs and S. N. Timasheff, eds. Academic Press, New York (1972), pp. 244–249.

Rose, S.P.R., Hambley, J., and Haywood, J. Neurochemical approaches to developmental plasticity and learning, in *Neural Mechanisms of Learning and Memory.* M.R. Rosenzweig and E.L. Bennett, eds. M.I.T. Press, Cambridge, Massachusetts (1976), pp. 293–310.

Shashoua, V.E. RNA metabolism in goldfish brain during acquisition of new behavioral patterns. *Proc. Nat. Acad. Sci. USA* 65, 160–167 (1970).

Shashoua, V.E. Dibutyryl adenosine cyclic 3':5'-monophosphate effects on goldfish behavior and brain RNA metabolism. *Proc. Natl. Aca. Sci. USA* 68, 2835–2838 (1971).

Shashoua, V.E. A multistage transduction model for information processing in the nervous system. *Int. J. Neurosci.* 3, 299–304 (1972).

Shashoua, V.E. RNA metabolism in the brain. *Int. Rev. Neurobiol.* 16, 183–231 (1974).

Shashoua, V.E. Identification of specific changes in the pattern of brain protein synthesis after training. *Science* 193, 1264–1266 (1976a).

Shashoua, V.E. Brain metabolism and the acquisition of new behaviors. I. Evidence for specific changes in the pattern of protein synthesis. *Brain Res.* 111, 347–364 (1976b).

Shashoua, V.E. Brain protein metabolism and the acquisition of new behaviors. II. Immunological studies of the α, β, and γ proteins of goldfish brain. *Brain Res.* 122, 113–124 (1977a).

Shashoua, V.E. Brain protein metabolism and the acquisition of new patterns of behavior. *Proc. Natl. Acad. Sci. USA* 74, 1743–1747 (1977b).

Shashoua, V.E. Ependymin β: A brain protein metabolically linked with behavioral plasticity in goldfish, in *Mechanisms, Regulation and Special Functions of Protein Synthesis in the Brain.* S. Roberts, A. Lajtha and W.H. Gispen, eds. Elsevier, Amsterdam (1977c), pp. 331–342.

Shashoua, V.E., and Moore, M.E. Effect of antisera to β and γ goldfish brain proteins on the retention of a newly acquired behavior. *Brain Res.* 148, 441–449 (1978).

Shashoua, V.E. Brain metabolism and the acquisition of new behaviors. III. Evidence for secretion of two proteins into the brain extracellular fluid after training. *Brain Res.* 166, 349–358 (1979).

Susor, W.A., Kochman, M., and Rutter, W.J. Heterogeneity of presumably homogeneous protein preparations. *Science* 165, 1260–1262 (1969).

Tanzi, E. Nel'odierna istologia de sistema nervoso. *Rivista Specimenal di Freniatria E. Medicina Lega* 19, 419–472 (1893).

Ueda, T., and Greengard, P. Adenosine 3':5'-monophosphate-regulated phosphoprotein system of neuronal membranes. *J. Biol. Chem.* 252, 5155–5163 (1977).

Vigh-Taichmann, I., and Vigh, B. Structure and function of the liquor-containing neurosecretory system, in *Aspects of Neuroendocrinology, V. International Symposium on Neurosecretion.* W. Bargman and B. Scharrer, eds. Springer, New York (1970), pp. 329–337.

Weiner, A.M., Platt, T., and Weber, K. Amino-terminal sequence analysis of proteins purified on a nanomole scale by gel-electrophoresis. *J. Biol. Chem.* 247, 3242–3251 (1972).

Werner, G., and Mountcastle, V.B. Neural activity in mechanoreceptive cutaneous afferents: stimulus-response relations, Weber functions, and information transmission. *J. Neurophysiol.* 28, 359–397 (1965).

PART III

Affective States

Copyright © 1982, Spectrum Publications, Inc.
The Neural Basis of Behavior

9

Affective Disorders: An Overview of Current Concepts and Ongoing Research

Morris A. Lipton

To the psychiatrist, affective disorders mean those illnesses whose primary manifestations involve major alterations in mood and subsequent or conmitant alterations in thinking and behavior, such as those found in depression or mania. In this regard, it is interesting to note that in the past twenty years probably the greatest advances in understanding and treatment of psychiatric illnesses have been in the area of affective disorders. There are many examples of success. Lithium effectively treats most patients with manic-depressive disorders, diminishing the amplitude and frequency of their recurrent mood swings. Lithium may also be effective in the prevention of recurrent depressions. The tricyclic antidepressants markedly accelerate the rate of recovery in about 75% of patients with severe depressions. More is being learned about the appropriate use of the monoamine oxidase inhibitors which are also powerful antidepressants. There have been major advances in understanding the psychobiology of depression, and there seems to be on the horizon the possibility of a biochemical classification of depressions that would permit a more selective approach to the utilization of the tricyclic antidepressants. However, just as all good research answers many questions and generates an equal number of different questions, so too do we have a large number of questions at the frontier of our knowledge about the affective disorders which will be the subject of the next three chapters.

As background material, let me begin with some definitions of terms which we all commonly use but rarely define precisely. First, the term "emotion" is derived from the Latin term "emovere" which means "to move away," "to disturb," or "to excite." It is a subjective state, a state of feeling, that may precede and generate motion or it may follow it as expressed in the James-Lange theory of emotion. Alternatively, emotion may be associated with motion in a complex interaction of thoughts and feelings as suggested by the work of the social psychologist, Stanley Schachter (1964).

The term "affect" is defined in the Diagnostic and Statistical Manual (1979) as "an immediately expressed and observed emotion." An emotion becomes an affect when it is expressed in observable behavior, such as overall demeanor, or tone and modulation of voice with or without attention to the content of the speech. Finally, there is the term "mood," and this is a "pervasive or sustained emotional state that markedly colors an individual's perceptions of the world." Affect is to mood as weather is to climate. In brief, emotion is that which is felt by an individual; affect is that which is noted by an observer because the emotion is expressed; and mood is the long-term set or attitude of an emotional state which influences one's feelings and behavior over prolonged periods of time.

The functions of emotions and of affects have been the subject of investigations for many years. Darwin, for example, devoted a good portion of his life's work to the study of the expression of emotion in man and animals and wrote a classic book on this subject (Darwin, 1855). From his work and that of others, it is clear that emotions have many functions. The first is communication with other individuals of the same or different species. What may be communicated is the need to mate, to protect one's territory or one's offspring, to warn of danger, to seek help, and so forth. This, of course, has great evolutionary significance to the individual and to the species. Emotions also serve to magnify and prolong reactions to behavioral stimulation. Emotions interact with memory in the sense that experiences that are emotionally laden are more likely to be remembered than those which are not. The emotional experiences associated with hunger and thirst contribute strongly to consumatory or ingestive behavior. The expression of emotion in the very young is perhaps the most effective mechanism for communication of needs to the mother or to older members of the tribe or herd. Emotions, as Darwin noted, are by no means limited to humans, and certainly occur in birds, reptiles, fish, and perhaps even lower species. Without emotions and their expression, the young and helpless would die and the species could not survive.

Schachter (1964) has suggested that in man emotion could best be described as a relatively non-specific state of physiological arousal accompanied by a much more specific cognitive state. Our vocabulary uses hundreds of words to describe emotional states. Thus, on a "pleasure-unpleasure" continuum, there is a graduation from hopelessness to despair, disappointment, sadness, neutrality, amusement, pleasure, euphoria, and ecstasy, all of which describe this continuum in different degrees and intensities. There are other terms which describe more complex and subtle emotions. Terms like pity, disgust, envy, and jealousy describe emotional states which have some physiological changes associated with arousal but have much more specific cognitive states which help to define and communicate the specific emotional state. It seems to me to be unlikely that there are hundreds of discrete physiological states, each of which is characteristic of a specific emotion. Rather there may be a state of generalized arousal involving the autonomic, cardiovascular, and endocrine systems, to which is added a cognition to give the arousal specificity as an emotion. If this is correct, the physiological changes associated with anger or rage may not differ greatly from those associated with equally intense emotions like sexual arousal or fright. Some differences may occur in specific organ systems and certainly major differences occur at the cognitive level. There is evidence to support this view. Schachter and Singer (1962), for example, administered adrenaline or placebo under blind conditions to a group of volunteers. They obtained and measured the characteristic effects of noradrenaline on the cardiovascular system. When the adrenaline was administered blindly in different settings in which the external stimuli were designed to generate fright, anger, or pleasure, they found that each one of these sensations was markedly amplified by the adrenaline as compared to the same stimuli when a placebo was given. Appropriate emotions and their expression are thus a means for recognizing internal and external stimuli and for communicating them. Emotional disorders occur when these subjective feelings and their expression as affects achieve their own autonomy and persist inappropriately under changing environmental circumstances. Thus, for example, clinically it is not difficult to find the circumstantial determinants of a first attack of mania or depression, but later attacks seem to come spontaneously and without any detectable environmental precepitants.

Goodwin (1977) has noted that it is conceptually useful to visualize affective disorders such as depression along a continuous spectrum. On one end there is sadness or the "blues" characterized by brief duration, lasting at most a few weeks. During such a period, functioning is still quite normal. In such cases the causative factors seem to be entirely environmental and generally no treatment is needed. The symptoms will subside spontaneously. On the other end of the spectrum, there are the depressions which have been called "endogenous" or "psychotic" and these are characterized by a long duration, lasting many months or even years, in which there is an inability to function. There are also symptom clusters which include alterations in mood, cognition, sleep, activity, energy level, appetite, and other physiological functions. These are the depressions which have generally been considered to be unresponsive to the environment. Work in the past decade has suggested that there is a biological and perhaps genetic predisposition to such depressions. These are the depressions for which drugs are most commonly employed. These are also the depressions which may be separable on clinical or even biochemical grounds. Thus, clinically one can separate the bipolar, or manic-depressive illnesses, from the unipolar, or recurring depressions in which there are no intervening episodes of mania. Apparently, the heredity of these two types of depression differs.

Depressions have been most carefully examined in regard to alterations in the functions of the neurotransmitters, norepinephrine and serotonin. For many years there appeared to be a geopolitical scientific conflict with American investigators emphasizing the role of norepinephrine while British and other European investigators emphasized the role of serotonin. It now appears that both may be correct. There appear to be norepinephrine depressions, characterized by a diminution in the urinary levels of 3-methoxy 4-hydroxyphenylglycol, the major metabolite of norepinephrine. There are other depressions, however, in which this metabolite is normal and instead there is a diminution in cerebrospinal fluid levels of the major metabolite of serotonin. If this proves to be correct, there will be a rationale for selecting tricyclic antidepressants which act primarily either on norepinephrine or on serotonin for the treatment of those cases which can be classified biochemically. This should improve therapeutics by offering greater specificity and probably will result in fewer adverse reactions. There is also research relating blood levels of tricyclic drugs to clinical response which may permit more accurate drug usage.

With the heavy emphasis on pharmacological intervention in depression, there has been a simultaneous diminution in interest in psychological treatments, even though there is general acceptance that psychosocial factors are significant determinants of at least initial onsets. This perspective has been further amplified by repeated failures to help depressed patients by psychological interventions alone. However, within the past few years, Beck and his associates (Beck, 1964; Beck, 1967; Beck, 1971; Beck, 1976; Kovacs and Beck, 1978; Rush and Beck; 1978) have introduced a psychological treatment called "cognitive therapy" which they claim is as effective as pharmacotherapy in depressed outpatients. Cognitive therapy differs from more traditional psychotherapies insofar as the cognitive therapist actively engages the patient in the treatment process. Thus, emphasis is placed upon teaching the patient to organize his behavior and to alter his cognitions about the stimuli in the external world. The content of the therapy is focused on the here-and-now, with little attention paid to childhood material. The therapist makes no interpretations of unconscious factors; a transferance neurosis is avoided. The goal of cognitive therapy is to change maladaptive thinking patterns and thus to treat the existing depression as well as to reduce vulnerability to future depressions. Beck's work makes sense if one visualizes depression as a spectrum disorder. However, it is not yet certain whether Beck's success can be replicated by other workers, nor is it yet certain whether his treatment will be effective in those severe depressions that are generally so unresponsive to the environment and which seem to be so biologically loaded. It may be that the patients most suited to Beck's cognitive therapy will fall in the middle of the continuum where they would be responsive to either pharmacotherapy or cognitive therapy. If this should be the case, then the combination of both treatments might be more effective than either alone, but this has yet to be investigated.

There are many questions which remain in the continued study of the affective disorders. For example, why is it that both depressive and manic states are limited in their duration, even without treatment, and why do they recur? Why do the drugs used in the treatment of depression take a month or more to be effective and why do their effects continue to be manifested for months after they are discontinued? The genetics of the affective disorders are gradually being unravelled, but much more needs to be done before there will be adequate understanding of the complex hereditary transmission of susceptibility to depressive disorders. Only within the past few years have the alterations in endocrine function associated with affective disorders

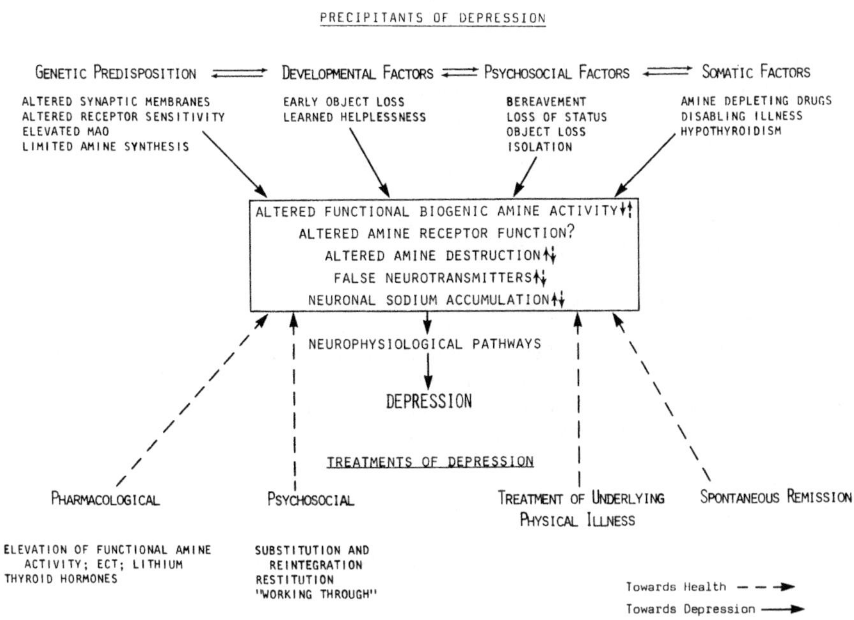

FIG. 1. A multivalent model of depression.

become the focus of the attention of investigators. It is becoming clear that there are indeed alterations in pituitary and hypothalamic function that are associated with these disorders. Whether these are state or trait dependent is not yet entirely clear, and the extent to which newer types of endocrine interventions will be therapeutically effective has yet to be determined. If we accept the concept that affective disorders occur as a result of interaction between a biological diathesis and environmental precipitants (see Fig. 1), then it should follow that the most effective treatments in the future will involve a combination of biological and psychosocial interventions. A beginning has been made to the study of combined therapies by Weissman and Klerman (Klerman et al., 1974; Weisman and Klermann, 1977) and combined treatment has yielded encouraging results, but much more needs to be done. Currently, there are as many different types of psychotherapy as there are drugs. Psychoanalysis, behavior modification, family therapy, and cognitive therapy are only a few of them. One of the major tasks of the future will be to select precisely the form of psychological therapy that should be interdigitated with a specific pharmacological intervention to maximize the therapeutic benefit of both.

REFERENCES

American Psychiatric Association. Diagnostic and Statistical Manual of Mental Disorders, 3rd edition. American Psychiatric Association, Washington, D.C. (1980).

Beck, A.T. Thinking and depression. I. Idiosyncratic content and cognitive distortions. *Arch. Gen. Psych.* 9, 324–333 (1964).

Beck, A.T. *Depression: Clinical, Experimental, and Theoretical Aspects.* Harper & Row, New York (1967).

Beck, A.T. Cognition, affect, and psychopathology. *Arch. Gen. Psych.* 24, 495–500 (1971).

Beck, A.T. *Cognitive Therapy and the Emotional Disorders.* International Universities Press, New York (1976).

Darwin, C.R. *The Expression of the Emotions in Man and Animals.* Philosophical Library, New York (1955).

Goodwin, F.K. Diagnosis of affective disorders, in *Psychopharmacology in the Practice of Medicine.* M.E. Jarvik, ed. Appleton-Century-Crofts, New York (1977), pp. 219–228.

Klerman, G.L., DiMascio, A., Weissman, M.M., Prusoff, B., and Paykel, E.S. Treatment of depression by drugs and psychotherapy. *Am. J. Psych.* 131, 186–191 (1974).

Kovacs, M., and Beck, A.T. Maladaptive cognitive structures in depression. *Am. J. Psych.* 135, 525–533 (1978).

Rush, A.J., and Beck, A.T. Cognitive therapy of depression and suicide. *Am. J. Psychother.* 32, 201–219 (1978).

Schachter, S. The interaction of cognitive and physiological determinants of emotional state, in *Advances in Experimental Social Psychology,* Vol. I. L. Berkowitz, ed. Academic Press, New York (1964), pp. 49–80.

Schachter, S., and Singer, J. Cognitive, social and physiological determinants of emotional state. *Psychol. Rev.* 69, 379–399 (1962).
Weissman, M.M., and Klerman, G.L. The chronic depressive in the community: unrecognized and poorly treated. *Comp. Psych.* 18, 523–532 (Nov-Dec 1977).

Copyright © 1982, Spectrum Publications, Inc.
The Neural Basis of Behavior

10

Neural Associations of the Limbic System

Walle J.H. Nauta
Valerie B. Domesick

Even in its most restrictive connotation, the term *limbic system* refers to the hippocampal formation and amygdala, together with the gyrus fornicatus (gyrus cinguli, retrosplenial cortex, and parahippocampal gyrus) which is associated with the hippocampal formation by both direct and indirect fiber connections. It is a logical question to ask how such very dissimilar telencephalic structures came to be integrated into a unitary concept. Whereas hippocampus and gyrus fornicatus are cortical structures—and quite different from each other at that—the amygdala (or at least the greater part of it) is unmistakably subcortical grey matter. For a proper understanding of how the notion came about, a brief historical summary may be useful.

The term limbic system (MacLean, 1952) has its origin in the name "grand lobe limbique" coined a century ago by Broca (1878) to denote the somewhat distinct region of cortex nearest the margin (limbus) of the cortical mantle, a region which in the mammalian brain fully encircles the hilus of the cerebral hemisphere. Broca's term referred to a detail of cerebral surface anatomy that comprised the hippocampus and gyrus fornicatus, but did not explicitly include the deep-lying amygdala. Neither was the amygdala mentioned in the classical paper in which Papez (1937) stressed the interconnectedness of hippocampus and gyrus fornicatus and suggested that this cortical aggregate, by the medium of its fornix projections to the hypothalamus, serves as a neural substrate of emotion. The amygdala became recognized as a limbic structure only when MacLean (1952) emphasized that it, like the hippocampal formation, is closely associated with the hypothalamus, and therefore should be considered to belong in a class with the hippocampus and the latter's superstructure, the gyrus fornicatus. For this category of telencephalic structures MacLean introduced the name *limbic system*, adding to it in his earlier publications the physiological sub-title, "visceral brain." On the basis of MacLean's unifying concept, the limbic system became in essence defined as a heterogeneous group of basal and medial telencephalic structures together composing that part of the cerebral hemisphere which is most directly associated with the hypothalamus.

MacLean's important concept was based for the most part on findings by himself and others in electrophysiological experiments by the then widely-used strychnine method. His own strychnine studies in collaboration with K.H. Pribram, as well as his clinical observations in cases of temporal-lobe epilepsy, led him to include in the "visceral brain" the posterior orbitofrontal cortex and the cortex of the temporal pole ("...[this] entire frontotemporal region fires into the amygdala and rostral hippocampus") (MacLean, 1952). At the time it was put forward, this notion could already lean on some anatomical evidence (briefly reviewed by Nauta, 1962) suggesting a direct projection from the posterior orbitofrontal cortex to the hypothalamus. Further support for it came from evidence that the orbitofrontal cortex is associated with the amygdala both by way of a direct amygdalo-orbitofrontal projection (Nauta, 1961) and more indirectly via an amygdalofugal pathway to the medial subdivision of the mediodorsal thalamic nucleus (Fox, 1949; Nauta, 1961, 1962; Krettek and Price, 1974); moreover, the inferior temporal cortex was found to have direct efferent (Whitlock and Nauta, 1956; Jones and Powell, 1970) and afferent (Nauta, 1961; Krettek and Price, 1974) connections with the amygdala. It is largely a matter of preference whether one wishes to include the posterior orbitofrontal and anterior temporal cortex in the limbic system, or to exclude them for the reason that they should first and foremost be considered part of the neocortical organization. Regardless of one's choice, it would seem reasonable to assume that a basal frontotemporal region of the neocortex represents a class of functions that is subserved at the next lower (i.e., distal) level by the complex of the hippocampus, amygdala, and gyrus fornicatus.

It is likewise a matter of preference whether or not to include in the concept of the limbic system (as MacLean [1952] did) the subcortical structures associated with the limbic telencephalon by generally reciprocal conduction pathways. Much can be said in favor of such inclusiveness, especially since the hypothalamus as a common projection target for certain telencephalic structures figured so prominently in the development of the limbic system concept. However, the objection could be raised that the projections from the limbic telencephalon are now known to involve not only the hypothalamus but also the so-called nucleus accumbens, a structure which by histological and histochemical criteria is unmistakably part of the striatum. This objection, of course, could be countered by the argument that the central nervous system is replete with examples of neural structures that form part of one "system" when considered from one particular point of view, but just as plainly appear to be part of another "system" when they are viewed from another perceptual angle. Such ambiguities seem distressing only because of our tendency to expect a degree of separateness of neural mechanisms that appears to be an exception rather than the rule in the more highly developed central nervous system.

These latter considerations are relevant to the next point of this survey, which concerns the question, how far into the brainstem is it possible to trace the ramifications of the limbic system? An examination of this question (Nauta, 1958) in the light of MacLean's then recent concept led to the notion that the limbic telencephalon is reciprocally connected with an uninterrupted continuum of subcortical grey matter that begins with the septum, continues from there caudalward over the preoptic region and hypothalamus, and extends beyond the latter over a paramedian zone of the mesencephalon that reaches caudally as far as the isthmus rhombencephali. The mesencephalic part of this continuum comprises the ventral tegmental area, the ventral half of the central grey substance (including the cell group now named dorsal raphe nucleus but then known as the fountain nucleus of Sheehan), the nucleus centralis tegmenti superior of Bechterew (now better known as the median raphe nucleus), the interpeduncular nucleus, and the dorsal and ventral tegmental nuclei of Gudden. To be sure, in the three species in which these studies were done (rat, cat, and monkey), few if any direct projections from either hippocampus or amygdala could be traced caudalward beyond the septum, preoptic region, and hypothalamus. The paramedian zone of the mesencephalon nonetheless became included in the subcortical limbic continuum as "limbic midbrain area" when in the guinea pig it was found to receive a substantial contingent of fornix fibers, and in the other three species turned out to be a common distribution area for direct and indirect projections descending from the septum, preoptic region, and hypothalamus. Such projections follow three fiber systems: a) the medial forebrain bundle, b) the route composed of stria medullaris and fasciculus retroflexus, and c) the mammillotegmental tract. Moreoever, the paramedian zone of the mesencephalon was found (Nauta and Kuypers, 1958) to be a main origin of projections ascending in the medial forebrain bundle and presumably linking up with known projections from the anterior hypothalamus and septum back to, respectively, the amygdala and the hippocampal formation. The combined evidence suggested a reciprocal connection ("limbic forebrain-midbrain circuit") between the amygdala and hippocampus at the rostral end and a paramedian zone of the midbrain at the caudal end, a circuit in which the continuum of the septum, preoptic region, and hypothalamus, as well as the habenular complex, occupied intermediate positions. The construct as formulated more than 20 years ago is illustrated schematically in Fig. 1.

In the past fifteen years or so, the initial and quite schematic construct of the "limbic forebrain-midbrain circuit" has become much expanded and differentiated, especially as a result of studies by the aid of several technical innovations. The autoradiographic fiber-tracing method (Cowan et al., 1972) has vastly increased the confidence with which fiber connections can be traced from their origin to their terminal distribution, in particular by eliminating the fiber-of-passage problem that has bedeviled and frustrated so many studies by the older fiber-degeneration methods. Together with the

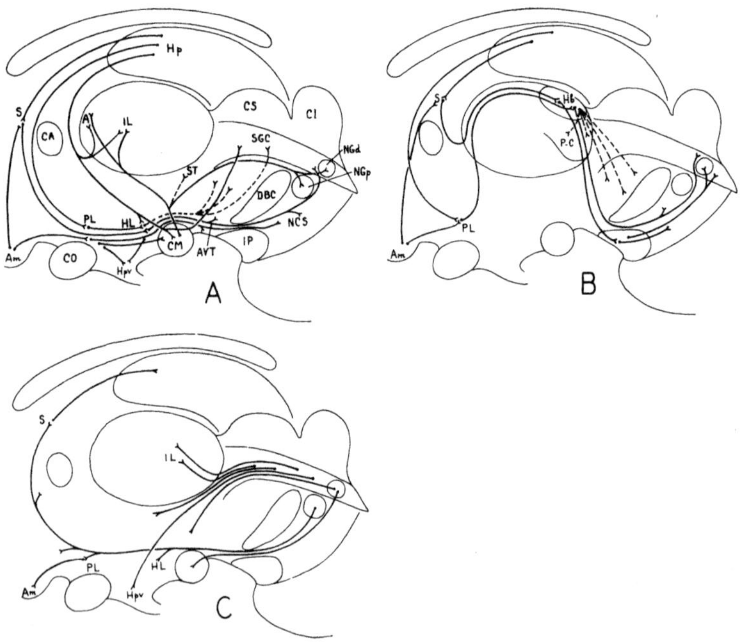

FIG. 1. The "limbic forebrain-midbrain circuit" as initially proposed. *A*: Descending pathways following medial forebrain bundle and mammillo-tegmental tract to the paramedian zone of the midbrain, and their suggested links with hippocampal and amygdalofugal projections. More laterally distributed components of medial forebrain bundle and mammillotegmental tract are indicated in broken lines. *B*: Descending conduction lines following stria medullaris and fasciculus retroflexus. *C*: Some ascending return links from the paramedian midbrain region to limbic forebrain structures; all of the lines ascending to hippocampus and amygdala were thought to be interrupted in the hypothalamo-preoptico-septal continuum. Reproduced from *Brain*, Vol. 81, 1958, by courtesy of MacMillan & Co., Ltd., London.

complementary and equally innovative method of retrograde labelling of cell bodies with horseradish-peroxidase (Kristensson et al., 1971; Lavail et al., 1973) this technique can be said to have revolutionized the traditional examples will be found of the remarkable capacity of these sophisticated histochemical methods to lift out from among bewilderingly complex neural networks chemically specified subcircuits that could not possibly be identified separately by any other anatomical technique now available.

In the remaining part of this review, some of the major modifications that now seem necessary in the original anatomical construct will be indicated. Both by intent and by constraints of space, this survey will be incomplete, and, like its 22-year-old ancestor, stripped of many important details concerning, among others, the patterns in which the various fiber systems are distributed within their areas of termination. For the most part it will be expressed in the form of schematic drawings based on a more or less standardized, sagittally oriented view of fore- and midbrain (Fig. 2). For practical reasons, this ground figure represents the primate brain, but it must be emphasized that the more recently identified components of the circuitry illustrated were discovered for the most part in non-primate species, the rat in particular, and thus far have not been corroborated in primates. Transcription of findings from a particular mammalian species to the class of mammals in general is, of course, done at a risk, especially since some inter-species differences (and even some inter-strain differences) in limbic circuitry have been reported from earlier studies (see Valenstein and Nauta, 1959). However, these same studies have suggested that such differences may relate more to the synaptic fractionation than to the overall deployment of the fiber systems in question.

To prevent visual overcrowding, it was necessary to limit structure identification by lettering in the circuit diagrams; for a complete listing of labels reference is made to Fig. 2.

DESCENDING COMPONENTS OF THE "LIMBIC FOREBRAIN-MIDBRAIN CIRCUIT"

Medial Forebrain Bundle

This complex longitudinal fiber system composes the basal of the two main limbic pathways leading to the mesencephalon. Rather than being a circumscript, compact fiber bundle, the medial forebrain bundle is a vaguely delineated fiber system that is interspersed throughout its extent with grey matter, in an arrangement characteristic of brainstem reticular formation. Thus, the lateral preoptic nucleus, lateral hypothalamic nucleus, ventral tegmental area, and other regions of the midbrain tegmentum can collectively be interpreted as interstitial nuclei of the medial forebrain bundle (cf. Millhouse, 1969), receiving fibers—or collateral axon branches—from the bundle, as well as adding fibers to it in either the caudal or rostral direction, or both. As a consequence of this complex grey-and-white composition, it is extraordinarily difficult to follow individual conduction lines through the length of the medial forebrain bundle, and impossible to express the true complexity of the system in a survey diagram. However, since the medial forebrain bundle has been found to contain also a considerable number of fibers that span much, or even all, of the distance between rostral forebrain levels and the ponto-mesencephalic transition, some statements about the origin and distribution of the system as a whole can be made with some confidence. It must, however, be emphasized that no complete accounting of its shorter components and their concatenations can as yet be given. Such more detailed data may gradually emerge from continued autoradiographic and histochemical exploration of the system.

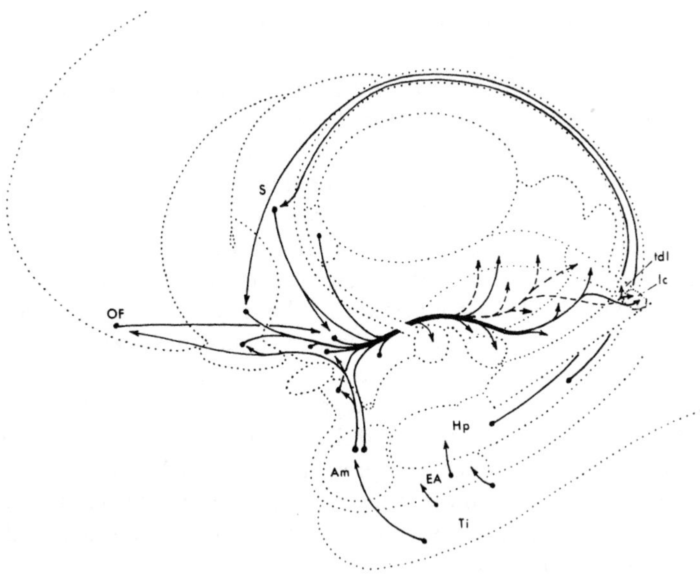

FIG. 3. Diagrammatic representation of the descending components of the medial forebrain bundle. Broken lines represent bundle's lateral division, distributed to nigral complex, central regions of the mesencephalic reticular formation, peripeduncular nucleus, and parabrachial region. Not indicated are those lateral-division fibers that arise from the hypothalamus and central amygdaloid nucleus and continue caudalward to the nucleus of the solitary tract, dorsal motor nucleus of the vagus, and lateral horn of the spinal grey matter (see text). Also included in the diagram are projections from the antero-inferior temporal cortex (Ti) to amygdala (Am) and—indirectly, by way of the entorhinal area (EA)—to hippocampus. For identification of structures left unlabelled see Figure 2.

As indicated schematically in Fig. 3, descending components of the medial forebrain bundle originate from a great variety of medial and basal forebrain structures. Most prominent, and longest recognized, among the contributors to this system are the septal region and the lateral preoptico-hypothalamic continuum. Variously sparser contributions are know to originate in the olfactory tubercle and piriform cortex (Lundberg, 1960, 1962), in the substantia innominata, in particular the basal nucleus of Meynert (Jones et al., 1976), in the nucleus accumbens (Swanson and Cowan, 1975; Conrad and Pfaff, 1976c; Powell and Leman, 1976; Nauta et al., 1978), amygdala (Krettek and Price, 1978; Hopkins and Holstege, 1978), bed nucleus of the stria terminalis (Swanson and Cowan, 1979), and orbitofrontal cortex (cf. Nauta, 1962; Beckstead, 1979). The medial forebrain bundle appears fully formed and most readily delineated in its sagittal passage through the lateral preopticohypothalamic zone. Throughout this part of its course, however, the bundle receives numerous further contributions not only from the lateral hypothalamic nucleus but also from more medial hypothalamic cell groups (Conrad and Pfaff, 1976a, b; Saper et al., 1976; Krieger et al., 1979).

Upon entering the ventral tegmental area, the medial forebrain bundle begins to spread out widely in the lateral direction. From here on caudalward, it can be subdivided somewhat arbitrarily into a) a medial division that maintains throughout its mesencephalic extent the sagittal orientation that characterized the hypothalamic trajectory of the medial forebrain bundle as a whole, and, b), a large lateral division composed of fibers that become deflected lateralward as they descend. It is mainly the medial subdivision that established the connection of the limbic forebrain structures with the paramedian zone of the midbrain ("limbic midbrain area"). As schematically indicated in Fig. 3 by continuous lines, its distribution involves the medial part of the ventral tegmental area, the interpeduncular nucleus, the median raphe nucleus, and the dorsal raphe nucleus along with other ventral regions of the central grey substance including the nucleus tegmenti dorsalis lateralis and the locus coeruleus (cf. Nauta, 1958; Conrad and Pfaff, 1976a, b; Swanson, 1976; Domesick, 1976; also unpublished observations in this laboratory).

The lateral subdivision of the medial forebrain bundle (indicated in Fig. 3 by broken lines), by contrast, spreads widely in the lateral direction as it descends through the gradually narrowing ventral tegmental zone (actually a caudal extension of the subthalamic region) that lies sandwiched between the medial lemniscus dorsally and the pars compacta of the substantia nigra ventrally. In this part of its course it forms a fairly compact stratum of laterally and caudally oriented fibers, scattered among which lie the neurons that compose the lateral, wing-like expansion of the dorsally outlying nigral dopamine cell group A10 of Dahlstrom and Fuxe (1964). (The larger part of this dopamine cell groups occupies a more medial region of the ventral tegmental area extending from the substantia nigra to the midline, and lies embedded among the more medial fibers of the medial forebrain bundle (Nauta and Domesick, 1978; Nauta, 1979). Throughout its course beneath the medial lemniscus the lateral division of the medial forebrain bundle issues fibers in three main directions: a) sparse fibers are deflected ventrally to be distributed to the pars compacta and the dorsal one-third of the pars reticulata of the substantia nigra (Swanson, 1976; Nauta and Domesick, 1978); b) others extend laterally to the peripeduncular nucleus, a region of medium-sized cells occupying most of the interval between the dorsolateral margin of the substantia nigra and the medial geniculate body, and bordered medially by the medial lemniscus, and c), a quite substantial fiber contingent curves sharply in the dorsomedial direction around the lateral margin of the medial lemniscus and along the lateral side of the red nucleus. These latter fibers traverse a wide central region of the midbrain tegmentum; most seem to terminate in this part of the midbrain reticular formation, but some longer fibers extend into the ventral half of the central grey substance, a region also invaded by fibers of the medial subdivision.

The fibers of the lateral division that remain after these various issues accumulate into a substantial fiber bundle that occupies a ventrolateral position in the midbrain tegmentum near the caudal pole of the substantia nigra. Embedded in this fiber group is a second outlying nigral cell aggregate, Dahlstrom and Fuxe's (1964) dopamine cell group A8 (Nauta and Domesick, 1978). At this point in its caudal course the lateral division of the medial forebrain bundle initiates a dorsomedial curve that leads it through a wide region of the caudal midbrain tegmentum, in particular the cuneiform and parabrachial nuclei. The longest of its fibers extend through the parabrachial nuclei into the caudal part of the central grey substance where they appear to converge with fibers of the medial division. From its gradual decrease in volume it can be assumed that the lateral division of the medial forebrain bundle distributes fibers to most or all of the tegmental regions that lie in the path of this caudal trajectory of the bundle.

Fiber degeneration techniques have consistently failed to reveal fibers of the medial forebrain bundle descending beyond the level of the locus coeruleus. Studies by anterograde and retrograde labelling methods, however, have revealed a direct hypothalamic projection to the nucleus of the solitary tract and the dorsal motor nucleus of the vagus in the medulla oblongata, as well as to the lateral horn of the spinal cord (Saper et al., 1976). Findings in retrograde-labelling experiments have indicated medial hypothalamic cell groups, in particular the paraventricular and dorsomedial nucleus, as the main origin of this direct hypothalamo-autonomic connection (Kuypers and Maisky, 1975; Saper et al., 1976); Hopkins and Holstege (1978), however, found it accompanied by numerous fibers from the central amygdaloid nucleus to the nucleus of the solitary tract and dorsal motor nucleus of the vagus (see below). It appears from Hopkins and Holstege's chartings that the connection is established largely by fibers of the lateral division of the medial forebrain bundle that continue caudally beyond the parabrachial region.

Hippocampal and Amygdaloid Contributions to the Medial Forebrain Bundle

Next to be considered is the question, at which points do the efferents from the telencephalic limbic structures (hippocampus, amygdala, gyrus fornicatus, and orbitofrontal cortex) lead into the medial forebrain bundle? The hippocampal formation projects by way of the precommissural fornix to all parts of the septum (even though heaviest by far to the lateral septal nucleus, the projection includes the nucleus of the diagonal band of Broca) and to the nucleus accumbens (Fig. 3). Its massive postcommissural fornix projection to the mammillary body, by contrast, forms part of a separate, though closely related line that leads over the lateral mammillary nucleus to both the dorsal and the ventral tegmental nucleus of Gudden by way of the mammillotegmental tract (Fig. 9).[1] The amygdalofugal lines are more complex, for the amygdala projects into the medial forebrain bundle (or, in some instances, to origins of the latter's descending fibers) by way of two fiber systems: the stria terminalis and the ventral amygdalofugal pathway. The stria terminalis (not illustrated) distributes itself to its bed nucleus, to the nucleus accumbens (de Olmos, 1972), and to medial preoptic and hypothalamic cell groups, prominently including the ventromedial hypothalamic nucleus (Heimer and Nauta, 1969; de Olmos and Ingram, 1972; Krettek and Price, 1978). Since these medial regions are now known to contribute substantially to the medial forebrain bundle (Conrad and Pfaff, 1976a and b; Saper et al., 1976; Krieger et al., 1979), they can be interpreted *in the present context* as intermediaries in a medial amygdalohypothalamic conduction line leading, in part at least, onto the larger limbic forebrain-midbrain channel. The amygdala has, however, additional and more direct access to this larger channel by way of the ventral amygdalofugal pathway, a

[1] It must be emphasized once more that the present description of subcortical limbic circuitry is based for the most part upon findings in the rat, and that not all its details may apply to all mammalian species. For example, fornix fibers passing beyond the mammillary body into the paramedian region of the midbrain appear to be very sparse or absent in the rat, cat, and monkey, but are quite numerous in the rabbit (Edinger and Wallenberg, 1902) and guinea pig (Valenstein and Nauta, 1959). Actually, it was the prominent mesencephalic extension of the guinea pig's fornix that first suggested the concept of a "limbic midbrain area."

complex fiber system intercalated in which, as a bed-nucleus, lie the cell groups composing the substantia innominata (a relationship far more evident in primates than in carnivores and rodents). The ventral amygdalofugal pathway contains numerous fibers that reciprocally connect the amygdala with the septo-preoptico-hypothalamic region (Nauta, 1961; Krettek and Price, 1978). In their comprehensive and detailed autoradiographic study in the rat, Krettek and Price found that it also contains fibers from at least one subdivision of the amygdaloid complex, the central amygdaloid nucleus, that projects beyond the hypothalamus to the midbrain. Similar findings in cat were reported by Hopkins and Holstege (1978). The chartings in both studies indicate that this direct amygdalomesencephalic projection follows the lateral division of the medial forebrain bundle, and both studies identify the parabrachial regions as its main target. Hopkins and Holstege (1978) emphasize, however, that the projection has further substantial distributions that involve central regions of the mesencephalic tegmentum and the central grey substance, and continues caudally beyond the isthmus to the lateral reticular formation of the pons and medulla oblongata, the nucleus of the solitary tract, and the dorsal motor nucleus of the vagus. The projection appears to be accompanied in its more rostral mesencephalic course by fibers to the peripeduncular nucleus from the basal nucleus of Meynert in the substantia innominata (Jones et al., 1976), and from the ventromedial hypothalamic nucleus (Saper et al., 1976; Krieger et al., 1979).

Other components of the ventral amygdalofugal pathway are distributed to the orbitofrontal cortex (Nauta, 1961, in the monkey), olfactory tubercle (Nauta, 1961; Krettek and Price, 1978) and nucleus accumbens (Krettek and Price, 1978), all of which have been reported to contribute fibers to the medial forebrain bundle. The fiber system also includes projections from the amygdala to the subcallosal region of the anterior cingulate cortex (Lammers and Lohman, 1957; Krettek and Price, 1977), as well as a return projection to the amygdala from the ventromedial nucleus of the hypothalamus (Krieger et al., 1979).

Stria Medullaris and Fasciculus Retroflexus

These two circumscript fiber bundles together compose an alternate pathway from the rostral diencephalon to the paramedian zone of the midbrain. In contrast to the medial forebrain bundle this conduction route leads over the dorsum of the thalamus, and it is the habenular complex, rather than the lateral preoptico-hypothalamic nucleus, that straddles its course.

The stria medullaris as originally thought to arise exclusively from medial and basal forebrain structures also gives origin to fibers of the medial forebrain bundle. More recently, however, it has been shown to include additional fibers that arise from the internal segment of the globus pallidus (Nauta, 1974). It thus appears that the habenular complex receives input not only of limbic but also of extrapyramidal origin. Some of the main anatomical features of the stria medullaris and its trans-synaptic extension, the fasciculus retroflexus, are shown diagrammatically in Fig. 4, and can be described as follows.

A main component of the stria medullaris that originates in the dorsal or supracommissural septum constitutes the medial division of the stria medullaris and terminates in the medial habenular nucleus. Further fibers of the stria arise more ventrally, mainly from the nucleus of the diagonal band of Broca and from the lateral preoptico-hypothalamic region. These fibers form part of the lateral division of the stria, which terminates in the lateral habenular nucleus with the exception of some fibers of hypothalamic origin that bypass the habenular complex and follow the faciculus retroflexus to the ventral tegmental area (for references see Herkenham and Nauta, 1977). A third main component originates in the internal segment of the globus pallidus (it must be stressed that in rodents and carnivores this segment does

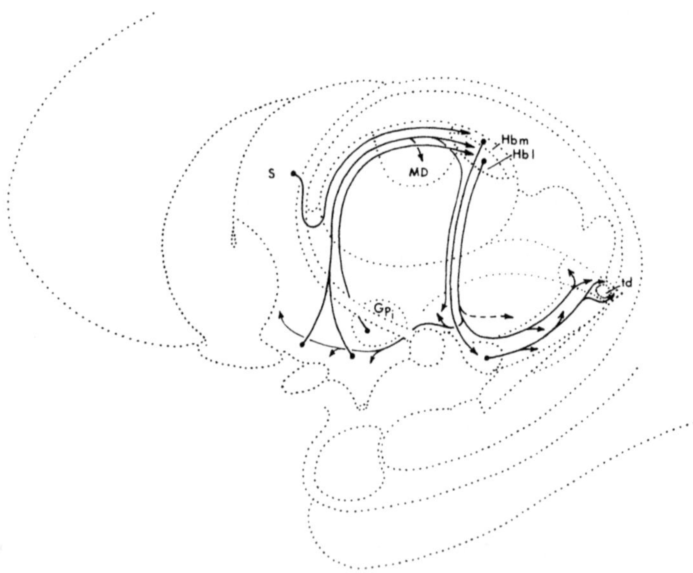

FIG. 4. Conduction pathways involving the habenular complex, as described in the text. Broken line indicates projections from lateral habenular nucleus (Hbl) to structures lateral to the paramedian "limbic midbrain area," in particular substantia nigra, pars compacta, and tegmental reticular formation. For identification of structures not labelled in this drawing see Fig. 2.

not form part of the structure labelled globus pallidus in atlases, and instead corresponds to the entopeduncular nucleus). Its fibers join the lateral division of the stria medullaris by arching dorsally through and around the rostral pole of the thalamus and terminate in a ventrolateral compartment of the lateral habenular nucleus (Nauta, 1974) in partial overlap with the limbic component of the lateral division.

The fasciculus retroflexus originates in both the medial and the lateral habenular nucleus, and is distributed mainly to the paramedian zone of the caudal mesencephalon. Those fibers of the bundle that arise in the medial habenular nucleus terminated almost exclusively in the interpeduncular nucleus, which in turn gives rise to a system of fine fibers, Ganser's "radiation of the ganglion interpedunculare," that is distributed to the median and the dorsal raphe nucleus, and in particular density to a zone of the central grey substance immediately surrounding the dorsal tegmental nucleus of Gudden. By contrast, habenular efferents to the paramedian zone of the midbrain that originate from the lateral habenular nucleus bypass the interpeduncular nucleus and are distributed directly to the median and the dorsal raphe nucleus. Finally, the fasciculus retroflexus continued a considerable number of fibers—apparently all from the lateral habenular nucleus—that either a) turn rostrally near the base of the midbrain to distribute themselves in the ventral tegmental area, hypothalamus, preoptic region and ventral parts of the septum, or b) sweep caudolaterally (broken lines in Figure 4) to 1) pars compacta of the substantia nigra and the lateral (sub-lemniscal) expanse of the ventral tegmental area, and 2) a medial region of midbrain reticular formation flanking the median raphe nucleus. These complex efferent relationships of the habenular complex, schematically indicated in Fig. 4, are described and illustrated in more detail elsewhere (Herkenham and Nauta, 1979).

By way of summary, the stria medullaris-fasciculus retroflexus route from the mediobasal forebrain to the midbrain can be described as comprising two distinct conduction lines. One of these, originating from the dorsal septal region—hence presumably transmitting first and foremost hippocampal outflow—leads over the medial habenular nucleus to the interpeduncular nucleus and thence to the raphe nuclei. A second, more diverse line originates in more ventral parts of the septum as well as in the lateral preoptico-hypothalamic region, and leads over the lateral habenular nucleus to the raphe nuclei, with side branches a) ascending in the medial forebrain bundle to the septo-preoptico-hypothalamic continuum, b) spreading laterally to the ventral tegmental area and the substantia nigra pars compacta, and c) descending into the medial mesencephalic reticular formation. Leading into this second conduction line at the level of the lateral habenular nucleus is a substantial extrapyramidal pathway originating in the internal pallidal segment. It is important to note that the two lines appear to remain largely if not entirely separate in their passage through the habenular complex, and thus seem to converge only in the region of the raphe nuclei. Cajal (1911) was the first to emphasize the apparent absence of both axonal connections and dendritic overlap between the medial and the lateral habenular nucleus (for further references see Herkenham and Nauta, 1979).

ASCENDING COMPONENTS OF THE "LIMBIC FOREBRAIN-MIDBRAIN CIRCUIT"

A detailed accounting of the various fiber systems ascending from the paramedian "limbic midbrain area" to the forebrain has thus far remained elusive, largely because only few of the likely sources of such fibers have been explored by appropriate combinations of anterograde and retrograde tracing methods. Important data, however, have come from studies by the histofluorescence method. This method provided the first evidence that several such projections, in part at least, affect the hippocampus, amygdala, and gyrus fornicatus directly rather than exclusively indirectly by way of the

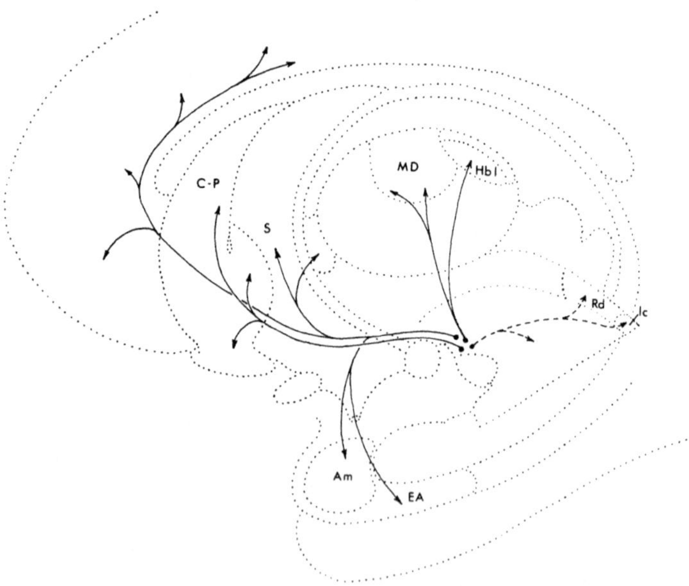

FIG. 5. Projections ascending from the ventral tegmental area, as described in the text. Broken line indicates descending projections to tegmental reticular formation and locus coeruleus. For identification of unlabelled structures see Fig. 2.

septo-preoptico-hypothalamic continuum as previously believed (Nauta, 1958; Nauta and Haymaker, 1969).

Projections Ascending from the Ventral Tegmental Area (VTA)

These projections are diagrammatically illustrated in Fig. 5. In histofluorescence studies Anden et al. (1966) and Ungerstedt (1971) identified dopamine cell group A10 in the VTA as the source of the dopamine fibers innervating the nucleus accumbens and olfactory tubercle. Ungerstedt added the observation that A10 projects also to the central nucleus of the amygdala, the bed nucleus of the stria terminalis and the septum; apparently on the strength of these additional connections (and perhaps the consideration that A10 projects to that part of the striatum that receives projections also from the hippocampal formation and amygdala) Ungerstedt introduced the term *meso-limbic system* to denote the ascending A10 projection. Additional support for the notion that A10 is closely associated with the limbic system came from later evidence of A10 projections to the anteromedial (i.e., frontocingulate) cortex (Fuxe et al., 1974; Lindvall et al., 1974; Beckstead, 1976) as well as to the entorhinal area (Lindvall and Bjorklund, 1974).

The ascending VTA projections first identified in histofluoresence studies by virtue of their content of dopamine fibers have subsequently been demonstrated also by anterograde (autoradiographic) and retrograde labelling methods. Studies by these latter methods have in some instances indicated a wider distribution of VTA efferents. For example, they have shown that the VTA projection to the striatum spreads beyond the nucleus accumbens over a considerable adjacent expanse of the striatum (Domesick et al., 1976; Fallon and Moore, 1978; Beckstead et al., 1979). They have also demonstrated VTA projections to the thalamus, in particular the lateral habenular nucleus and a circumferential zone of the mediodorsal nucleus (Herkenham and Nauta, 1977; Beckstead et al., 1979), as well as (broken lines in Fig. 5) to the midbrain reticular formation (Domesick et al., 1976; Beckstead et al., 1979), dorsal raphe nucleus and locus coeruleus (Simon et al., 1979). Since the methods used to demonstrate these additional VTA projections can supply no information whatever about the chemical characteristics of the neurons they label, it cannot *a priori* be concluded that VTA projections to striatal regions outside the nucleus accumbens, to the midbrain and to the thalamus, are dopaminergic.

Projections Ascending from the Raphe Nuclei

A projection ascending the medial forebrain bundle from the paramedian zone of the caudal midbrain—the location of the major mesencephalic raphe nuclei—to the hypothalamus, preoptic area, and septum was noted first in fiber-degeneration studies (Nauta and Kuypers, 1958). However, it was the monoamine-histofluorescence method that supplied the first evidence that the projection is composed, in part at least, of serotonin fibers whose distribution extends beyond the septo-preopticohypothalamic continuum to the limbic structures of the cerebral hemisphere (Dahlstrom and Fuxe, 1964). Figure 6, in which the connections of the mesencephalic raphe nuclei with the forebrain are schematically indicated, is based upon these histochemical findings as well as upon later studies by anterograde labelling methods (Conrad et al., 1974; Bobillier et al., 1975; Moore et al., 1978; Azmitia and Segal, 1978).

As indicated in the diagram, the ascending projections from the raphe nuclei are comparable to those from the ventral tegmental area in the sense that both are distributed to the striatum as well as to limbic structures. However, the raphe projections directly affect a much greater expanse of the limbic hemisphere than do the VTA projections. The latter appear not to extend beyond the amygdala, the entorhinal area, and the anterior half of the medial cortex (Fig. 5), whereas raphe projections have been traced to the

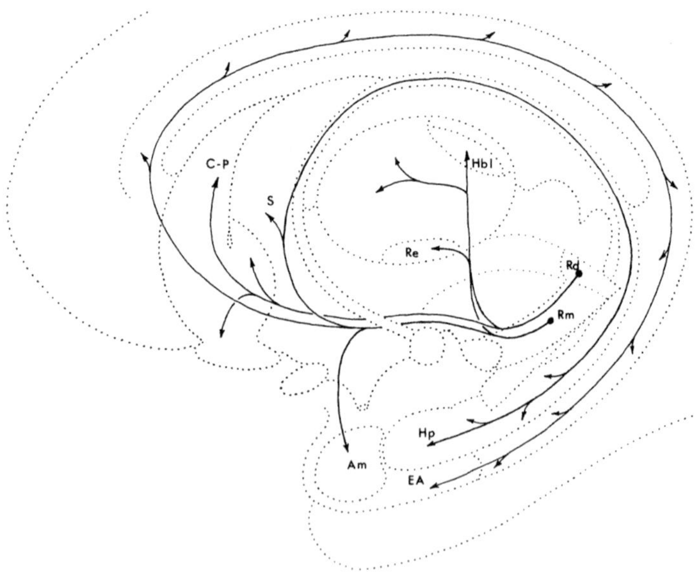

FIG. 6. Projections ascending from the median (Rm) and dorsal (Rd) raphe nuclei of the midbrain, as described in the text. For identification of structures not labelled in this figure, see Fig. 2.

amygdala, the hippocampus, and the length of the gyrus fornicatus, including the entorhinal area. Like the VTA projection, the ascending raphe projection in addition involves the lateral habenular nucleus, but it also spreads to various other thalamic cell groups (Conrad et al., 1974; Bobillier et al., 1975; Moore et al., 1978; Azmitia and Segal, 1978).

Non-Monoaminergic Projections Ascending from the Limbic Midbrain Area

It is still an open question whether the projections ascending from the ventral tegmental area and from the raphe nuclei are composed of monoamine fibers entirely or only in part. The difficulty is that the histofluorescence method demonstrates exclusively monoamine fibers, whereas the autoradiographic technique—the most sensitive anterograde fiber-tracing method currently available—allows no distinction to be made between monoamine and non-monoamine fibers. It is possible that future histochemical studies will show the ascending VTA and raphe projections to include non-monoaminergic sub-systems, each identified by an individual

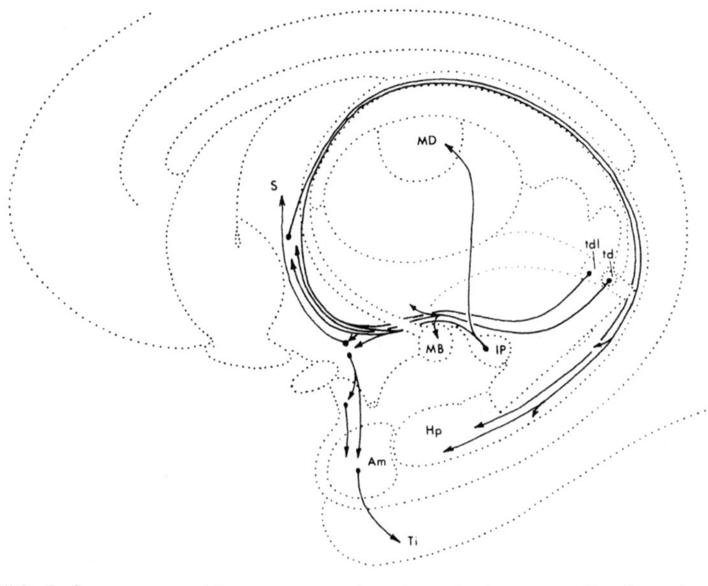

FIG. 7. Some presumably non-monoaminergic projections ascending from the paramedian zone of the midbrain, more in particular from dorsal tegmental nucleus of Gudden (td) and interpeduncular nucleus (IP). Both cell groups project directly to the hippocampus; their efferent relationship to the amygdala is uncertain, but has been assumed to be indirect, by way of the hypothalamus and/or preoptic area. Also indicated is the amygdalofugal projection to the inferior temporal cortex.

histochemical characteristic. However, even if matters should turn out otherwise, it is virtually certain that the ascending limb of the limbic forebrain-midbrain circuit is not exclusively monoaminergic. A projection ascending the medial forebrain bundle to the septum and hippocampus has recently been traced from the interpeduncular nucleus in the rat and cat (Stofer and Edwards, 1978; Baisden et al., 1979; Riley et al., 1979; Wyss et al., 1979). The interpeduncular nucleus is not know to contain monoamine neurons. Neither is the dorsal tegmental nucleus of Gudden, from which a projection ascends in the mammillary peduncle to the lateral mammillary nucleus; beside fibers reciprocating the mammillotegmental connection, this ascending projection includes fibers that bypass the mammillary body and continue forward in the medial forebrain bundle as far rostrally as the medial septal nucleus (Morest, 1961). Some of these fibers terminate in the supramamillary region, which projects in turn to both the hippocampus (Segal and Landis, 1974) and amygdala (Pretorius et al., 1979). Furthermore, Riley et al. (1979) have reported evidence of a direct projection from the nucleus tegmenti dorsalis lateralis to the hippocampus; this connection likewise seems unlikely to originate from monoamine neurons.

Finally, non-monoaminergic fibers are likely to be contained also in the dorsal longitudinal fasciculus of Schutz. In fiber-degeneration experiments (Nauta and Kuypers, 1958; Morest, 1961; Chi, 1970) ascending components of this fine-fibered system have been traced to posterior and dorsal regions of the periventricular and medial hypothalamic zones, but thus far neither the origin nor the distribution of the dorsal longtiudinal fasciculus appear to have been determined by the aid of present-day labelling methods.

Projections to the Limbic Forebrain from Lateral Brainstem Structures

In recent years, evidence has emerged of projections to the limbic forebrain that arise not from the paramedian "limbic midbrain area" but, instead, from more lateral parts of the pontine and mesencephalic tegmentum, in particular the parabrachial regions and the peripeduncular nucleus. The parabrachial region of the isthmus was found by Norgren (1976) to project not only to the thalamic gustatory nucleus but also to the central amygdaloid nucleus and the bed nucleus of the stria terminalis. According to Koh and Ricardo (1978), the two last-mentioned projections arise primarily from a dorsolateral part of the parabrachial region that receives secondary-sensory afferents mainly from the caudal, more exclusively visceroceptive division of the nucleus of the solitary tract, and only more sparsely from the rostral, predominantly gustatory part of the nucleus. McBride and Sutin (1977) have reported evidence that a more anteiror part of the parabrachial region projects directly to the ventromedial hypothalamic nucleus.

The peripeduncular nucleus has only very recently become identified as a source of fibers ascending to the limbic forebrain. In an autoradiographic study, Jones et al. (1976) traced fibers from this lateral tegmental structure to the amygdala, and Pretorius et al. (1979) reported retrograde cell labelling in the peripeduncular nucleus by horseradish peroxidase injected into the amygdala.

Projections to the Limbic Forebrain from the Rhombencephalon

The first unequivocal evidence of a direct projection to the limbic forebrain from levels below the ponto-mesencephalic transition was reported by Ricardo and Koh (1978) in the form of a projection from the caudal third of the nucleus of the solitary tract to a remarkable diversity of mediobasal forebrain structures: the bed nucleus of the stria terminalis, the paraventricular, dorsomedial, and arcuate nuclei of the hypothalamus, and the medial preoptic nucleus. This direct solitario-hypothalamic connection could be viewed as a sensory counterpart of sorts to the direct hypothalamo-autonomic projection demonstrated by Saper et al. (1976).

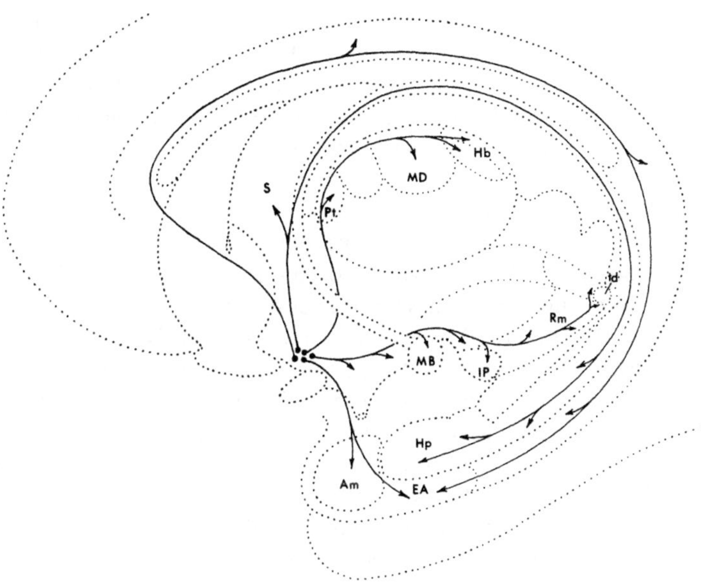

FIG. 8. The widespread projections of the nucleus of the diagonal band of Broca, as reported by Domesick (1976).

Projections from the Nucleus of the Diagonal Band

Although a systematic account of the known efferent connections of each individual limbic forebrain structure lies outside the scope of this article, the projections from the nucleus of the diagonal band deserve separate mention for their extraordinarily wide distribution. As schematically indicated in Fig. 8, this cell group gives origin to fibers that spread to virtually all of the telencephalic, most of the diencephalic, and several of the mesencephalic components of the limbic system (Domesick, 1976; Swanson and Cowan, 1979). It seems likely that its distribution to the hippocampus forms part of the acetylcholinergic septohippocampal projection (Lewis and Shute, 1967), but this, as well as the histochemical nature of the remainder of the projection, remains to be established. The distribution of this remarkably widespread system is somewhat comparable to that of the projections ascending from the raphe nuclei, except that it appears to exclude the striatum.

LIMBIC CIRCUITS INVOLVING THE THALAMUS

Several limbic connections associated with the thalamus have been schematically indicated in Fig. 9. Most familiar are those composing the so-called Papez circuit: hippocampal projections—originating from the subiculum hippocampi rather than from the CA fields (Swanson and Cowan, 1977)—pass to the anterior thalamic nucleus both directly (Gudden, 1881; Nauta, 1956) and by way of the mammillary body and mammillothalamic tract; the anterior thalamic nucleus projects, largely by way of the fasciculus cinguli, to the cingulate cortex, retrosplenial cortex and presubiculum (Domesick, 1973); the presubiculum in turn projects to the entorhinal area (Shipley, 1974) from which the massive perforant pathway to the hippocampus originates. A somewhat comparable circuit involving the amygdala is established by a massive projection from the amygdala to the medial division of the mediodorsal thalamic nucleus (cf. Nauta, 1961, 1962; Krettek and Price, 1977) which in turn projects to the orbitofrontal cortex; the latter is reciprocally associated with the inferior temporal cortex (broken line in Fig. 9), from which arise projections to the amygdala; an alternative orbitofronto-amygdaloid connection (not illustrated) is likely to lead by way of the medial forebrain bundle over the preoptic area and hypothalamus.

Two further thalamic connections are indicated in Fig. 9. One of these is a substantial projection from the nucleus reuniens by way of the fasciculus cinguli to the full extent of the gyrus fornicatus, including the entorhinal area. At the level of the retrosplenial cortex this projection spreads into the hippocampus where it terminates profusely and selectively in the stratum

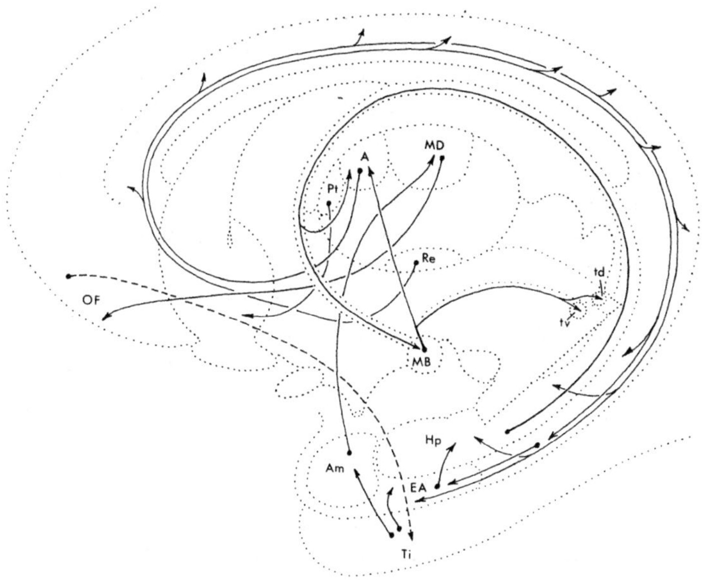

FIG. 9. Limbic circuitry associated with the thalamus, as discussed in the text.

lacunosummoleculare of field CA 1 (Herkenham, 1978). The projection is of interest especially as it establishes the only direct thalamohippocampal connection known at present. The information conveyed by it is as uncertain as are the afferent connections of the nucleus reuniens; of the latter little is known beyond the suggestion that they include fibers from the septum, subiculum hippocampi, antero-medial cortex, and mesencephalic raphe nuclei (cf. Herkenham, 1978). Last to be mentioned is a projection to the nucleus accumbens from the parataenial nucleus of the thalamus (Cowan and Powell, 1955; Swanson and Cowan, 1975); this thalamic nucleus has been reported to receive a sparse reciprocating projection from the nucleus accumbens (Conrad and Pfaff, 1976c; Nauta et al., 1978), as well as afferents from the nucleus of the diagonal band (Domesick, 1976) and from the ventromedial hypothalamic nucleus (Krieger et al., 1979).

DISCUSSION

General Considerations

On the basis of its efferent connections the limbic system could be defined as an array of forebrain structures whose descending efferent channels in whole or in part course along the medial side of the internal capsule and cerebral peduncle (more in particular in the fornix, stria terminalis and medial forebrain bundle), and thereby invade or traverse the septo-preoptico-hypothalamic continuum. Among the most remarkable findings made possible by the autoradiographic fiber-tracing method is the evidence that structures meeting this criterion are even more diverse than was originally believed. In addition to the initially recognized components of the limbic system (hippocampal formation, gyrus fornicatus and amygdala), these structures have been reported to include an anterior, ventromedial part of the striatum called nucleus accumbens, and the latter's ventral expansion that forms the core of the olfactory tubercle. The inclusion of a striatal district among the constituents of the limbic telencephalon might seem paradoxical, but would seem less so if it were assumed that a fundamental subdivision into a large lateral expanse and a narrower zone at the medial margin (limbus) is not absolutely characteristic of the cortical mantle, but affects also—though perhaps less overtly—the central core of the cerebral hemisphere, the corpus striatum. According to this assumption, the (ontogenetically derived) medio-lateral coordinate of any given telencephalic region would determine whether its descending efferents follow the lateral forebrain bundle (Edinger's term for the efferent fiber systems of the corpus striatum, augmented and complicated in later evolution by the intrusion of the corticofugal cerebral peduncle) or the medial forebrain bundle (the term in this context could be widened to refer not only to the fiber system known by that name, but also to the closely related fornix and stria terminalis).[2] Cerebral structures straddling the critical latitude could be expected to project into both the lateral and the medial forebrain bundle. Examples of such dual trajectories are found in the descending projections of the orbitofrontal cortex which follow both the medial forebrain bundle and the cerebral peduncle, and also in those of the nucleus accumbens, for the latter are not confined to the medial forebrain bundle but also include a massive projection to the external segment of the globus pallidus that is comparable to the striatopallidal connection arising from the large remainder of the striatum.

Cross-Links of Limbic System and Corpus Striatum

Several of the connections mentioned in the foregoing account can be viewed as efferent limbic channels bridging over to the striatum either directly or by way of structures known to project to the striatum. Direct limbico-striatal projections arise from the hippocampal formation,

[2] It is of incidental interest that a similar determining role of the medio-lateral coordinate, to some extent overriding cytoarchitectonic patterning, recently as been noted in the organization of the thalamocortical projection to the frontal lobe (Kievit and Kuypers, 1977).

amygdala, and cingulate cortex. Those from hippocampus and amygdala together appear to involve an anteroventral part of the striatum considerably larger than the nucleus accumbens as conventionally demarcated from the large remainder of the striatum (for a brief discussion of the problem of de-limiting the nucleus accumbens see Nauta et al., 1978). The cingulate cortex projects to a narrow mediodorsal zone of the striatum; only its most anteroventral, infralimbic region entrains, in addition, a quite substantial projection to the nucleus accumbens (Beckstead, 1979).

An even larger part of the striatum—if not indeed its entire expanse—could be affected by the limbic system more indirectly, by way of the substantia nigra and the dorsal raphe nucleus. The entire nigral dopamine complex, including the outlying cell group A10 and A8, lies within the distribution area of preoptic and hypothalamic efferents descending in the medial forebrain bundle (Nauta and Domesick, 1978), and cell groups A10 and A9 receive additional limbic afferents by way of the lateral habenular nucleus (Herkenham and Nauta, 1979). The raphe nuclei, likewise, can be assumed to receive inputs from limbic forebrain structures by way of both the medial forebrain bundle and the fasciculus retroflexus.

Connections oriented in the opposite direction—from the striatum to the limbic system—appear to be more limited in number. The only direct striato-limbic connection thus far reported is established by a rather sparse projection from the nucleus accumbens to the lateral amygdaloid nucleus (Nauta et al., 1978). More indirect channels of striato-limbic communication, however, are potentially numerous. From the nucleus accumbens fibers have been traced not only to the substantia nigra (Swanson and Cowan, 1975) but also to the lateral septal nucleus, bed-nucleus of the stria terminalis, various hypothalamic cell groups, and ventral tegmental area (Conrad and Pfaff, 1976c; Nauta et al., 1978). Longer accumbens efferents have been reported to follow the mesencephalic course of the medial forebrain bunde and to be distributed much like the larger number of fibers descending from the septo-preoptico-hypothalamic continuum. This striato-mesencephalic projection originates not only from the nucleus accumbens as conventionally defined but also from more lateral parts of the ventral striatal region (Nauta et al., 1978). It seems certain to be distributed in part at least to the ventral tegmental area and other paramedian regions from which projections ascend to limbic forebrain structures.

A somewhat similar, although more restricted, confluence of efferent limbic channels with the circuitry of the extrapyramidal system takes place in the lateral habenular nucleus (Nauta, 1974; Herkenham and Nauta, 1977; 1979). In this instance it is not the striatum but the pallidum (more specifically its internal segment) that gives rise to an extrapyramidal cross-bridge into the circuitry of the limbic system.

The "Limbic Forebrain-Midbrain Circuit"

It is plain from the foregoing survey that recent anatomical analyses have added much detail to the previously elaborated picture of subcortical limbic connections. None of these newer findings, however, appears to contradict the initial impression (Nauta, 1958; Nauta and Haymaker, 1969) that these connections in part compose a circuit reciprocally linking the limbic structures of the cerebral hemisphere with a continuum of subcortical grey matter extending from the olfactory tubercle and septal region caudalward over the preoptic region, the hypothalamus, and the paramedian zone of the midbrain. The most important revision of the original construct is dictated by the evidence that the ascending limb of the circuit is composed in part at least of fibers, especially of the monoamine variety, that directly invade the limbic structures of the cerebral hemisphere. In the initial report the ascending return loop of the circuit was assumed to be quantitatively interrupted in the septo-preoptico-hypothalamic continuum.

A Second "Limbic Forebrain-Midbrain Circuit"

A further and more fundamental modification of the original notion of a reciprocal limbico-mesencephalic connection has become necessary, for data now available indicated the existence of a second limbic forebrain-midbrain circuit not identified in the earlier studies by the fiber-degeneration method. This circuit, in contrast to the aforementioned one, involves *lateral* tegmental cells groups rather than the paramedian "limbic midbrain area", and appears to form part of the lateral rather than the medial division of the medial forebrain bundle (Fig. 10). Its descending limb is composed of a) fibers from the central nucleus of the amygdala to the parabrachial region (Krettek and Price, 1978), and b) fibers to the peripeduncular nucleus originating from the basal nucleus of Meynert in the substantia innominata (Jones et al., 1976) as well as from the ventromedial hypothalamic nucleus (Saper et al., 1976; Krieger et al., 1979). The ascending limb of this lateral circuit includes a) fibers from the parabrachial region to the central nucleus of the amygdala, bed nucleus of the stria terminalis (Koh and Ricardo, 1978) and ventromedial hypothalamic nucleus (McBride and Sutin, 1977) and b) a projection from the peripeduncular nucleus to the amygdala (Jones et al., 1976; Pretorius et al., 1979) and possibly to other limbic forebrain structures. It is interesting to note that this circuit at its rostral end involves the amygdala as well as several structures known to be closely associated with the amygdala: the basal nucleus of Meynert, the bed nucleus of the stria terminalis, and the ventromedial hypothalamic nucleus. Of further interest is that the dorsolateral part of the parabrachial region, the central amygdaloid nucleus and the bed nucleus of

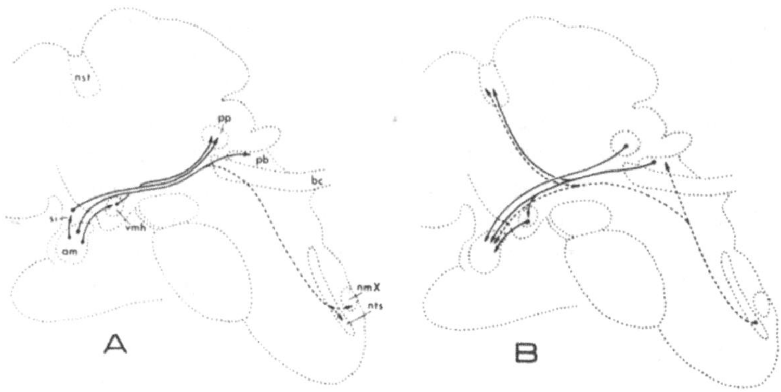

FIG. 10. The lateral limbic forebrain-midbrain circuit as described in the text. *A*: Descending components, leading from central nucleus of the amygdala (*am*) to the parabrachial region (*pb*), and from ventromedial hypothalamic nucleus (*vmh*) and substantia innominata (*si*) to the peripeduncular nucleus (*pp*). The direct amygdalofugal projection to dorsal motor nucleus of the vagus (*nmX*) and nucleus of the solitary tract (*nts*) (Hopkins and Holstege, 1978) is indicated in broken line. Other labels: *bc*: brachium conjunctivum; *nst*: bednucleus of stria terminalis. *B*: Ascending components of the lateral circuit. Broken lines indicate projections from nucleus of the solitary tract to parabrachial region, central amygdaloid nucleus, and bed nucleus of stria terminalis (Ricardo and Koh, 1978).

the stria terminalis have all been found to receive direct projections from the caudal part of the nucleus of the solitary tract (Ricardo and Koh, 1978). This appears to suggest that the lateral limbic forebrain-midbrain circuit is closely involved in the monitoring of neural inputs from viscera innervated by the vagus and glossopharyngeal nerves. The close proximity of visceral- to gustatory afferent channels in the circuit, not only at the level of the nucleus of the solitary tract but also in the parabrachial region (Koh and Ricardo, 1978), raises the question whether perhaps the lateral limbic forebrain-midbrain circuit is involved more in particular in the visceral and motivational mechanisms underlying the selection and intake of food.[3]

The Action Radius of the Limbic System

It is perhaps unnecessary to emphasize that the connection of the limbic system with the ponto-mesencephalic tegmentum is not defined by the forebrain-midbrain circuits mentioned above. A large contingent of

[3] Its close afferent relationship with the vagus nerve suggests, however, that the lateral circuit may be involved in a host of further visceral functions. Moreover, McBride and Sutin's (1977) report indicates that the parabrachial projection to the ventromedial hypothalamic nucleus originates from cells situated far enough laterally to lie within the path of the lateral lemniscus, and may thus convey auditory information to the hypothalamus.

descending medial-forebrain-bundle fibers is distributed to the wide expanse of central midbrain reticular formation that lies between the medial and the lateral circuit. The available data indicate that this limbic projection to the central midbrain tegmentum originates largely in the preoptic region and hypothalamus (Nauta, 1958; Conrad and Pfaff, 1976a and b; Swanson, 1976; Saper et al., 1979) and receives lesser contributions from the central amygdaloid nucleus (Hopkins and Holstege, 1978); nucleus accumbens (Nauta et al., 1978) and bed nucleus of the stria terminalis (Swanson and Cowan, 1979); other basal forebrain structures may eventually be found also to contribute to it. A similar, although more restricted distribution to tegmental regions lateral to the "limbic midbrain area" has been found to characterize those fibers of the fasciculus retroflexus that originate from the lateral half of the lateral habenular nucleus (Herkenham and Nauta, 1979). It thus seems that the limbic forebrain can convey its influence to a wide cross-sectional area of the midbrain reticular formation by way of both the medial forebrain bundle and the conduction routes involving the lateral habenular nucleus. Both these descending pathways presumably synapse in the midbrain with the upper links of a generally polysynaptic descending reticular pathway ultimately affecting, among other structures, preganglionic visceral motor neurons of the brainstem and spinal cord. This putative transreticular supranuclear component of the central visceromotor system is paralleled by the direct hypothalamo- and amygdalo-autonomic projections reported by Saper et al. (1976) and Hopkins and Holstege (1978), respectively.

These connections doubtless form part of the anatomical substratum for the visceromotor functions of the limbic system. However, by its aforementioned wide access routes to the pontomesencephalic reticular formation, the limbic system seems likely to also modulate the effects of the reticular formation upon the forebrain. These effects are exerted largely, it seems, over reticular pathways ascending to the subthalamic region and intralaminar thalamic nuclei. Recent findings have suggested a further, and shorter, path by which the limbic system could affect the forebrain, in this instance the cerebral cortex in particular. In retrograde-lebelling experiments, Divac (1975) and Kievit and Kuypers (1975) have demonstrated a projection originating from large neurons in the nucleus of the diagonal band, preoptico-hypothalamic region, and substantia innominata that spreads to most or all of the neocortex. Judging from their very wide distribution, both this fiber system of basal-forebrain origin and the pathways ascending from the pontomesencephalic reticular formation seem likely to convey to the cerebral cortex non-specific forms of information that affect the functional state of the cortex as a whole, rather than that of any cortical area in particular. However, in the monkey, anatomical evidence has been found of several limbico-neocortical connections that have a more limited distribution, and therefore seem likely to have a more selective function. All of these originate from the amygdala and are directed at the frontal and inferior temporal cortex. One is composed of fibers from the amygdala directly to the inferior temporal region (Nauta, 1961; Krettek and Price, 1974) (Fig. 7). A second one is a direct projection from the amygdala to the dorsal half of the convexity of the frontal cortex (Jacobson and Trojanowski, 1975), whereas a third one is a dual amygdalo-orbitofrontal projection that is in part direct (Nauta, 1961; Porrino and Goldman, 1979) (Fig. 3) and in part indirect, by way of the mediodorsal nucleus of the thalamus (Fig. 9). The collective distribution of these more circumscript limbico-cortical projections is of considerable interest, for it corresponds, in part at least, to those cortical regions which are most heavily converged upon by the concatenated cortico-cortical conduction lines that lead away from each of the primary sensory areas of the cortex (Jones and Powell, 1970). From various parts of these same fronto- temporal convergence regions[4], direct or indirect projections have been traced in return to the amygdala (Whitlock and Nauta, 1956; Jones and Powell, 1970; Herzog and Van Hoesen, 1976) and also to the entorhinal area (Van Hoesen and Pandya, 1975; Van Hoesen et al., 1975) (Fig. 3). The amygdalocortical connections mentioned above could thus be viewed as limbico-cortical projections reciprocating, part at least, the flow of multisensory information from the cortex to the limbic system. In the light of these connections, the limbic system could be viewed as a neural mechanism that not only monitors the sensory processes of the cerebral cortex, but can also reach out to intervene in these processes. It could thus be suspected, even on the basis of no more than anatomical data, that the functional set of the limbic system affects not only, as generally acknowledged, the organism's visceral and endocrine functions and its motivational state, but also the sensory and associative mechanisms involved in its perceptions and ideational processes.

ACKNOWLEDGEMENTS

This survey is based in part on studies made possible by USPHS Grants NB 06542 and MH 25515, and by NSF Grant 76-81227.

[4] The term "convergence" refers here to cortical regions, not necessarily to cortical neurons or even to particular neuronal assemblies such as those composing cortical columns.

REFERENCES

Anden, N.-E., Dahlstrom, A., Fuxe, K., Larsson, K., Olson, L., and Ungerstedt, U. Ascending monamine neurons to the telencephalon and diencephalon. *Acta Physiol. Scand.* 67, 313–326 (1966).

Azmitia, E.G., and Segal, M. An autoradiographic analysis of the differential ascending projections of the dorsal and median raphe nuclei in the rat. *J. Comp. Neurol.* 179, 641–688 (1978).

Baisden, R.H., Hoover, D.B., and Cowie, R.J. Retrograde demonstration of hippocampal afferents from the interpeduncular and reuniens nuclei. *Neurosci. Letters* 13, 105–109 (1979).

Beckstead, R.M. Convergent thalamic and mesencephalic projections to the anterior medial cortex in the rat. *J. Comp. Neurol.* 166, 403–416 (1976).

Beckstead, R.M. An autoradiographic examination of cortico-cortical and subcortical projections of the mediodorsal-projection (prefrontal) cortex in the rat. *J. Comp. Neurol.* 184, 43–62 (1979).

Beckstead, R.M., Domesick, V.B., and Nauta, W.J.H. Efferent connections of the substantia nigra and ventral tegmental area in the rat. *Brain Res.* 175, 191–217 (1979).

Bobillier, P., Petitjean, F., Salvert, D., Ligier, M., and Seguin, S. Differential projections of the nucleus raphe dorsalis and nucleus raphe centralis as revealed by autoradiography. *Brain Res.* 85, 205–210 (1975).

Broca, P. Anatomie comparee des circonvolutions cerebrales. Le grand lobe limbique et la scissure limbique dans la serie des mammiferes. *Rev. d'Anthrop.* Ser. 2, 1, 285–498 (1878).

Cajal, S.R.y. Histologie du Systeme Nerveux de l'Homme et des Vertebres. Vol. II. Maloine, Paris (1911).

Chi, C.G. An experimental silver study of the ascending projections of the central grey substance and adjacent tegmentum in the rat with observations in the cat. *J. Comp. Neurol.* 139, 259–272 (1970).

Conrad, L.C.A., Leonard, C.M., and Pfaff, D. Connections of the median and dorsal raphe nuclei in the rat: an autoradiographic and degeneration study. *J. Comp. Neurol.* 156, 179–205 (1974).

Conrad, L.C.A., and Pfaff, D.W. Efferents from medial basal forebrain and hypothalamus in the rat. I. An autoradiographic study of the medial preoptic area. *J. Comp. Neurol.* 169, 185–220 (1976a).

Conrad, L.C.A., and Pfaff, D.W. Efferents from medial basal forebrain and hypothalamus in the rat. II. An autoradiographic study of the anterior hypothalamus. *J. Comp. Neurol.* 169, 221–262 (1976b).

Conrad, L.C.A., and Pfaff, D.W. Autoradiographic tracing of nucleus accumbens efferents in the rat. *Brain Res.* 113, 589–596 (1976c).

Cowan, W.M., Gottlieb, D.I., Hendrickson, A.E., Price, J.L., and Woolsey, T.A. The autoradiographic demonstration of axonal connections in the central nervous system. *Brain Res.* 37, 21–51 (1972).

Cowan, W.M., and Powell, T.P.S. The projections of the midline and intralaminar nuclei of the thalamus of the rabbit. *J. Neurol. Neurosurg. Psychiat.* 18, 266–279 (1955).

Dahlstrom, A., and Fuxe, K. Evidence for the existence of monoamine-containing neurons in the central nervous system. I. Demonstration of monoamines in the cell bodies of brainstem neurons. *Acta Physiol. Scand.* 62, Suppl. 232, 1–55 (1964).

Divac, I. Magnocellular nuclei of the basal forebrain project to neocortex, brain stem, and olfactory bulb. Review of some functionâl correlates. *Brain Res.* 93, 385–398 (1975).

Domesick, V.B. Thalamic projections in the cingulum bundle to the para-hippocampal cortex of the rat. *Anat. Rec.* 175, 308 (1973).

Domesick, V.B. Projections of the nucleus of the diagonal band of Broca in the rat. *Anat. Rec.* 184, 391-392 (1976).

Domesick, V.B., Beckstead, R.M., and Nauta, W.J.H. Some ascending and descending projections of the substantia nigra and ventral tegmental area in the rat. *Neurosci. Abs.* II, Part 1, 61 (1976).

Edinger, L., and Wallenberg, A. Untersuchungen uber den Fornix und das Corpus mammillare. *Arch. f. Psychiat.* 35, 1-21 (1902).

Fallon, J.H., and Moore, R.Y. Catecholamine innervation of the basal forebrain. IV. Topography of the dopamine projection to the basal forebrain and neostriatum. *J. Comp. Neurol.* 180, 545-580 (1978).

Fox, C.A. Amygdalo-thalamic connections in Macaca mulatta. *Anat. Rec.* 103, 537-538 (1949).

Fuxe, K., Hokfelt, T., Johansson, O., Jonsson, G., Lidbrink, P., and Ljungdahl, A. The origin of the dopamine nerve terminals in limbic and frontal cortex. Evidence for meso-cortical dopamine neurons. *Brain Res.* 82, 349-355 (1974).

Gudden, B. von. Beitrag zur Kenntniss des Corpus mammillare und der sogenannten Schenkel des Fornix. *Arch. f. Psychiat. Nervenkr.* 11, 428-452 (1881).

Heimer, L., and Nauta, W.J.H. The hypothalamic distribution of the stria terminalis in the rat. *Brain Res.* 13, 284-297 (1969).

Herkenham, M. The connections of the nucleus reuniens thalami: evidence for a direct thalamo-hippocampal pathway in the rat. *J. Comp. Neurol.* 177, 589-610 (1978).

Herkenham, M., and Nauta, W.J.H. Afferent connections of the habenular nuclei in the rat. A horseradish peroxidase study, with a note on the fiber-of-passage problem. *J. Comp. Neurol.* 173, 123-146 (1977).

Herkenham, M., and Nauta, W.J.H. Efferent connections of the habenular nuclei in the rat. *J. Comp. Neurol.* 187, 19-48 (1979).

Herzog, A.G., and Van Hoesen, G.W. Temporal neocortical afferent connections to the amygdala in the rhesus monkey. *Brain Res.* 115, 57-69 (1976).

Hopkins, D.A., and Holstege, G. Amygdaloid projections to the mesencephalon, pons and medulla oblongata in the cat. *Exp. Brain Res.* 32, 529-547 (1978).

Jacobson, S., and Trojanowski, J.Q. Amygdaloid projections to prefrontal granular cortex in rhesus monkey demonstrated with horseradish peroxidase. *Brain Res.* 100, 132-139 (1975).

Jones, B.E., and Moore, R.Y. Ascending projections of the locus coeruleus in the rat. II. Autoradiographic analysis. *Brain Res.* 127, 23-53 (1977).

Jones, E.G., Burton, H., Saper, C.B., and Swanson, L.W. Midbrain, diencephalic and cortical relationships of the basal nucleus of Meynert and associated structures in primates. *J. Comp. Neurol.* 167, 385-420 (1976).

Jones, E.G., and Powell, T.P.S. An anatomical study of converging sensory pathways within the cerebral cortex of the monkey. *Brain* 93, 793-820 (1970).

Kievit, J., and Kuypers, H.G.J.M. Subcortical afferents to the frontal lobe in the rhesus monkey studied by means of retrograde horseradish peroxidase transport. *Brain Res.* 85, 261-266 (1975).

Kievit, J., and Kuypers, H.G.J.M. Organization of the thalamo-cortical connexions to the frontal lobe in the rhesus monkey. *Exp. Brain Res.* 29, 299-322 (1977).

Koh, E.T., and Ricardo, J.A. Afferents and efferents of the parabrachial region in the rat: evidence for parallel ascending gustatory versus visceroceptive systems arising from the nucleus of the solitary tract. *Anat. Rec.* 190 (2), 449 (1978).

Krettek, J.E, and Price, J.L. A direct input from the amygdala to the thalamus and the cerebral cortex. *Brain Res.* 67, 169-174 (1974).

Krettek, J.E., and Price, J.L. Projections from the amygdaloid complex to the cerebral cortex and thalamus in the rat and cat. *J. Comp. Neurol.* 172, 687-722 (1977).

Krettek, J.E., and Price, J.L. Amygdaloid projections to subcortical structures within the basal forebrain and brainstem in the rat and cat. *J. Comp. Neurol.* 178, 225–254 (1978).

Krieger, M.S., Conrad, L.C.A., and Pfaff, D.W. An autoradiographic study of the afferent connections of the ventromedial nucleus of the hypothalamus. *J. Comp. Neurol.* 183, 785–816 (1979).

Kristensson, K., Olsson, Y., and Sjostrand, J. Axonal uptake and retrograde transport of exogenous proteins in the hypoglossal nerve. *Brain Res.* 32, 339–406 (1971).

Kuypers, H.G.J.M., and Maisky, V.A. Retrograde axonal transport of horseradish peroxidase from spinal cord to brain stem cell groups in the cat. *Neurosci. Letters* 1, 9–14 (1975).

Lammers, H.J., and Lohman, A.H.M. Experimenteel anatomisch onderzoek naar de verbindingen van piriforme cortex en amygdalakernen bij de kat. *Nederl. Tijdschr. Geneesk.* 101 (13), 1–2 (1957).

Lavail, J.H., Winston, K.R., and Tish, A. A method based on retrograde intraaxonal transport of protein for identification of cell bodies of origin of axons terminating within the CNS. *Brain Res.* 58, 470–477 (1973).

Lewis, P.R., and Shute, C.C.D. The cholinergic limbic system: projections to hippocampal formation, medial cortex, nuclei of the ascending cholinergic reticular system, and the subfornical organ and supra-optic crest. *Brain* 90, 22–54 (1967).

Lindvall, O., and Bjorklund, A. The organization of the ascending catecholamine neuron systems in the rat brain as determined by the glyoxylic acid fluorescence method. *Acta Physiol. Scand.*, Suppl. 412, 1–48 (1974).

Lindvall, O., Bjorklund, A., Moore, R.Y., and Stenevi, U. Mescencephalic dopamine neurons projecting to neocortex. *Brain Res.* 81, 325–331 (1974).

Lundberg, P.O. Cortico-hypothalamic connexions in the rabbit. *Acta Physiol. Scand.*, Suppl. 171, 1–80 (1960).

Lundberg, P.O. The nuclei gemini. Two hitherto undescribed nerve cell collections in the hypothalamus of the rabbit. *J. Comp. Neurol.* 119, 311–316 (1962).

MacLean, P.D. Some psychiatric implications of physiological studies on frontotemporal portion of limbic system (visceral brain). *Electroenceph. Clin. Neurophysiol.* 4, 407–418 (1952).

McBride, R.L., and Sutin, J. Amygdaloid and pontine projections to the ventromedial nucleus of the hypothalamus. *J. Comp. Neurol.* 174, 377–396 (1977).

Millhouse, O.E. A Golgi study of the descending MFB. *Brain Res.* 15, 341–363 (1969).

Moore, R.Y., Halaris, A.E., and Jones, B.E. Serotonin neurons of the midbrain raphe: Ascending projections. *J. Comp. Neurol.* 180, 417–438 (1978).

Morest, D.K. Connexions of the dorsal tegmental nucleus in rat and rabbit. *J. Anat.* (Lond.) 95, 246–299 (1961).

Nauta, W.J.H. Evidence of a pallidohabenular pathway in the cat. *J. Comp. Neurol.* 156, 19–28 (1974).

Nauta, W.J.H. An experimental study of the fornix system in the rat. *J. Comp. Neurol.* 104, 247–271 (1956).

Nauta, W.J.H. Hippocampal projections and related neural pathways to the midbrain in the cat. *Brain* 81, 319–340 (1958).

Nauta, W.J.H. Fibre degeneration following lesions of the amygdaloid complex in the monkey. *J. Anat.* 95, 515–531 (1961).

Nauta, W.J.H. Neural associations of the amygdaloid complex in the monkey. *Brain* 85, 505–520 (1962).

Nauta, W.J.H. Expanding borders of the limbic system concept, in *Functional Neurosurgery*. T. Rassmussen and R. Marino, eds. Raven Press, New York (1979), pp. 7–23.

Nauta, W.J.H., and Domesick, V.B. Crossroads of limbic and striatal circuitry: hypothalamonigral connections, in *Limbic Mechanisms*. K.E. Livingston and O. Hornykiewicz, eds. Plenum Publishing Corporation, New York & London (1978), pp. 75–93.

Nauta, W.J.H., and Haymaker, W. Hypothalamic nuclei and fiber connections, in *The Hypothalamus*. W. Haymaker et al., eds. Charles C. Thomas, Inc., Springfield, Illinois (1969), pp. 136–209.

Nauta, W.J.H., and Kuypers, H.G.J.M. Some ascending pathways in the brain stem reticular formation, in *Reticular Formation of the Brain*. H.H. Jasper et al., eds. Little, Brown and Co., Boston & Toronto (1958), pp. 3–30.

Nauta, W.J.H., Smith, G.P., Faull, R.L.M., and Domesick, V.B. Efferent connections and nigral afferents of the nucleus accumbens in the rat. *Neuroscience* 3, 385–401 (1978).

Norgren, R. Taste pathways to hypothalamus and amygdala. *J. Comp. Neurol.* 166, 17–30 (1976).

Olmos, J.S. de. The amygdaloid projection field in the rat studied with the cupric-silver method, in *The Neurobiology of the Amygdala*. B.E. Eleftheriou, ed. Plenum Press, New York & London (1972), pp. 145–204.

Olmos, J.S. de, and Ingram, W.R. The projection field of the stria terminalis in the rat brain. An experimental study. *J. Comp. Neurol.* 146, 303–333 (1972).

Papez, J.W. A proposes mechanism of emotion. *Arch. Neurol. Psychiat.* Chicago, 38, 725–743 (1937).

Porrino, L.J., and Goldman, P.S. Selective distribution of projections from amygdala to prefrontal cortex in rhesus monkey. *Soc. Neurosci. Abs.* 5, 280 (1979).

Powell, E.W., and Leman, R.B. Connections of the nucleus accumbens. *Brain Res.* 105, 389–403 (1976).

Pretorius, J.K., Phelan, K.D., and Mehler, W.R. Afferent connections of the amygdala in rat. *Anat. Rec.* 193, 657 (1979).

Ricardo, J.A., and Koh, E.T. Anatomical evidence of direct projections from the nucleus of the solitary tract to the hypothalamus, amygdala, and other forebrain structures in the rat. *Brain Res.* 153, 1–26 (1978).

Riley, J.N., Marchand, E.R., and Moore, R.Y. Diencephalic and brainstem afferents to the hippocampal formation of the rat. *Soc. Neurosci. Abs.* 5, 281 (1979).

Saper, C.B., Loewy, A.D., Swanson, L.W., and Cowan, W.M. Direct hypothalamo-autonomic connections. *Brain Res.* 177, 305–312 (1976).

Saper, C.B., Swanson, L.W., and Cowan, W.M. The efferent connections of the ventromedial nucleus of the hypothalamus of the rat. *J. Comp. Neurol.* 169, 409–422 (1976).

Saper, C.B., Swanson, L.W., and Cowan, W.M. An autoradiographic study of the efferent connections of the lateral hypothalamic area in the rat. *J. Comp. Neurol.* 183, 689–706 (1979).

Segal, M., and Landis, S. Afferents to the hippocampus of the rat studied with the method of retrograde transport of houseradish peroxidase. *Brain Res.* 78, 1–15 (1974).

Shipley, M.T. Presubiculum afferents to the entorhinal area and the Papez circuit. *Brain Res.* 67, 162–168 (1974).

Simon, H., Le Moal, M., Stinus, L., and Calas, A. Anatomical relationships between the ventral mesencephalic tegmentum-A10 region and the locus coeruleus as demonstrated by anterograde and retrograde tracing techniques. *J. Neural Transmission* 44, 77–86 (1979).

Stofer, W.B., and Edwards, S.B. Organization and efferent projections of the interpeduncular complex in the cat. *Soc. Neurosci. Abs.* 4, 228 (1978).

Swanson, L.W. An autoradiographic study of the efferent connections of the preoptic region in the rat. *J. Comp. Neurol.* 167, 227–256 (1976).

Swanson, L.W., and Cowan, W.M. A note on the connections and development of the nucleus accumbens. *Brain Res.* 92, 324–330 (1975).

Swanson, L.W., and Cowan, W.M. An autoradiographic study of the organization of the efferent connections of the hippocampal formation in the rat. *J. Comp. Neurol.* 172, 49–84 (1977).

Swanson, L.W., and Cowan, W.M. The connections of the septal region in the rat. *J. Comp. Neurol.* 186, 621–656 (1979).

Ungerstedt, U. Stereotaxic mapping of the monoamine pathways in the rat brain. *Acta Physiol. Scand.* 197, Suppl. 367, 1–48 (1971).

Valenstein, E.S., and Nauta, W.J.H. A comparison of the distribution of the fornix system in the rat, guinea pig, cat, and monkey. *J. Comp. Neurol.* 113, 337–363 (1959).

Van Hoesen, G.W., and Pandya, D.N. Some connections of the entorhinal (area 28) and perirhinal (area 35) cortices of the rhesus monkey. I. Temporal lobe afferents. *Brain Res.* 95, 1–24 (1975).

Van Hoesen, G.W., Pandya, D.N., and Butters, N. Some connections of the entorhinal (area 28) and perirhinal (area 35) cortices of the rhesus monkey. II. Frontal lobe afferents. *Brain Res.* 95, 25–38 (1975).

Whitlock, D.G., and Nauta, W.J.H. Subcortical projections from the temporal neocortex in Macaca mulatta. *J. Comp. Neurol* 106, 183–212 (1956).

Wyss, J.M., Swanson, L.W., and Cowan, W.M. A study of subcortical afferents to the hippocampal formation in the rat. *Neurosci.* 4, 463–476 (1979).

Copyright © 1982, Spectrum Publications, Inc.
The Neural Basis of Behavior

11

Peptides in Affective Disorders

A.J. Prange, Jr.
P.T. Loosen

The affective disorders are mania and depression. Depression, more than mania, has been subject to a variety of systems of subclassification (Schatzberg, 1976). Since both mania and depression tend notoriously to recur, it is often possible in a given patient to base diagnosis on life history (Mazure and Gershon, 1979). Thus, one may speak of a depressed patient as showing either the bipolar or the unipolar form of the disorder; respectively, the patient has or has not suffered a previous manic attack. "Mania" almost always implies bipolar affective disorder, for mania without diagnosable episodes of depression, i.e., unipolar mania, is rare. This simple classification, now generally accepted, corresponds reasonably well to an assortment of biological findings (Goodwin and Potter, 1976) and treatment responses (Schildkraut et al., 1976). Whenever possible, we shall use it in the discussion that follows.

Intensive biological research in the affective disorders has coincided roughly with the availability, for about 25 years, of effective anti-depressant drugs and more recently with the availability of lithium salts for the treatment of mania. Information about the biochemical properties, presumably the modes of action, of these drugs has contributed prominently to concepts of the pathophysiology of the affective disorders. It is generally held that catecholamines (Goodwin and Potter, 1976; Schildkraut et al., 1976) and indolamines (Coppen et al., 1972) or distorted relationships between them (Prange et al., 1974) play an important role. Nevertheless, amine theories can readily be criticized, perhaps not so much for inaccuracy as for insufficiency.

Psychoendocrinology antedates psychopharmacology. It is sometimes said to have been born with the observation of Berthold (1849) concerning the changes in behavior of roosters after castration. Psychoendocrinology experienced a renaissance about 1970 with the description of hypothalamic hypophysiotropic hormones and with the spreading application of radioimmunoassay techniques. These advances were rapidly applied to the affective disorders, perhaps because of dissatisfaction with aminergic theories of cause and perhaps because of the venerable notion that hormone changes, as in menopause, play a role in the cause of some affective disorders (Prange et al., 1977). In any case, it would be an error, on prima facia grounds, to set aminergic and endocrine theories in opposition. They should, we think, be complementary. Thyroid hormone-catecholamine interactions, for example, have been recognized since 1918 (Goetsch, 1918) and from time to time have been reappraised (Waldstein, 1966). Furthermore, it is now clear that the peptidergic cells of the hypothalamus receive aminergic input and serve as transducers between the nervous system and the endocrine system.

Just as psychoendocrine research is venerable so is its use of peptides as independent or dependent variables. This is no less true in research addressed to affective disorders than to other disorders. Of course, not all hormones are peptides and not all peptides are hormones. Nevertheless, nearly all newly discovered hormones are peptides and increasingly these have become, in one way or another, important focal points for research. In the paragraphs that follow we shall review the salient features of this body of work.

MANIA

Behavioral Studies

There are many fewer biological studies of mania than of depression. There are fewer manic patients and they are more troublesome to study, due to their behavior. Psychoendocrine studies generally are sparse and so, specifically, are studies involving peptides.

Thyrotropin-releasing hormone (TRH)

TRH is pyro-Glu-His-Pro-NH_2 (Boler et al., 1969; Burgus et al., 1969). It releases from the anterior pituitary gland thyrotropin (TSH), prolactin (PRL) and, in certain conditions, growth hormone (GH) (Bowers et al., 1971; Maeda et al., 1975; Sawin and Hershman, 1976). There is increasing evidence that TRH exerts effects on the brain that are independent of its endocrine effects. These matters have been discussed in detail (Plotnikoff et al., 1974; Prange et al., 1975, 1976b, 1978b).

Huey et al. (1975) gave TRH (0.5 mg IV) or saline to five euthyroid manic men in a double-blind, cross-over trial. The peptide produced favorable changes significantly more often than the comparison substance. Endocrine changes produced by TRH were not reported. Physostigmine, a cholinesterase inhibitor, has produced prompt behavioral improvement in manic patients (Davis et al., 1978). TRH appears to have potent, central cholinomimetic actions (Yarbrough, 1976). Whether this property accounts for its apparent antimanic action is uncertain.

Endocrine Studies

TRH

Kirkegaard and his coworkers (1978) injected TRH in 14 manic patients, 19 patients with unipolar depression, 12 with bipolar depression, and five with mixed manic depressive disorders. The TSH responses were decreased in all of these groups as compared to normal controls, though not always significantly. Manic patients showed a significant reduction in baseline T_3 and free T_3-Index. Takahashi et al. (1974) also reported somewhat diminished TSH response in some manic patients.

DEPRESSION

Behavioral Studies

TRH

In a double-blind crossover study ten women with unipolar depression were treated with TRH, 0.6 mg, given as an IV bolus. The peptide produced a rapid, though brief and partial, improvement. Patients improved in both observer and self-rating assessments within a few hours. Maximum improvement was about 50 percent as measured by the Hamilton Rating Scale for Depression (Hamilton, 1960) and less than full remission. It occurred the day after treatment. Patients relapsed to baseline severity within one week (Prange et al., 1972b,c).

Other investigators have studied the efficacy of TRH as an efficient remedy for depression. These data are summarized in Table 1. In general, the results are disappointing. We have reviewed this mass of data in detail (Prange et al., 1978a,b). Generalizations about the many studies performed are difficult; size of dose, frequency, and route of administration and population characteristics have varied greatly. Pecknold et al. (1977), alone among all others, repeated our original experiment and obtained substantially the same results. Furlong et al. (1976) have suggested that differences in results might be attributed to the existance of endocrinologically distinct types of depression.

Table 1. Behavioral Studies of TRH in Depression

Studies	*Positive*	*Negative*
Oral TRH		
Single Blind	1 (1 patient)	0
Double Blind	1 (4 patients)	4 (66 patients)
Total	2 (5 patients)	4 (66 patients)
Intravenous TRH		
Single Blind	5 (188 patients)	6 (61 patients)
Double Blind	6 (43 patients)	8 (109 patients)
Total	11 (231 patients)	14 (170 patients)

Recent data from our laboratory (Loosen et al., unpublished data) indicate that the behavioral response after TRH in depression is highly sensitive to ambient levels of thyroid hormones. Pretreatment with a single small dose of thyroid hormones attenuated the behavioral response seen after TRH without such pretreatment.

Luteinizing Hormone Releasing Hormone (LHRH)

LHRH is pGlu-His-Trp-Ser-Tyr-Gly-Leu-Arg-Pro-Gly-NH_2 (Guillemin, 1978; Schally, 1978). It releases the gonadotropins, LH and FSH, from the anterior pituitary gland. Eighty percent of LHRH is localized in the hypothalamus with the remaining 20 percent in the circumventricular organs (Brownstein et al., 1976). As mentioned above anent TRH, there is evidence that LHRH has direct effects on the brain that are independent from its endocrine effects (Moss, 1975; Moss and McCann, 1973).

Benkert (1975; Benkert et al., 1974) gave LHRH, TRH, or saline, in crossover design to a small group of depressed patients. Both hormones were somewhat more effective than saline, though not statistically significantly.

Melanocyte Stimulating Hormone Release Inhibiting Factor (MIF-I)

The identification of endogenous peptides that inhibit the release of MSH from the intermediate lobe of the pituitary is still controversial (Vale et al.,

1977). Two such peptides have been identified: MIF-I and MIF-II (Nair et al., 1971, 1972). MIF-I is Pro-Leu-Gly-NH_2 and has been used in psychiatric patients.

Ehrensing and Kastin (1974) treated 18 depressed women in a double-blind study. Six received MIF-I, 60 mg/day p.o.; six received 150 mg; six received placebo capsules. There was a marked prompt improvement from the lower dose of the hormone. In a second double-blind, placebo-controlled study the same authors treated 24 patients with either bipolar or unipolar depression (Ehrensing and Kastin, 1978). Patients received MIF-I orally, 75 or 750 mg per day, or placebo. Again, only the smaller dose of the tripeptide was found to produce a significant antidepressant effect.

Adrenocorticotropic Hormone (ACTH)

ACTH is a 39-membered amino acid chain (Daughaday, 1974). It resembles the larger molecule, β-lipotropin, fragments of which contain the amino acid sequences of α, β, and γ-endorphin as well as methionine-enkephalin but not leucine-enkephalin (DeWied and Gispen, 1977). The first 13 amino acids of ACTH occur in the same sequence as the 13 amino acids that comprise the molecule of α-MSH. There is increasing evidence that ACTH is localized in the brain as well as in the anterior pituitary (Krieger et al., 1977). The main physiologic role of ACTH is its stimulation of the adrenal cortex (Daughaday, 1974).

Endroczi (1972) conducted clinical studies with $ACTH_{1-10}$. Apparently his patients bore the primary diagnosis of schizophrenia but showed prominent traits of depression. He summarized his findings as follows: ". . . . in extreme depressive states (schizophrenia patients) daily treatment with 3–6 mg of the ACTH fragment resulted in elimination of the depressive state, increase in communication, and mood elevation. These effects were observed within 5–7 days."

Thyroid Stimulating Hormone (TSH)

As mentioned above, there is evidence that ACTH is localized in the anterior pituitary as well as in the brain (Krieger et al., 1977). In a recent report, Moldow and Yalow (1978) demonstrated that TSH occurs in the hypothalamus as well as the anterior pituitary of man and is even more widely distributed in rat brain. The pituitary does, however, appear to be the only site of synthesis. TSH is a polypeptide that contains two peptide chains, an alpha chain with eight amino acids and a beta chain with 113 amino acids. Hormonal specificity of the complete molecule is conferred by the beta chain, while the role of the alpha chain is uncertain. The major physiological role of TSH is its stimulation of the thyroid gland.

In a double-blind, placebo-controlled study, we ascertained whether bovine TSH, 10 IU administered IM, would accelerate the antidepressant effects of imipramine in depressed women (Prange et al., 1970). Patients who received imipramine plus TSH improved more rapidly than those who received imipramine plus saline. It is possible that TSH may have exerted an antidepressant affect independent of its endocrine effects. However, it is also possible that imipramine potentiation was the consequence of enhanced thyroid hormone secretion prompted by TSH. This interpretation is consistent with earlier findings that indicate that oral administration of T_3 accelerates the therapeutic action of imipramine in depressed women (Prange et al., 1969; Wilson et al., 1970).

Prolactin (PRL)

PRL is a large polypeptide produced by the anterior pituitary gland. When administered to animals, it influences parental behavior (Prange et al., 1978b). It has not been used as an independent variable in psychiatric research. Its use as a dependent variable will be discussed below.

Growth Hormone (GH)

GH is a 191-membered amino acid chain. It bears resemblance to human chorionic somatomammotropin and prolactin (Daughaday, 1974). GH influences many metabolic processes, a description of which goes beyond the scope of this presentation. In man, it has well documented anabolic and diabetogenic effects (Daughaday, 1974).

It has been shown recently that human GH tends to heal stress ulcers in patients with neoplasms (Winawer et al., 1975). Direct mucosal effects provide a sufficient explanation for this observation. However, possible CNS effects of GH cannot be excluded, especially since stress ulcers can occur in a variety of conditions, including cerebral lesions.

GH has not been given to depressed patients. However, it is important to note that in the diencephalic syndrome of children, there is an overabundant secretion of GH, and the children often show euphoria (Reichlin, 1974).

Vasopressin (VP) and Oxytocin (OXT)

The posterior lobe of the pituitary gland secretes two peptides, VP and OXT, both of which are elaborated in brain. VP, synthesized mostly in the supraoptic nucleus, reduces water excretion by the kidney and increases smooth muscle tone (Kleeman and Vorhen, 1974). VP is also called antidiuretic hormone. OXT, synthesized largely in the paraventricular nucleus, facilitates milk ejection (Kleeman and Vorhen, 1974). It is commonly used as a therapeutic agent to produce uterine contraction. VP contains eight amino acid residues arrange with a free member S-S bonded ring and a tail composed of three amino acids (Leaf and Coggins, 1974). OXT differs from VP in only two locations on the molecule.

DeWied and his colleagues (DeWied, 1973; DeWied and Gispen, 1977; DeWied et al., 1975) have evaluated the role of VP and related substances in learning and memory processes in animals. Pedersen and Prange (1979) showed that OXT, given centrally to virgin female rats in the presence of pups, will promptly induce maternal behavior.

To our knowledge, neither VP nor OXT has been administered to depressed patients. Forizs, however, found VP useful in schizophrenic patients in early, uncontrolled studies (Forizs et al., 1954).

Recently, Gold et al. (1978) have proposed a possible role for VP in affective disorders. Briefly, they think that VP can influence several processes that are at issue in affective illness, namely "alterations in memory, changes in pain sensitivity, synchronization of biological rhythms, the timing and quality of rapid eye movement sleep, and the regulation of fluid and electrolyte balance."

Opiate Related Substances

A striking advance in neurobiology was the demonstration that the nervous system and other tissues contain peptides that mimic, more or less closely, the actions of opiate alkaloids (Costa and Trabucchi, 1978; Goldstein, 1976; Verebey et al., 1978, for a review). These peptides are the penta-peptides, leu- and met-enkephalin, and the larger endorphins. In general, the enkephalins are heterogenously distributed in the CNS whereas the endorphins are found mainly in the pituitary gland. Blume et al. (1977) have discovered an endogenous opiate-like substance that is not a peptide.

Two major strategies have been employed to evaluate the functional role of opiate-like peptides in affective disorders: administration of opiate-like peptides; and administration of opiate antagonists.

In an uncontrolled study, Kline et al. (1977) injected various doses of β-endorphin (1.5–8 mg IV) in three depressed and three schizophrenic patients. All schizophrenic patients showed rapid improvement as regards cognitive impairment, and two of the depressed patients exhibited improvement in mood. On second injection, larger doses of β-endorphin were administered, but no objective or subjective changes were noted.

Davis and his coworkers (1977) injected naloxone (0.4 to 10 mg) in five patients with affective disorders in a double-blind study. There was no improvement in mood as assessed either by the patients themselves or by the physicians. Terenius and Wahlstrom (1978) and Terenius et al. (1977) administered naloxone (0.4–0.8 mg tid) to five depressed patients. No mood changes occurred.

Insulin

Insulin was the first peptide used in psychiatry for therapeutic purposes. In 1928, Schmidt systematically studied the effects of insulin in schizophrenic patients. Beneficial effects were noted, even when insulin administration was accompanied by carboyhydrate administration to prevent hypoglycemia, and this phenomenon has been confirmed in many later studies (Rinkel and Himwich, 1959, for a review). Cowie et al. (1924) gave small dose of insulin along with glucose to depressed patients and noted no significant behavioral improvement.

Glutathione

Glutathione, a tripeptide (γ-glutamyl-cysteinyl-glycine), plays an important role in oxidation-reduction systems of cells. It is widely distributed in both animals and plants. Several enzymes related to carbohydrate and lipid metabolism depend on glutathione for their activity (Meister and Tate, 1976).

In 1957, Altschule et al. injected glutathione, 0.5 mg/kg, in five mentally ill patients. One patient, diagnosed as "psychoneurotic, depressive reaction" did not show behavioral improvement. However, three patients diagnosed as "manic depressive psychosis, depressed phase," showed clinical improvement after tripeptide injection. In two of these patients, a remission of depressive symptoms occurred, while one patient reported increased "feeling of relaxation." Moreover, one patient diagnosed as a paranoid schizophrenic improved after several infusions of glutathione. Since all patients showed changes in carbohydrate metabolism after glutathione injection, it is difficult to assess whether a direct effect of glutathione accounted for the behavioral changes observed.

Endocrine Studies

TRH

TRH causes the release from the anterior pituitary gland of TSH, PRL, and, in certain conditions, GH (Bowers et al., 1971; Maeda et al., 1975; Sawin and Hershman, 1976). Thus the administration of the tripeptide allows the observation of both behavioral and endocrine responses.

There is now broad agreement that some euthyroid depressed patients show grossly blunted TSH responses (Table 2). This event has not yet been

Table 2. TRH-Induced TSH Response in Affective Disorders

Authors	N	
		Depression
Prange et al. (1972)	10	All responses borderline low or absent. Thyroid state normal.
Kastin et al. (1972)	5	Four showed diminished responses.
Shopsin et al. (1973)	2	Responses normal.
Coppen et al. (1974)	16	Four showed no response. Thyroid state normal.
Chazot et al. (1974)	30	Fifteen showed diminished responses.
Ehrensing et al. (1974)	8	Three showed diminished responses.
Hutton (1974)	1	Baseline TSH as well as TSH response diminished.
Takahashi et al. (1974)	36	Twelve showed diminished responses.
Dimitrikoudi et al. (1974)	2	Responses normal.
van den Burg et al. (1975)	10	Mean TSH response diminished. Thyroid state normal.
Kirkegaard et al. (1975)	15	Mean response diminished in depression as compared to recovery; diminished response related to early relapse.
Widerlov and Sjostrom (1975)	10	Baseline TSH as well as TSH responses lower than in hospitalized, non-depressed controls.
Maeda et al. (1975)	13	Mean response diminished as compared to controls.
Pecknold et al. (1976)	6	Diminished in all patients. All patients euthyroid.
Loosen et al. (1976)	23	Six showed diminished responses. No correlation with age, severity of illness, clinical subtypes, or clinical remission.
van den Burg et al. (1976)	10	Responses normal. TRH infused during 4 hr period, possibly masking blunting.
Gold et al. (1977)	23	TSH responses lower in unipolar than in bipolar patients or controls. Negative correlation of CSF-5HIAA and baseline TSH.
Gregoire et al. (1977)	19	TSH response to TRH diminished in depression, normalized after clinical remission.
Vogel et al. (1977)	15	Baseline TSH as well as response to TRH diminished.
Loosen et al. (1978)	7	TSH blunting related to serum cortisol elevation.
Kirkegaard et al. (1978)	74	Mean TSH response diminished in manic depressive disease; normal in neurotic and reactive depression.
		Mania
Takahashi et al. (1974)	8	TSH response somewhat diminished.
Kirkegaard et al. (1978)	14	Tendency toward diminished response.

convincingly linked to any demographic or subdiagnostic feature (Loosen et al., 1976; Prange, 1976a). It appears not to be the result of hyperthyroidism or of thyroidal activation. Indeed, Takahashi et al. (1974) showed that patients with the lowest thyroid indices may show the greatest blunting. In some patients blunting may be related to elevated cortisol (Loosen et al., 1978a,b). Many authors, however, have found TSH blunting in patients in remission (Coppen et al., 1974; Kirkegaard et al., 1975; Loosen et al., 1977; Maeda et al., 1975), when cortisol is usually normal.

TSH blunting occurs not only in depression, but also in alcoholism (Loosen and Prange, 1979b; Loosen et al., 1979). Thus two important questions emerge: does TSH blunting sometimes reflect genetic predispostion; does the phenomenon represent a biological link between some depressed

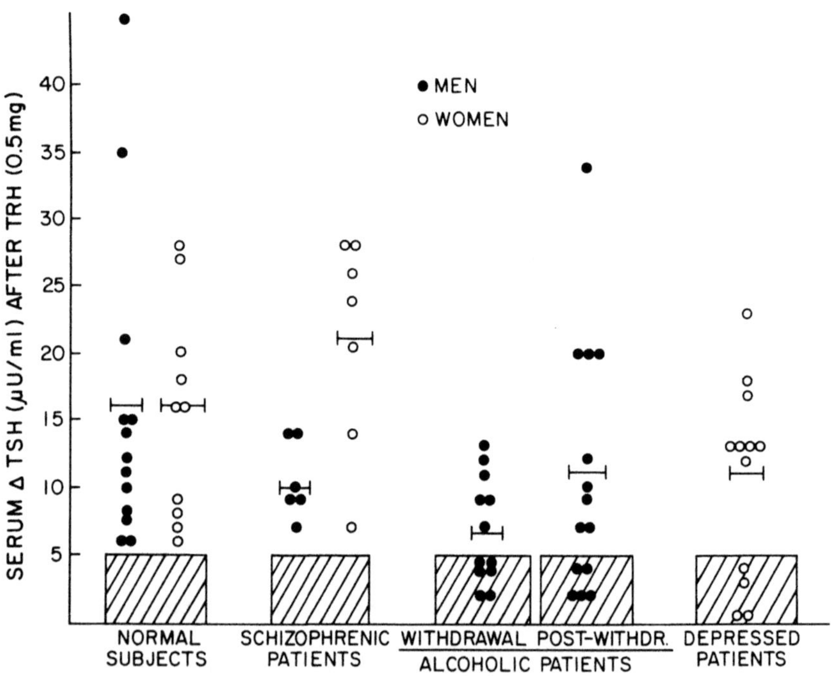

FIG. 1. Using the same technique in all cases, we injected TRH, 0.5 mg IV in one minute, in patients in various diagnostic groups or in control subjects matched for age and sex. Alcoholic patients were in acute alcohol withdrawal or the postwithdrawal state one week later, when all symptoms of acute withdrawal had disappeared. TSH was measured in serum at baseline and at regular intervals after injection. For each patient and subject, the baseline value was subtracted from the peak response, yielding a difference score (Δ). Mean values are indicated for sexes within diagnostic groups. Some depressed and some alcoholic patients (but not schizophrenic patients) showed blunted TSH responses ($\Delta < 5$ μU/ml TSH).

and some alcoholic patients? Here it is important to note that TSH blunting is not seen in schizophrenic patients, indicating that the fault is not a non-specific attribute of mental illness (Fig. 1).

LHRH

LHRH releases LH and FSH from the anterior pituitary gland which in turn induce gonadal stimulation.

Ettigi and Brown (1978) injected LHRH in a group of depressed patients. They found a significantly increased LH response in men with secondary depression as compared to men with primary unipolar depression. Since sexual disturbances usually occur in depression, the lack of investigations of the hypothalamic-pituitary-gonadal axis in this condition is striking.

MIF-I

MIF-I inhibits release by the anterior pituitary gland of MSH (Vale et al., 1977). It is of interest to note that the structure of MIF-I occurs as the side chain of the OXT molecule (Nair et al., 1972). Ehrensing and Kastin (1974, 1978) studied the behavioral effects of this tripeptide in depression but did not report endocrine effects.

ACTH

ACTH stimulates the secretion of glucocorticoids from the adrenal cortex (Daughaday, 1974). It is now an established finding of psychoendocrinology that about 40 percent of patients with depression show findings in the hypothalamic-pituitary-adrenal axis reminiscent of diencephalic Cushing's disease (Carroll and Mendels, 1976).

The best evidence that these derangements are based in central disinhibition of the axis is the poor suppressibility of the anterior pituitary secretion, ACTH, by dexamethasone. After dexamethasone, cortisol is poorly suppressed or, if suppressed, escapes early, indicating that the adrenal cortex has continued to receive stimulation from higher centers. The circadian profiles of cortisol in diencephalic Cushing's disease and in depression can be remarkably similar, and hormonal elevations are often similar in degree (Sachar et al., 1973b). It is interesting to note, however, that the physical stigmata of Cushing's disease have not yet been reported in depressed patients. Whatever the fault in the hypothalamic-pituitary-adrenal axis in depression, it seems to be limited to the state of depression and cannot be observed in remission (Carroll and Mendels, 1976).

TSH

The resting TSH levels are usually normal in depressed patients (Coppen et al., 1974; Kirkegaard et al., 1975; Loosen et al., 1978a; Maeda, 1975), as are the thyroid responses to TSH injection (Prange et al., 1970). However, Weeke and Weeke (1978) have shown that in severe endogenous depression there is loss of diurnal rhythmicity of TSH, due mainly to loss of the nocturnal TSH elevation. The TSH response to TRH, on the other hand, as described above, is often blunted in depressed patients.

PRL

In depressed patients PRL secretion has been studied in response to TRH (Ehrensing et al., 1974; Maeda et al., 1975) and L-Dopa (Sachar et al., 1973A). PRL response to TRH was found to be diminished (Ehrensing et al., 1974) or increased (Maeda et al., 1975). After L-Dopa, depressed patients showed a normal PRL suppression (Sachar et al., 1973a). Basal PRL concentration in depressed patients was found to be increased in one study (Sachar et al., 1973a) and normal in another (Arana et al., 1977). Here it should be kept in mind that elevated PRL may reflect diminished central dopaminergic activity.

GH

While GH has not been given to depressed patients it has been employed as a dependent variable, after insulin administration. Thus, one peptide, insulin, has been used to evoke the response of another, GH, just as TRH has been used to evoke TSH responses.

The response of GH to insulin-induced hypoglycemia was found to be diminished in depressed patients (Gruen et al., 1975, Mueller et al., 1972, Sachar et al., 1971, 1973a). Since estrogens potentiate the GH response, and since estrogens decline after menopause, Gruen and his colleagues (1975) tested the possibility that the finding might have been an artifact of postmenopausal women being overly represented in depressed groups. However, the finding persisted when postmenopausal women with unipolar depression were compared to postmenopausal controls.

Heninger and his colleagues (1976) performed insulin hypoglycemia testing (insulin tolerance test, ITT) in 40 depressed patients before and during treatment with amitriptyline when "most of their symptoms had decreased." They found a mean decrease in resting GH levels upon second testing. In addition, these authors reported "several correlations between increased symptomatology and decreased GH responsiveness in the ITT."

VP

VP is noted here as a possible dependent variable in psychoendocrine research in depression because of the theoretical considerations submitted by Gold et al. (1978). Data pertaining to these concepts have not yet appeared.

Opiate Related Substance

Terenius and Wahlstrom (1978) and Terenius et al. (1977) measured opiate-like activity in CSF from psychiatric and chronic pain patients. Two fractions (I and II) with opiate-like activity were isolated from human CSF. Control values from healthy volunteers fell within narrow limits whereas psychotic patients showed a broad range of values. Patients with depression had higher levels of Fraction I and II. After administration of naloxone (0.4–0.8 mg, three times per day) to five depressed patients (Terenius et al., 1977), Fraction I levels decreased in depressed patients but not in controls.

Insulin

As described above, insulin has been used to test the integrity of the GH response to hypoglycemia in depressed patients.

Glutathione

As described above, Altschule (1975) noted that glutathione usually tended to correct putative faults in carbohydrate metabolism when given to psychiatric patients.

COMMENT

To understand the behavioral effects of peptides in affective disorders one must look outside the affective disorders, both to other human disorders and to animal behavioral studies.

From animal studies two generalizations emerge. First, nearly all the peptides mentioned in this review exert behavioral effects in animals. Second, in animals at least some of the behavioral effects of most peptides have been shown to be independent of the peptide's endocrine effects. In studies of TRH, for example, hypophysectomy has not interfered with, and administration of TSH or thyroid hormones has not mimicked, behavioral effects. The demonstration of such effects in animals increased the plausibility of behavioral effects in man though such effects must, of course, be demonstrated directly.

For one peptide (TRH) a beneficial effect in mania has been claimed, and for five peptides (TRH, MIF-I, ACTH, β-endorphin, and glutathione) a beneficial effect in depression has been claimed. Animal models for depression exist, but they have not been used systematically to evaluate peptides. Pharmacologic screening procedures for putative antidepressant drugs also exist, and these have been used to some extent in peptide investigations. Thus, both TRH and MIF-I enhance the activation produced by parygline-L-DOPA in aggregated male mice, while TRH, but not MIF-I, is active in a similar test involving I-5-hydroxytryptophan (Prange et al., 1978b).

Human studies in conditions other than affective disorders provide another persepctive to the behavioral actions of peptides in affective disorders. Both TRH and MIF-I have been used in Parkinson's disease, and both have been reported to elevate mood and to increase the sense of well-being of these patients (Prange et al., 1978b). Furthermore, TRH has been reported in three consecutive double-blind studies to produce mild euphoria in normal subjects (Betts, 1976; Wilson et al., 1973; Wilson et al., unpublished data). These findings, like the findings in screening tests for antidepresant drugs, support the notion that the tripeptides are behaviorally active in depression.

Studies of other human disorders are also informative. Just as TRH has been reported to produced brief and partial improvement in depressed patients and in manic patients, it has also been reported to produce similar benefits in some schizophrenics (Prange et al., 1978a, b, 1979) and in depressed alcoholics (Lossen and Prange, 1979b; Loosen et al., 1979). MIF-I has not been used in mental disorders other than depression, but β-endorphin appears to confer at least as much benefit in schizophrenia as in depression (Kline et al., 1977). These findings, taken together, suggest that the behavioral effects of peptides are not specific to affective disorders. Indeed, they are probably not specific to any disease entity. We think that these endogenous substances probably contribute to the regulation of adaptive processes, dysfunction of which cut across diagnostic lines. At the present state of research, behavioral studies of peptides in affective disorders have taught us at least as much about peptides as about affective disorders.

Peptides have been used more often to elucidate the endocrine state of patients with affective disorders than to alter their clinical condition. Evidence from this and related work has established beyond reasonable doubt that in depression, there is often a state of dysregulation in the hypothalamus and possibly in higher centers as well. The strongest evidence for this conclusion comes from studies of the hypothalamic-pituitary adrenal axis, wherein central disinhibition seems often to occur. The blunted TSH response to TRH seen in some depressed patients may also be regarded as evidence of central dysregulation when it cannot be regarded as secondary to elevated cortisol (as in patients in remission) or as a consequence of thyroid activation.

The influence of cortisol on the TSH response to TRH suggest two considerations for future psychoendocrine research. The first is the need to study relationships between the various hypothalamic-pituitary target gland axes rather than merely events within a single axis. The second consideration is the need for longitudinal studies to sort out possible causal events from events that may only reflect the fact of established illness.

Endocrine changes in affective disorders have often been employed to construct inferences about biogenic amine function. Used in this way, they tend generally to support findings from psychopharmacology. Thus, for example, disinhibition of ACTH supports the concept that in depression central noradrenergic systems are hypoactive, for such systems appear to inhibit ACTH secretion (McCann and Ojeda, 1976). Such generalizations, of course, are tenuous, for a given pituitary hormone may be influenced by more than one hypothalamic hormone, and each of them may be influenced by the activity of several transmitters as well as by possible feedback influences from the endocrine system itself (Daughaday, 1974; Reichlin, 1974). Another scheme for formulating some endocrine data is apparent if, as we have suggested in this review, at least some hypothalamic releasing factors exert behavioral effects. One might then formulate results in terms of releasing factors rather than in terms of the aminergic systems that influence them. For example, diminished GH response to insulin is evidence for increased activity of the tetradecapeptide, GH inhibiting hormone (GHIH). In a similar way, a diminished TSH response to TRH can be taken as evidence for the same change, when other explanations are absent, for GHIH is known to inhibit this response (Vale et al., 1973). One may postulate, then, excess GHIH activity in depression; indeed, in animal systems GHIH exerts a variety of behavioral effects which are consistent with this view (Prange et al., 1978a,b), insofar as animal models can be instructive about this complex human disorder. Formulations of this kind, of course, must be regarded as no less tentative than formulations that are directed toward the further explication of biogenic amine changes. What does appear clear is that at least some hormones endogenous to brain, like some hormones of peripheral origin (Loosen and Prange, 1979a; Prange and Lipton, 1972a), can alter behavioral states. It is quite likely that they do so by altering the function of neurons that employ biogenic amines as transmitters. Additional research may clarify the points of communication between the two great communication systems of the organisms, the nervous system and the endocrine system.

ACKNOWLEDGEMENTS

This research was supported by grants from the National Institute of Mental Health, MH33127 and MH22536 (a Career Scientist Award to AJP)

REFERENCES

Altschule, M.D., Siegal, E.P., and Hennemann, D.H. Carbohydrate metabolism in brain disease: VII. The effect of glutathione on carbohydrate intermediary metabolism in schizophrenic and manic-depressive psychoses. *AMA Arch. Int. Med.* 99, 22–27 (1957).

Arana G., Boyd, A.E., Reichlin, S., and Lipsitt, D. Prolactin levels in depression. *Psychosom. Med.* 39, 193–197 (1977).

Benkert, O. Studies on pituitary hormones and releasing hormones in depression and sexual impotence, in *Hormones, Homeostasis and the Brain, Progress in Brain Research* 42, W.H. Gispen, Tj. B. van Wimersma Greidanus, B. Bohus, and D. deWied, eds. Elsevier, Amsterdam (1975), pp. 25–36.

Benkert, O., Gordon, A., and Martschke, D. The comparison of thyrotropin releasing hormone, luteinising hormone-releasing hormone and placebo in depressive patients using a double-blind cross-over technique. *Psychopharmacologia* (Berl.) 40, 191–198 (1974).

Berthold, A.A. Transplantation der hoden. *Arch. Anat. Physiol. Wiss. Med.* 16, 42 (1849).

Betts, T.A., Smith, J., Pidd, S., Mackintosh, J., Harvey, P., and Funicane, J. The effects of thyrotropin-releasing hormone on measures of mood in normal women. *Brit. J. Clin. Pharmacol.* 3, 469–473 (1976).

Blume, A.J., Sharr, J., Finberg, J.P.M., and Spector, S.S. Binding of the endogenous nonpeptide morphine-like compound to opiate receptors. *Proc. Natl. Acad. Sci. USA* 74(11), 4931 (1977).

Boler, J., Enzmann, F., Folkers, K., Bowers, C.Y., and Schally, A.V. The identity of chemical and hormonal properties of the thyrotropin releasing hormone and pyroglutamyl-histidyl-proline-amide. *Biochem. Biophys. Res. Commun.* 37, 705 (1969).

Bowers, C.Y., Friesen, N.G., Hwang, P., Guyda, H.Y., and Folkers, K. Prolactin and thyrotropin release in man by synthetic pyroglutamyl-histidyl-prolinamide. *Biochem. Biophys. Res. Commun.* 45, 1033–1041 (1971).

Brownstein, M.J., Palkovits, M., Saavedra, J.M., and Kizer, J. Distribution of hypothalamic hormones and neurotransmitters within the diencephalon, in *Frontiers in Neuroendocrinology*. L. Martini, and W.F. Ganong, eds. Raven Press, New York (1976), pp. 1–23.

Burgus, R., Dunn, T.F., Desiderio, D., and Guillemin, R. Structure moleculaire de facteur hypothalamique hypophysiotrope TRH d'origine ovine: Mise en evidence par spectrometrie de masse de la sequence PCA-His-Pro-NH_2. *C.R. Acad. Sci. (Paris)*, 269, 1870–1873 (1969).

Carroll, B.J. and Mendels, J. Neuroendocrine regulation in affective disorders, in *Hormones, Behavior and Psychopathology*. E.J. Sacher, ed. Raven Press, New York, (1976), pp. 41–68.

Chazot, G., Chalumeau, A., Aimard, G., Mornes, R., Garde, A., Schott, B., and Girard P.F. Thyrotropin releasing hormone and depressive states: from agroagonines to TRH. *Lyon Medical* 231, 831–836 (1974).

Coppen, A., Montgomery, S., Peet, M., and Bailey, J. Thyrotropin-releasing hormone in the treatment of depression. *Lancet* ii, 433–434 (1974).

Coppen, A., Prange, A.J., Jr., Whybrow, P.C., and Noguera, R. Abnormalities of indoleamines in affective disorders. *Arch. Gen. Psychiat.* 26, 474–478 (1972).

Costa, E., and Trabucchi, M. *The Endorphins.* Raven Press, New York (1978).

Cowie, D., Parsons, J.P., and Raphael, T. Insulin and mental depression. *Arch. Neur. Psych.* 12, 522 (1924).

Daughaday, W.H. The adenohypophysis, in *Textbook of Endocrinology.* R.H. Williams, ed. W.B. Saunders Co., Philadelphia (1974).

Davis, K.L., Berger, P.A., Hollister, L.E., and Defraites, E. Physostigmine in mania. *Arch. Gen. Psychiat.* 35, 119–122 (1978).

Davis, G.C., Bunney, W.E., Jr., Defraites, E.G., Kleinman, J.E., van Kammen, D.P., and Wyatt, R.J. Intravenous naloxone administration in schizophrenia and effective illness. *Science* 197, 74–77 (1977).

DeWied, D. The role of the posterior pituitary and its peptides on the maintenance of conditioned avoidance behavior, in *Hormones and Brain Function.* K. Lissak, ed. Plenum Press, New York (1973).

DeWied, D., and Gispen, W.H. Behavioral effects of peptides, in *Peptides in Neurobiology.* H. Gainer, ed. Plenum Press, New York (1977).

DeWied, D., Bohus, B., Urban, I., van Wimersma Greidnus, Tj.B., and Gispen, W.H. Pituitary peptides and memory, in *Peptides: Chemistry Structure and Biology.* R. Walter and J. Meienhofer, eds. Ann Arbor Publishers, Ann Arbor, Michigan (1975).

Dimitrikoudi, M., Hanson-Norty, E., and Jenner, F.A. T.R.H. in psychoses. *Lancet* i, 456 (1974).

Ehrensing, R.H., and Kastin, A.J. MSH release-inhibiting hormone as an antidepressant. *Arch. Gen. Psychiat.* 30, 63–65 (1974).

Ehrensing, R.H. and Kastin, A.J. Dose-related biphasic effect of prolyl-leucyl-glycinamide (MIF-I) in depression. *Am. J. Psychiat.* 135, 562–566 (1978).

Ehrensing, R.H., Kastin, A.J., Schalch, D.S., Friesen, H.G., Vargas, J.R., and Schally, A.V. Affective state and thyrotropin and prolactin responses after repeated injections of thyrotropin-releasing hormone in depressed patients. *Am. J. Psychiat.* 131(6), 714–718 (1974).

Endroczi, E. Pavlovian conditioning and adaptive hormones, in *Hormones and Behavior.* S. Levine, ed. Academic Press, New York (1972), pp. 173–208.

Ettigi, P.G., and Brown, G. TSH and LH responses in subtypes of depression. *Annual Meeting, American Psychosomatic Society*, Washington, D.C., (March 1978).

Forizs, L., Vitols, E., and Vitols, M. Combined pitressin and electric shock in schizophrenia. *Dis. Nerv. Syst.* 15, 176–179 (1954).

Furlong, F.W., Brown, G.M, and Beeching, M.R. Thyrotropin-releasing hormone: Differential antidepressant and endocrinological effects. *Am. J. Psychiat.* 133, 1187–1190 (1976).

Goetsch, E. Newer methods in the diagnosis of thyroid disorders: Pathological and clinical. *N.Y. State J. Med.* 18, 259–267 (1918).

Gold, P.W., Goodwin, F.K., and Reus, V.I. Vasopressin in affective illness. *Lancet* i, 1233–1236 (1978).

Gold, P.W., Goodwin, F.K., Wehr, T., and Rebar, R. Pituitary thyrotropin response to thyrotropin-releasing hormone in affective illness: Relationship to spinal fluid amine metabolites. *Am. J. Psychiat.* 134(9), 1028–1031 (1977).

Goldstein, A. Opioid peptides in pituitary and brain. *Science* 193, 1081–1086 (1976).

Goodwin, F.K., and Potter, W.Z. The biology of affective illness: Amine neurotransmitters and drug response, in *Depression, Biology, Psychodynamics and Treatment.* J.O. Cole, A.F. Schatzberg, and S.H. Frazier, eds. Plenum Press, New York (1976).

Gregoire, F., Brauman, H., de Buck, R., and Corvilain, J. Hormone release in depressed patients before and after recovery. *Psychoneuroendocrinology* 2, 303–312 (1977).

Gruen, P.H., Sachar, E.J., Altman, N., and Sassin, J. Growth hormone responses to hypoglycemia in postmenopausal depressed women. *Arch. Gen. Psychiat.* 32, 31–33 (1975).

Guillemin, R. Peptides in the brain: The new endocrinology of the neuron. *Science* 202, 390–402 (1978).

Hamilton, M. A rating scale for depression. *J. Neurol. Neurogsurg. Psychiat.* 23, 56–62 (1960).

Heninger, G.R., Mueller, P.S., and Davis, L.S. Responsivness of endocrine-energy metabolism systems in depression and schizophrenia: Relationships to symptomatology, in *Hormones, Behavior and Psychopathology*. E.J. Sachar, ed. Raven Press, New York (1976), pp. 237–242.

Huey, L.Y., Janowsky, D.S., Mandell, A.J., Judd, L.L., and Pendery, M. Preliminary studies on the use of thyrotropin releasing hormone in manic states, depression, and the dysphoria of alcohol withdrawal. *Psychopharmacol. Bull.* 11(1), 24–27 (1975).

Hutton, W.N. Thyrotropin-releasing hormone in depression. *Lancet* ii, 53 (1974).

Kastin, A.J., Ehrensing, R.H., Schalch, D.S., and Anderson, M.S. Improvement in mental depression with decreased thyrotropin response after administration of thyrotropin-releasing hormone. *Lancet* ii, 740–742 (1972).

Kirkegaard, C., Bjorum, N., Cohn, D., and Lauridsen, U.B. TRH stimulation test in manic depressive disease. *Arch. Gen. Psychiat.* 35, 1017–1023 (1978).

Kirkegaard, C., Norlem, N., Lauridsen, U.B., Bjorum, N., and Christiansen, C. Protirelin stimulation test and thyroid function during treatment of depression. *Arch. Gen. Psychiat.* 32, 1115–1118 (1975).

Kleeman, C.R., and Vorhen, H. Water metabolism and the neurophypophyseal hormones, in *Duncan's Diseases of Metabolism: Endocrinology* 7th ed. P.K. Bondy, and L.E. Rosenberg, eds. W.B. Saunders, Co., Philadelphia (1974).

Kline, N.S., Li, C.H., Lehmann, H.E., Lajtha, A., Laski, E., and Cooper, T. β-Endorphin-induced changes in schizophrenic and depressed patients. *Arch. Gen. Psychiat.* 34, 1111–1113 (1977).

Krieger, P.T., Liotta, A., and Brownstein, M.J. Presence of corticotropin in brain of normal and hypophysectomized rats. *Proc. Natl. Acad. Sci. USA* 74, 648–652 (1977).

Leaf, A., and Coggins, C.H. The neurohypophysis, in *Textbook of Endocrinology*. R.H. Williams, ed. W.B. Saunders, Philadelphia (1974), pp. 80–94.

Loosen, P.T., and Prange, A.J., Jr. Psychoendocrinology: A brief survey, in *Psychiatric Complications of Medical Drugs*. R.I. Shader, ed. Raven Press, New York (1979a).

Loosen, P.T., and Prange, A.J., Jr. Thyrotropin response to thyrotropin releasing hormone: Findings in depressed and alcoholic patients, in *Alcoholism and Affective Disorders*. D.W. Goodwin, and C.K. Erickson, eds. Spectrum Publications, New York (1979b) pp. 145–155.

Loosen, P.T., Prange, A.J., Jr., and Wilson, I.C. Influence of cortisol on TRH induced TSH response in depression. *Am. J. Psychiat.* 135, 244–246 (1978a).

Loosen, P.T., Prange, A.J., Jr., and Wilson, I.C. The TSH response to TRH in psychiatric patients: Relation to serum cortisol. *Prog. Neuropsychopharmacol.* 2, 479–486 (1978b).

Loosen, P.T., Prange, A.J., Jr., and Wilson, I.C. Thyrotropin releasing hormone (TRH) in depressed alcoholic men: Behavioral changes and endocrine responses. *Arch. Gen. Psychiat.* 36, 540–547 (1979).

Loosen, P.T., Wilson, I.C., and Prange, A.J., Jr. Behavioral changes in depression after TRH: Antagonism by pretreatment with thyroid hormones (unpublished data).

Loosen, P.T., Prange, A.J., Jr., Wilson, I.C., and Lara, P.P. Pituitary responses to thyrotropin releasing hormone in depressed patients: A review. *Pharmacol. Biochem. Behav.* (Suppl. 1), 5, 95–101 (1976).

Loosen, P.T., Prange, A.J., Jr., Wilson, I.C., Lara, P.P., and Pettus, C. Thyroid stimulating hormone response after thyrotropin releasing hormone in depressed, schizophrenic and normal women. *Psychoneuroendocrinology* 2, 137–148 (1977).

Maeda, K., Kato, Y., Ohgo, S., Chihara, K., Yoshimoto, Y., Yamaguchi, N., Kuromaru, S., and Imura, H. Growth hormone and prolactin release after injection of thyrotropin releasing hormone in patients with depression. *J. Clin. Endocrin. Metab.* 40, 501–505 (1975).

Mazure, C., and Gershon, E.S. Blindness and reliability in lifetime psychiatric diagnoses. *Arch. Gen. Psychiat.* 36, 521–525 (1979).

McCann, S.M. and Ojeda, S.R. Synaptic transmitters involved in the release of hypothalamic releasing and inhibitory hormones, in *Reviews Neuroscience*, Vol. 2. S. Ehrenpreis and I.J. Kopin, eds. Raven Press, New York (1976), pp. 91–110.

Meister, A., and Tate, S.S. Glutathione and related f-glutamyl compounds: Biosynthesis and utilization. *Ann. Rev. Biochem.* 45, 559–603 (1976).

Moldow, R.L., and Yalow, R.S. Extrahypophyseal distribution of thyrotropin as a function of brain size. *Life Sciences* 22, 1859–1864 (1978).

Moss, R.L. Relationship between the central regulation of gonadotropin and mating behavior in female rats, in *Reproductive Behavior*. W. Montagna and W.A. Sadler, eds. Plenum Press, New York (1975), pp. 55–76.

Moss, R.L., and McCann, S.M. Induction of mating behavior in rats by luteinizing hormone-releasing factor. *Science* 181, 177–179 (1973).

Mueller, P.S., Heninger, G.R., and McDonald, R.K. Studies on glucose utilization and insulin sensitivity in affective disorders, in *Recent Advances in the Psychobiology of the Depressive Illness*. T.A. Williams, M.M. Kata, and J.A. Shield, Jr., eds. U.S. DHEW Publication 70–9053, U.S. Government Printing Office, Washington, D.C. (1972), pp. 235–248.

Nair, R.M.G., Kastin, A.J., and Schally, A.V. Isolation and Structure of hypothalamic MSH release-inhibiting hormones. *Biochem. Biophys. Res. Commun.* 43, 1376–1381 (1971).

Nair, R.M.G., Kastin, A.J., and Schally, A.V. Isolation and structure of another hypothalamic peptide possessing MSH-release inhibiting activity. *Biochem. Biophys. Res. Commun.* 47, 1420–1425 (1972).

Pecknold, J.C., and Ban, T.A. TRH in depressive illness. *Pharmacopsychiatry* 12, 166–173 (1977).

Pedersen, C.A., and Prange, A.J., Jr. Two hour induction of full maternal behavior in intact virgin rats after intracerebroventricular administration of oxytocin. Tenth Annual Meeting of the International Society for Psychoneuroendocrinology, Park City, Utah, August 8–10, (1979) (Abstract).

Plotnikoff, N.P., Prange, A.J., Jr., Breese, G.R., Anderson, M.S., and Wilson, I.C. The effects of thyrotropin-releasing hormone on DOPA response in normal, hypophysectomized and thyroidectomized animals, in *The Thyroid Axis, Drugs, and Behavior*. A.J. Prange, Jr., ed. Raven Press, New York (1974), pp. 103–114.

Prange, A.J., Jr. Patterns of pituitary responses to thyrotropin releasing hormone in depressed patients: A review, in *Phenomenology and Treatment of Depression*. W.E. Fann, I. Karacan, A. Pokorny, and R.L. Williams, eds. Spectrum Publications, New York (1976a), pp. 1–15.

Prange, A.J., Jr., and Lipton, M.A. Hormones and behavior: Some principles and findings, in *Psychiatric Complications of Medical Drugs*. R.I. Shader, ed. Raven Press, New York (1972a), pp. 213–249.

Prange, A.J., Jr., and Wilson, I.C. Thyrotropin releasing hormone (TRH) for the immediate relief of depression: A preliminary report. *Psychopharmacologia* 26, 82 (1972b).

Prange, A.J., Jr., Loosen, P.T., and Nemeroff, C.B. Peptides: Application to research in nervous and mental disorders, in *New Frontiers of Psychotropic Drug Research*. S. Fielding, ed. Futura Publishing Co., Inc., Mt. Kisco, New York (1979), pp. 117–189.

Prange, A.J., Jr., Nemeroff, C.B., and Loosen, P.T. Behavioral effects of hypothalamic peptides, in *Centrally Acting Peptides*. J. Hughes, ed. MacMillan Press, Ltd., Basingstoke, England (1978a), pp. 99–118.

Prange, A.J., Jr., Breese, G.R., Wilson, I.C., and Lipton, M.A. Brain-behavioral effects of hypothalamic releasing hormones: A generic hypothesis, in *Anatomical Neuroendocrinology*. W.E. Stumpf and L.D. Grant, eds. S. Karger, Basel (1976b), pp. 357–367.

Prange, A.J., Jr., Lipton, M.A., Nemeroff, C.B., and Wilson, I.C. The role of hormones in depression. *Life Sciences* 20, 1305–1318 (1977).

Prange, A.J., Jr., Wilson, I.C., Breese, G.R., and Lipton, M.A. Behavioral effects of hypothalamic releasing hormones in animals and man, in *Hormones, Homeostasis and the Brain, Progress in Brain Research*, Vol. 42. W.H. Gispen, Tj. B. van Wimersma Greidanus, B. Bohus, and D. deWied, eds. Elsevier, Amsterdam (1975), pp. 1–9.

Prange, A.J., Jr., Wilson, I.C., Rabon, A.M., and Lipton, M.A. Enhancement of imipramine antidepressant activity by thyroid hormone. *Am. J. Psychiat.* 126, 457–469 (1969).

Prange, A.J., Jr., Nemeroff, C.B., Lipton, M.A., Breese, G.R., and Wilson, I.C. Peptides and the central nervous system, in *Handbook of Psychopharmacology*, Vol. 13. L.L. Iversen, S.D. Iversen, and S.H. Snyder, eds. Plenum Press, New York (1978b), pp. 1–107.

Prange, A.J., Jr., Wilson, I.C., Knox, A., McClane, T.K., and Lipton, M.A. Enhancement of imipramine by thyroid stimulating hormone: Clinical and theoretical implications. *Am. J. Psychiat.* 127(2), 191–199 (1970).

Prange, A.J., Jr., Wilson, I.C., Lara, P.P., Alltop, L. B., and Breese, G.R. Effects of thyrotropin releasing hormone in depression. *Lancet* ii, 999–1002 (1972c).

Prange, A.J., Jr., Wilson, I.C., Lynn, C.W., Alltop, L.B., and Stikeleather, R.A. L-tryptophan in mania: Contribution to a permissive hypothesis of affective disorders. *Arch. Gen. Psychiat.* 30, 56–62 (1974).

Reichlin, S. Neuroendocrinology, in *Textbook of Endocrinology*. R.H. Williams, ed. W.B. Saunders, Philadelphia (1974), pp. 774–831.

Rinkel, M., Himwich, H.E. *Insulin Treatment in Psychiatry*. Philosophical Library, New York, (1959).

Sachar, E.J., Finkelstein, J., and Hellman, J. Growth hormone responses in depressive illness. *Arch. Gen. Psychiat.* 25, 263–269 (1971).

Sachar, E.J., Frantz, A.G., Altman, N., and Sassin, J. Growth hormone and prolactin in unipolar and bipolar depressed patients: Responses to hypoglycemia and L-DOPA. *Am. J. Psychiat.* 130, 1362–1367 (1973a).

Sachar, E.J., Hellman, L., Roffwarg, H., Halpern, F., Fukushima, D., and Gallagher, T. Disrupted 24 hour patterns of cortisol secretion in psychiatric patients. *Arch. Gen. Psychiat.* 23, 289–298 (1973b).

Sawin, C.T., and Hershman, J.M. Clinical use of thyrotropin-releasing hormone. *Pharmac. Ther. C.* 1, 351–366 (1976).

Schally, A.V. Aspects of hypothalamic regulation of the pituitary gland. *Science* 202, 18–28 (1978).

Schatzberg, A.F. Classification of depressive disorders, in *Depression, Biology, Psychodynamics and Treatment*. J.O. Cole, A.F. Schatzberg, and S.H. Frazier, eds. Plenum Press, New York (1976), pp. 13–40.

Schildkraut, J.J., Orsulak, P.J., Gudeman, J.E., Schatzberg, A.F., Rohde, W.A., Labrie, R.A., Cahill, J.R., Cole, J.O., and Frazier, S.H. Norepinephrine metabolism in depressive disorders: Implications for classification of depression, in *Depression, Biology, Psychodynamics and Treatment*. J.O. Cole, A.F. Schatzberg, and S.H. Frazier, eds. Plenum Press, New York (1976), pp. 75–101.

Schmidt, P. Uber organtherapie und insulinbehandlung bei endogenen geistesstorungen. *Klin. Woch.* 7, 839 (1928).

Shopsin, B., Shenkman, L., Blum, M., and Hollander, C. T_3 and TSH response to TRH: Newer aspects of lithium-induced thyroid disturbances in men. *Psychopharm. Bull.* 9, 29 (1973).

Takahashi, S., Kondo, H., Yoshimura, M., and Ochi, Y. Thyrotropin responses to TRH in depressive illness: relation to clinical sub-types and prolonged duration of depressive episode. *Folia Psychiat. Neurol. Jap.* 28, 355–365 (1974).

Terenius, L. and Wahlstrom, A. Physiological and clinical relevance of endorphins, in *Centrally Acting Peptides.* J. Hughes, ed. MacMillan Press, Ltd., London (1978), pp. 161–178.

Terenius, L., Wahlstrom, A., and Agren, A. Naloxone (Narcan) treatment in depression: Clinical observations and effects on CSF endorphin and monoamine metabolites. *Psychopharmacology* 54, 31–33 (1977).

Vale, W., Rivier, C., and Brown, M. Regulatory peptides of the hypothalamus. A review. *Physiology* 39, 473–527 (1977).

Vale, W., Brazeau, P., Rivier, C., Rivier, J., Grant, G., Burgus, R., and Guillemin, R. Inhibitory hypophysiotropic activities of hypothalamic somatostatin. *Fed. Proc.* 32, 211 (1973).

Van den Burg, W., van Praag, H.M., Box, E.R.H., Piers, D.A., van Zanten, A.K., and Doorenbos, H. TRH as a possible quick-acting but short-lasting antidepressant. *Psycholog. Med.* 5, 404–412 (1975).

Van den Burg, W., van Praag, H.M., Box, E.R.H., Piers, D.A., van Zanten, A.K., and Doorenbos, H. TRH by slow, continuous infusion: an antidepressant. *Psycholog. Med.* 6, 393–397 (1976).

Verebey, K., Volavka, J., and Clovet, D. Endorphins in psychiatry. *Arch. Gen. Psychiat.* 35, 877–888 (1978).

Vogel, H.P., Benkert, O., Illig, R., Mueller-Oerlinghausen, B., and Poppenberg, A. Psychoendocrinological and therapeutic effects of TRH in depression. *Acta Psychiat. Scand.* 56, 223–232 (1977).

Waldstein, S.S. Thyroid-catecholaminic interrelations. *Am. Rev. Med.* 17, 123–132 (1966).

Weeke, A., and Weeke, J. Disturbed circadian variation of serum thyrotropin in patients with endogenous depression. *Acta Psychiat. Scand.* 57, 281–289 (1978).

Widerlov, E., and Sjostrom, R. Effects of thyrotropin releasing hormone on endogenous depression. *Nordisk Psychiatrisk Tidskrift* 29, 503–512, (1975).

Wilson, I.C., Prange, A.J., Jr., and Loosen, P.T. Behavioral effects of TRH in normal women: antagonism by pretreatment with thyroid hormones (unpublished data).

Wilson, I.C., Prange, A.J., Jr., McClane, T.K., Rabon, A.M., and Lipton, M.A. Thyroid hormone enhancement of imipramine in non-retarded depression. *N. Engl. J. Med.* 282, 1063–1067 (1970).

Wilson, I.C., Prange, A.J., Jr., Lara, P.P., Alltop, L.B., Stikeleather, R.A., and Lipton, M.A. TRH (lopremone): psychobiological responses of normal women: (I) subjective experience. *Arch. Gen. Psychiat.* 29, 15–32 (1973).

Winawer, S.J., Sherlock, P., Sonnenberg, M., and Vaneamee, P. Beneficial effect of human growth hormone on stress ulcers. *Arch. Intern. Med.* 135, 569–572 (1975).

Winokur, A., and Utiger, R.D. Thyrotropin-releasing hormone: Regional distribution in rat brain. *Science* 185, 265–266 (1974).

Yarbrough, G.G. TRH potentiates excitatory actions of acetylcholine in cerebral cortical neurons. *Nature* 263, 523–524 (1976).

Copyright © 1982, Spectrum Publications, Inc.
The Neural Basis of Behavior

12

Brain Catecholamines in Relation to Afffect

Susan D. Iversen
Paul J. Fray

The Oxford dictionary defines affect as "feeling, emotion, desire especially as leading to action" and emotion as "instinctive feeling as opposed to reason." Within these definitions are the germs of several ideas to be highlighted in this chapter. First, although affect is a felt experience and thus dependent on the nature of sensory input, it leads to behavior. Second, behavior labelled as emotional manifests itself through response patterns. Third, emotional behavior is to be distinguished from reasoning. This distinction suggests that there may be different processes and different brain systems involved in the expression of emotion and reason.

THE RELATIONSHIP BETWEEN EMOTION AND MOTIVATION

Emotion is a major component of the fabric of normal behavior. Darwin (1890, reprinted 1965) was the first to recognize the immense survival value of well-defined emotional responses to new and challenging environmental events.

In emotional behavior we are dealing with responses which, in operational terms, are largely predetermined by genetics, developmental history and learning experience; responses to stimuli which signal events crucial to survival. The implication is that there may be less room for maneuver than with more cognitive behavior, which allows appraisal of new, unpredictable, and changing aspects of the environment. Distinctions of this kind are useful because they focus attention to the extremes of the functional mode. Clearly integration between affect and reason is crucial if behavior is to be influenced by present and past experience. Language and thought are the pillars of the reasoning process and are heavily dependent on the thalamo-cortical circuitries of the forebrain. Emotion, on the other hand, is linked with activity in the limbic forebrain and its strong connections to homeostatic centers of hypothalamus and brain stem. The latter areas of brain have been studied for decades in the context of emotional behavior. In any text book of physiological psychology, reviews can be found of the progress made in such studies, correlating various areas of the limbic system with the expression of emotional behaviors. Opinion differs as to how many emotional states can be identified, but one might be tempted to seek an anxiety circuit, an aggression circuit, one for ecstacy, and so on. In fact it is clear that although a given structure may contribute a specific aspect of behavioral expression, it will be implicated in a broad range of different emotional behaviors, and the task now is to define the general levels of integration capable of involvement in a wide range of emotional behaviors. This leads us to the question of the relationship between emotion and the homeostatic behavioral process of motivation. If an animal is hungry, thirsty, or sexually active, it is said to be "motivated" to behave in order to satisfy its needs. A hungry rat is motivated to press a lever to obtain food. One would not say that such a rat is "emotional," although in terms of our first definition (feeling, especially as leading to action), it is difficult to understand why we do not. Motivation is described in mechanistic terms as an increase in arousal, and it seems reasonable to suggest that emotion and motivation are distinguished, not by the kind of stimuli and responses associated with the two states, but by an intensity continuum. Consider a hungry rat that finds a food source with ease and consider one in direct competition with other animals for a limited source. The behavioral profile will be different in the two animals; the first would be described as motivated and the second as showing emotional behavior, possibly involving aggression or fear, as well as feeding behavior.

Several dynamic models of emotional behavior have been proposed which arrange a number of generally accepted and distinguishable emotional behavior patterns or experienced emotional states on different intensity continua. Such models (illustrated in Fig. 1B) are useful because they stress the following ideas:

(i) groups of emotional behaviors are linked together;

(ii) intensity is an important variable in a model of emotion;

(iii) motivation and emotion can be accommodated within a single model; and

(iv) emotion is a homeostatic mechanism which allows the animal to find the most appropriate level of behavioral output to deal with its present environment.

In Fig. 1B, concentric circles have been added to imply that when relatively low levels of activity are recorded on the three axes, it may be appropriate to describe the behaviors as motivated. When environmental stimuli result in a more dramatic shift in one direction or another, then we are dealing with behavior patterns designated as emotional. Many theorists have discussed emotion in the context of arousal theories. The classical U-shaped relationship between arousal and behavioral efficiency is shown at the left of Fig. 1. It is assumed that as the environment elicits behavior, in-

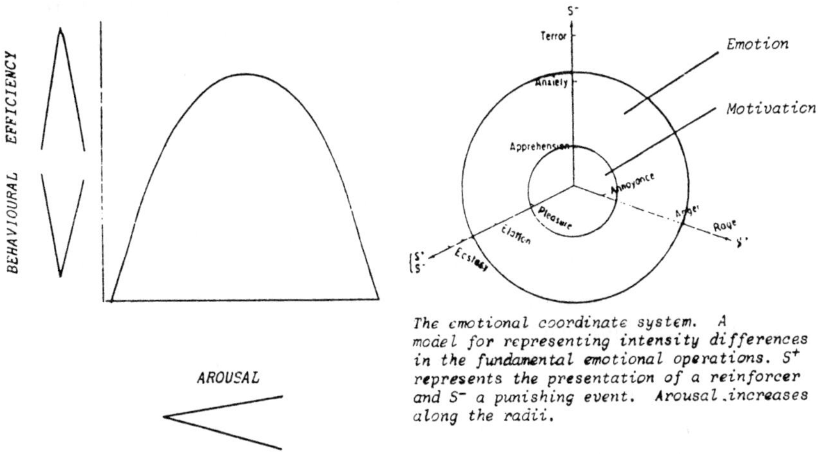

FIG. 1. This figure (*right*) is reproduced from Millenson (1967) illustrating an emotional coordinate system. The authors added the concentric circles to suggest an intensity continuum which could relate motivational and emotional states (*left*). Stylized graph illustrating the relationship between arousal and behavioral efficiency.

creasing efficiency is associated with increasing arousal. Within the rising phase of this curve may be accommodated motivated behavior and organized and directed emotional responses. When arousal reaches very high levels, behavioral disorganization is seen.

In this arousal continuum, we are dealing with a core integrative system of the forebrain that is essential for survival. Major classes of psychiatric illness, such as manic depression, involve distortion of affect and emotional responsiveness; others such as senile dementia result in profound cognitive disruption and loss of reasoning power; and yet others may involve disruption of the cross-talk between affect and reason. Thus, in trying to understand how the emotional arousal system works and communicates with cortical mechanism lies a challenge, but one of potential value in understanding mental illness.

Now to the title of the paper—"Brain catecholamines in relation to affect." With publication of the first results obtained with the histofluorescence method developed for staining catecholamine- and indoleamine-containing neuronal systems of brain *in situ,* it was apparent that there exists rich norepinephrine (NE), dopamine (DA), and serotonin (5HT) innervation or cortex, limbic system, and the forebrain subcortical output system (the striatum). Thus it was assumed that these chemical transmitters play a functional role in these structures. Indeed it was striking that the forebrain areas implicated in motivational and emotional behavior were particularly rich in their neurochemical monoamine innervation. This fact, coupled with the growing body of evidence that a number of disorders of mood and affect in man involved catecholamine dysfunction and could be normalized by pharmacological manipulation of catecholamine systems, has led to direct investigation of the role of forebrain NE and DA innervations in normal motivated behavior. There have, as yet, been few systematic excursions into what we have described as emotional response patterns in this chapter. However, the purpose of the introduction has been to stress the close behavioral relationship between motivation and emotion and to emphasize the belief that studies of brain mechanisms fundamental to motivational processes may also prove to be relevant to the understanding of affect.

Forebrain DA pathways have been most directly implicated in motivational processes. In this review, we concentrate on the two forebrain DA pathways and explore the hypothesis that one modulates information flow in limbic areas, to focus behavior on the most biologically relevant stimuli in the environment (processing largely, but not exclusively, *interoceptive* stimuli), and the other modulates information, much of it from cortex and thus *exteroceptive,* resulting in the appropriate sensorimotor integration for well-directed behavioral responses to occur. Both of these processes are, in a sense, attentional. These two DA pathways are termed mesolimbocortical and nigro-striatal, reflecting their different areas of innervation in the forebrain.

RECENT ANATOMICAL FINDINGS ON THE DISTRIBUTION OF DA PROJECTIONS IN FOREBRAIN

Typical stylized diagrams of the dopamine-containing neurons of the ventral mesencephalon differentiate two groups of cell bodies; one is localized to the zona-compacta of the substantia nigra (SN z.c.) and the other is located more medially as a separate group of neurons surrounding the interpeduncular nucleus (IPN). In fact, these two cell groups are clearly separated only in their posterior extent and in the more anterior region; the DA neurons form a continuous sheet of cells extending from the lateral SN to the IPN (Fig. 2). In gross topography, therefore, it is not easy to distinguish the neurons forming the nigro-striatal pathway from those providing the innervation of the limbic and cortical areas. In a number of laboratories, modern anatomical tracing techniques, combined with radioautography, have been used in a parallel with histofluorescence methods in an effort to redefine the projections of the mesencephalic DA neurons and describe their topographical organization. Originally unsuspected degrees of organization have been revealed in these studies (Fallon and Moore, 1978). Starting with the neurons in the most lateral part of the SN z.c. (A9 cells), we see the lateral and posterior extent of the nigro-striatal pathway to striatum; as we move medially along the SN z.c., the projection encompasses the central body of the striatum. What is interesting and new is that the medial part of the SN has projections which extend more medially than the striatum and innervate some of the ventral elements of the limbic system. However, the SN does not extend its innervation to the most medial limbic and cortical areas including the septum and medial frontal cortex. As we continue towards the midline, the A10 neurons of the ventral tegmental area (VTA) are shown to project to the more medial parts of the striatum, but most strongly to the limbic and cortical areas. Thus we have in the A10 and A9 neurons two dissociable but overlapping projections with only the dorsal and medial limbo-cortical areas receiving a pure A10 innervation and the lateral and posterior striatum a pure A9 innervation. However, although

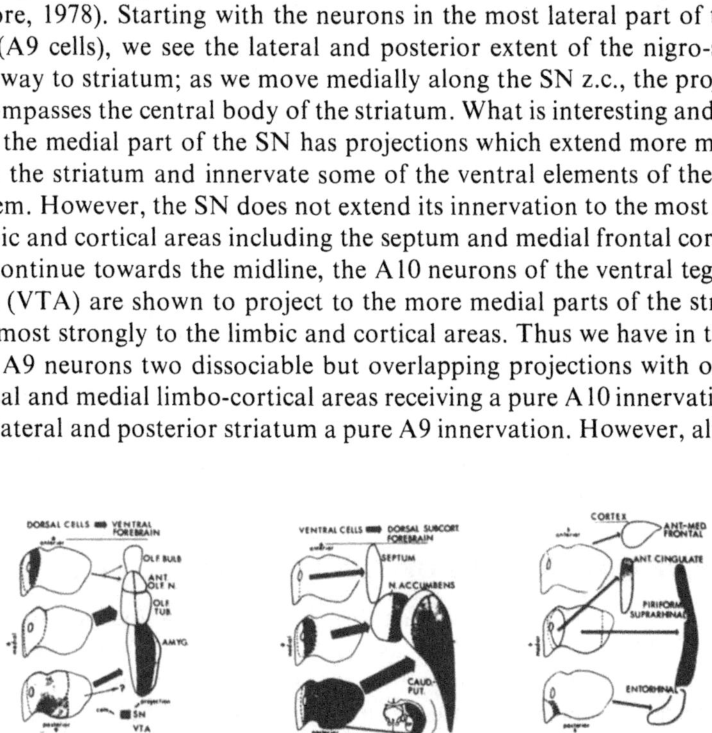

FIG. 2. Collation of the summary diagrams from Fallon and Moore's (1978) description of the topographical projections of the DA neurons to striatal, limbic, and cortical areas. On the left of each panel is shown a dorsal view of the sheet of DA neurons in the ventral mesencephalon of the right side of the brain. In the case of the limbic and striatal innervation (*left panel and middle*) there is a strict medial-to-medial and lateral-to-lateral topography in the innervation pattern (i.e., most medial VTA A10 DA neurons to most medial nucleus accumbens (NAS) and more lateral VTA to more lateral NAS). This is equally true of the SN A9 DA neuron innervation of caudate and putamen. The topography has a further feature with the most dorsal DA neurons projecting to the ventral aspect of the structures innervated, whereas the ventral DA neurons innervate the more dorsal aspects of the structures. There is also an indication of anterior-to-anterior and posterior-to-posterior organization. The situation with the cortical innervation (*right panel*) is less clear; anterior-posterior organization is the most obvious feature of these trajectories.

in gross topographical organization the distinction between a nigro-striatal and a mesolimbo-cortical projection appears blurred, it has been re-established in another form of dissociation. Fallon et al. (1978) have described two different types of DA neurons in the SN z.c., which differ in their neuronal architecture. Using Golgi techniques to visualize the profiles of the DA neurons, they find within the zona compacta some neurons with distinct dendritic fields extending ventrally into the zona reticulata of SN. Others of a fusiform shape have no such projections, but dendritic processes which extend laterally. It is suggested that the former neurons give rise to the axons of the nigro-striatal system, and that their anatomy is appropriate for the known striato-nigral feedback control to the zona reticulata. The fusiform-shaped neurons may give rise to the limbo-cortical DA projection; in this system a direct feedback control system to VTA from the DA terminal areas of forebrain has not been observed, which could be consistent with the lack of ventrally projecting dendritic fields in this second type of DA neuron.

Two important points in this new anatomy should be stressed:

(i) the SN zona compacta contains more than those neurons giving rise to the classical nigro-striatal tract, and

(ii) the structure delineated as striatum includes an anterior ventral portion which is more strongly innervated by A10 or non-striatal DA neurons than by the classical nigro-striatal pathway. This area of striatum requires anatomical and functional redefinition.

EXPERIMENTAL STUDIES OF THE FOREBRAIN DA PATHWAYS

How does one go about studying the functional significance of these forebrain DA pathways? The task seems simple enough; selectively eliminate one or other of the pathways, but how? A number of pharmacological tools have been used with varying success. For example, drugs exist which prevent the synthesis of DA. But systemic treatment with these invariably affects DA in all areas of brain, not just the forebrain, and also influences related amines such as NE. Other drugs interfere with DA transmission at the synapse. Some of these, such as the neuroleptic chlorpromazine, affect NE as well as DA receptors, whereas others that have been produced in recent years, such as haloperidol, are remarkably potent and selective at blocking DA receptors.

Unfortunately, biochemical knowledge of DA receptors had begun to advance even more rapidly than the development of new drugs. We now know that given areas of forebrain contain at least two different types of DA receptor, with differential responsiveness to agonist and antagonist drugs. Thus, even with intracerebral injection technique, it is now difficult to manipulate DA receptors pharmacologically in a unitary fashion at a given site. These problems of drug selectively are compounded by the spread of the drug from site of injection, a difficult, although not insurmountable, problem.

Lesions provide an alternative approach. Classical electrolytic or radio frequency lesions are accompanied by undesirable non-specific damage to nearby structures and pathways. Selective toxins have provided a breakthrough in this area. 6-hydroxydopamine (6OHDA), a drug closely related to DA and NE, was found to selectively destroy NE and DA neurons when injected locally into brain and, if used in appropriate dosages, non-specific damage may be kept at an acceptable minimum. With injection of this toxin into the cell bodies, trajectory, or the dense terminal innervation of the catecholamine pathways, a 99 percent depletion of DA or NE can be achieved. The uptake of the toxin into catecholamine neurons involves the membrane re-uptake inactivation process by which catecholamines are normally removed from the synapse. Certain antidepressant drugs selectively block this process in NE, but not in DA, neurons. Thus, by combining desmethylimipramine with local injections of 6OHDA into brain, a very useful tool for studying the function of the DA pathways has been developed. 6OHDA may also be injected stereotaxically in medullary and pontine areas to destroy NE neuron groups. A similar toxin exists for 5HT neurons (5,7-dihydroxytryptamine) and yet another toxin, kainic acid, is being investigated, as it appears to destroy neurons bearing glutamate receptors, rather than the catecholamine terminals, on the cell bodies.

Even selective neurochemical lesions have their problems. For example, in selecting a dose to avoid non-specific damage, it is often difficult to achieve substantial damage to catecholamine systems. Unfortunately, in these catecholamine systems, partial lesions do not result in partial deficits. On the contrary, a partial lesion may result in functional levels greater than normal. Two compensatory processes have been recognized which could account for such observations. First, the remaining neurons on a damaged pathway have been found to show higher than normal levels of biochemical turnover of the transmitter. Second, catecholamine receptors become supersensitive to agonists after denervation; thus very little DA released onto such receptors could account for virtually normal functional capacity. These findings are fascinating, but they create problems for the experimentalist trying to functionally inactivate a pathway.

Factors outside the DA pathways may also complicate the picture. It seems likely, for example, that receptors vacated by the degeneration of one chemical input pathway may result in enhanced growth of other inputs to this part of brain, thus creating the possibility of functional compensation mediated by a different pathway. Behavioral and general environmental experience during the post-lesion period may also modify the development of these compensatory processes. Therefore, after placing a lesion, it is very important to control both the time interval after which behavioral observations are made and the general experience of the animal.

THE EFFECT OF LESIONS IN DA PATHWAYS

Despite these problems, much has been learned by the judicious use of lesions of catecholamine pathways in brain. In early studies, bilateral infusions of 6OHDA were made into the SN of rats that probably destroyed a large part of both the A9 and A10 cell groups. These animals were essentially devoid of all behavior, including eating and drinking, and soon died (Ungerstedt, 1970). Whereas such massive lesions and accompanying deficits are difficult to interpret, recent studies utilizing more selective lesions to sectors of the DA projections have provided a finer analysis.

Lesions of the Mesolimbocortical System

The fabric of behavior is remarkably resilient in the face of CNS damage, and it is only when the animal is challenged that deficits appear.

First attempts to define the function of the mesolimbocortical DA system employed a useful pharmacological tool, amphetamine. This stimulant drug produces dose-dependent changes in behavior in many species. For example, in rats, low does induce a characteristic form of behavioral arousal involving movement and an increase in some behavioral elements normally associated with exploration of the environment. A wealth of *in vitro* and *in vivo* biochemical data (Moore, 1978) suggest that this behavioral effect is mediated primarily by brain dopamine, and this has been confirmed by lesion studies.

Substantial infusions of 6OHDA into the SN prevented the subsequent emergence of amphetamine-induced locomtor behavior, whereas lesions to either the ascending dorsal NE pathway or the ventral NE pathway had no such effect. Within the DA pathways, it was possible to show that lesions of the terminal areas of the mesolimbocortical DA system achieved by 6OHDA infusion into the nucleus accumbens (NAS) abolished the amphetamine arousal, whereas equivalent lesions to the body of the striatum did not (Kelly, 1978).

Lesions to the mesolimbocortical pathway also block spontaneous investigatory behavior (E. Joyce, unpublished results). The open field is commonly used to induce high levels of patterned investigatory behavior in the rat. After bilateral 6OHDA lesions focused on the NAS, rats show reduced behavior in such an apparatus and in locomotor cages which generate high levels of activity in normal animals. This lack of locomotor behavior associated with exploratory investigation can lead to highly abnormal behavior in certain situations. For example, upon entering a cage in which food is made available, normal rats investigate for a long period before eating. Lesioned animals, who do not investigate, eat immediately on entering the cage and often consume abnormally large amounts of food (Fig. 3).

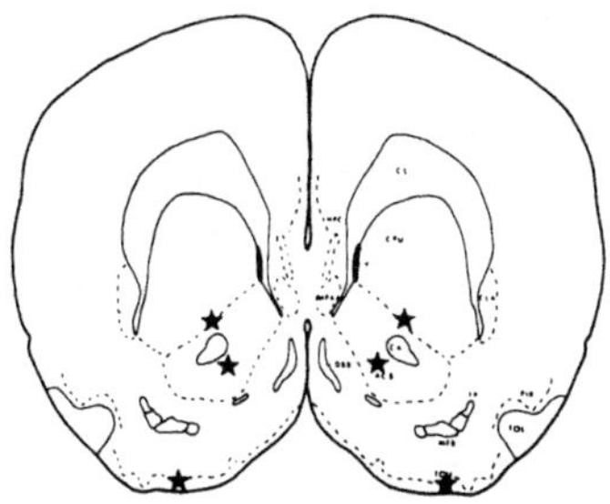

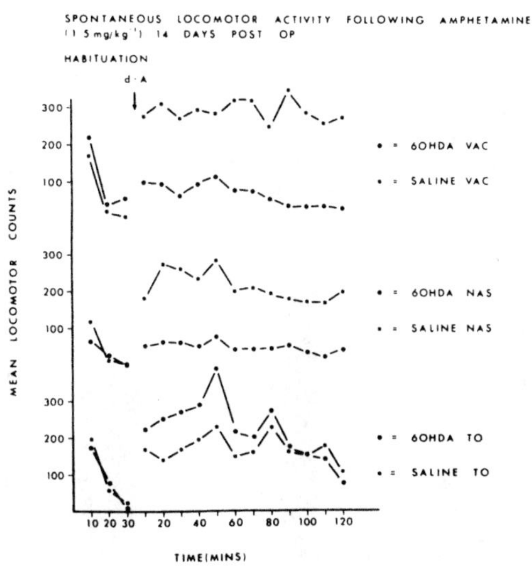

790933

FIG. 3. Rats with bilateral 6OHDA lesion were compared to controls in an open field situation containing bowls of six different food stuffs (familiar lab chow and five novel foods). During a ten-minute test period, the latency to eat, amount eaten, and preference for different foods were measured.

There is no independent evidence that they are more hungry; it is not that they are incapable of generating behavior, but merely that their pattern of behavior in response to the environment is abnormal. It would not be correct to say that these animals are not motivated; it is more accurate to say that the behavioral system is unbalanced. This has been shown dramatically in some recent studies with the same lesion. Rats were trained in a 16-hole box to retrieve four sugar pellets, placed in the same pattern of holes on each trial. Normal rats quickly learned an efficient strategy of hole visits. DA lesioned animals were reluctant to behave and totally unwilling to eat the novel sugar pellets. It took several days of training outside the test apparatus ot encourage them to sample and finally eat this novel food. Having learned to accept the reward, they then proceeded to show highly abnormal hole explorations. They could not be described as without motivation, as very large numbers of holes were visited, indeed significantly more than that visited by normal rats. Again, the investigatory pattern was disrupted and abnormal.

It seems that, when the world changes in a meaningful way, these DA lesioned animals are slow to appreciate the change and, even when change is responded to, they are slow to bring their behavior into appropriate balance. This was shown by the same lesioned animals when the diurnal

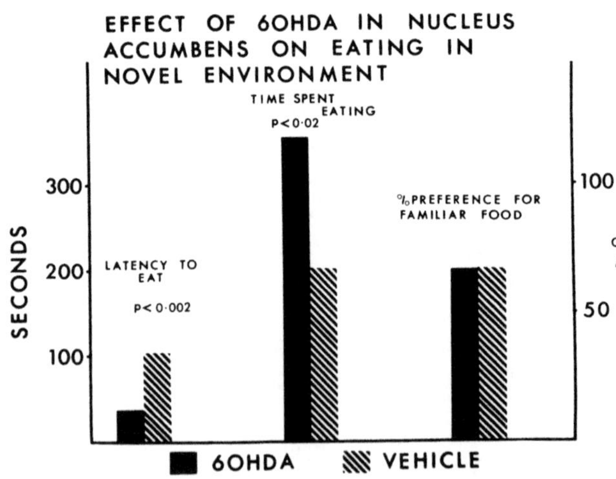

FIG. 4. Coronal section of the rat brain (upper) with stars illustrating the three different 6OHDA lesion groups. Most dorsal site = ventral anterior striatum (VAC); middle site = nucleus accumbens (NAS); bottom site = tuberculum olfactorium (TO). Eight g 6OHDA was injected bilaterally for each lesion group. In the lower figure, spontaneous activity levels (over 30 minutes) and the response to amphetamine (1.5 mg/kg) are presented for the three lesion groups and their control (Joyce and Iversen, unpublished results).

variations in spontaneous activity were measured. In daytime, the mesolimbic-cortical lesioned animal was hypokinetic, as mentioned. In the dark phase, however, when normal rats shifted from relative inactivity to activity, the lesioned animals also shifted and surprisingly became much *more active* than controls (Fig. 4). Again, their motivational arousal was not lacking, but unbalanced; the environment no longer elicited the normal profile of behavior.

The problems of interpreting lesion-induced dysfunction lead many to place more emphasis on studying the involvement of chemical pathways in ongoing behavior. Excellent examples of this approach are to be found in the description of tail-pinch-induced behavior and intracranial self-stimulation in a later section of the chapter.

Amphetamine-induced behavior is investigated, and considered particularly interesting, because in man amphetamine abuse leads eventually to a form of psychotic behavior which, in its acute phase, is indistinguishable from paranoid schizophrenia. Such people rapidly develop schizophrenic systoms if administered amphetamine under laboratory conditions. Furthermore, amphetamine is known to exacerbate the florid symptoms in schizophrenic patients (Iversen and Iversen, 1975).

Thus, in studying the brain areas and circuitries involved in the expression of acute amphetamine effects, we believe that we may be unravelling mechanisms of fundamental importance in schizophrenia. This optimism is reinforced by the fact that the major class of drug used for controlling the acute symptoms of schizophrenia acts to block DA and NE receptors, and that some of the more recent drugs which are said to be even more potent as anti-schizophrenic agents block DA receptors selectively. Such drugs also block amphetamine-induced behavior in animals.

FURTHER LOCALIZATION OF THE SITE OF STIMULATORY ACTION OF AMPHETAMINE IN FOREBRAIN

It yet remains that two of the most useful tools for exploring the functions of the DA pathways are amphetamine and the direct DA receptor agonist, apomorphine. The recent anatomy has led us to try to define more precisely the critical focus of the DA lesion which abolishes amphetamine arousal. The original lesion studied in our laboratory focused on the nucleus accumbens, -ut resulted in substantial DA loss from the tuberculum olfactorium (TO) and medial frontal cortex (probably also from the septum and amygdala, although these sites remain largely uninvestigated in our biochemical assay work). However, in independent studies, we have not been able to block amphetamine effects with direct 6OHDA injections into medial frontal cortex, despite substantial depletions of DA in this area.

Bilateral lesions of the tuberculum olfactorium have similarly been found to be without effect. It seems that 6OHDA lesions to the NAS or total destruction of the DA cell bodies in the VTA are the only lesions reported to block amphetamine-induced arousal. However, it has been our experience that NAS lesions sometimes fail to abolish amphetamine responses. The depletion of DA is usually substantially in the NAS, TO, and frontal cortex in these preparations. It now seems likely that the crucial variation between these groups of NAS-lesioned animals lies in the involvement or sparing of the area in the ventral anterior striatum which receives overlapping A10 and A9 innervation.

To pursue this hypothesis Eileen Joyce and I have compared three different 6OHDA lesions focused (i) on ventral anterior striatum (VAS group), (ii) a little lower in the nucleus accumbens (NAS group), and (iii) in the tuberculum olfactorium (TO group). The response to a low dose of amphetamine and apomorphine was tested two weeks after surgery, when depletion should have been maximal. Both the NAS and VAS group showed complete attenuation of the amphetamine response and an enhanced locomotor response to apomorphine (Fig. 5).

Both lesions involved loss of DA in NAS and VAS, although the profiles of depletion differed. Interestingly, the TO lesion, despite some spread to

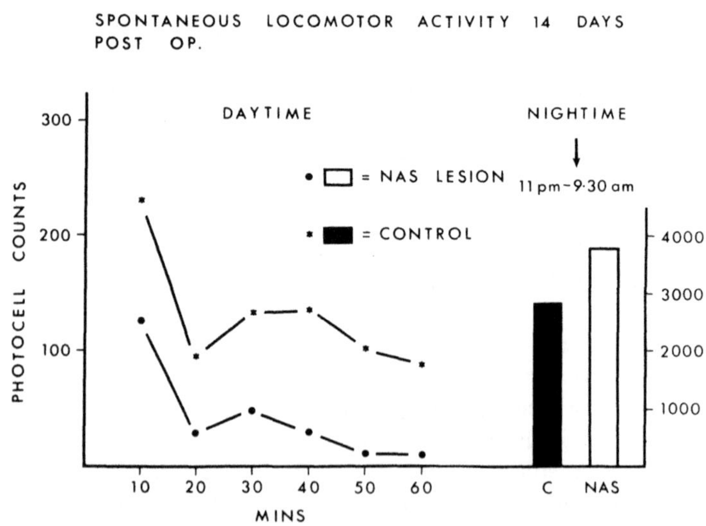

FIG. 5. Spontaneous locomotor activity (measured in photocell cages) of rats with bilateral lesions of the NAS and their controls tested for 1 hour during the daytime and for 10.5 hours during the dark. Hypoactivity during daylight is superseded by marked hyperactivity during dark time.

NAS and loss of DA at this site, did not block the amphetamine response. This is in agreement with our earlier finding (Creese and Iversen, 1974). However, the TO group did show apomorphine supersensitivity, but the behavior enhanced was a particularly interesting form of licking which we have not observed in any of our DA lesioned animals previously. Does the DA projection to the TO region represent a functionally distinct part of the dopamine limbic projection? Probably not. Accordingly to Heimer and Wilson (1975), the TO forms neuronal bridges with the VAS, and together with the NAS, these three areas form the "ventral striatum." It is suggested that the "ventral striatum" including the TO is involved in investigatory behavior, a correlate of behavioral arousal. The NAS and VAS are concerned with the full body movement, a major component of investigatory behavior. The TO, with its sensory input dominated by olfaction, is concerned with responses associated with nose and mouth investigatory behavior. This is not a new idea. Herrick coined the term "olfactostriatum" and described it as a region concerned with "the correlation of olfactory and tactual and other exteroreceptive stimuli...concerned chiefly with locomotor and *facial reflexes* involved in feeding."

PARALLEL ANATOMICAL AND NEUROCHEMICAL CIRCUITRY ASSOCIATED WITH THE MESOLIMBOCORTICAL AND NIGRO-STRIATAL DA PROJECTIONS

The definition of the *ventral striatum (VS)* as a system and its distinction from the *dorsal striatum (DS)* have focused interest again on the input and output relationships of these two discrete forebrain areas. Heimer and Wilson (1975) point out that just as the allo-cortex (hippocampus and pyriform cortex) projects to the VS, so the neocortex projects to dorsal striatum. Discrete output pathways can be identified (Fig. 6). The VS projects to the ventral pallidum and the DS to the dorsal pallidum. These projections involve the same structures but are localized to different sectors of those structures. Bjorklund has recently provided a neurochemical coding of two striatal systems (Fig. 7), which shows clearly that parallels exist here as well. The general organization involves cortical, glutamate projections to the striatum, DA innervation of striatum, gamma-aminobutyric acid (GABA), and substance P (SP) output to the dopamine cell body areas. There are some differences between the dorsal and ventral striatal systems; for example, SP in the dorsal striatal system arises from anterior striatum and projects to SN, whereas in the ventral striatal system, SP arises mainly from the medial habenular nucleus and projects to the lateral part of the interpeduncular nucleus. In the dorsal system, the pathway from the lateral habenular to the SN has not yet been chemically coded. Despite a number of gaps in our knowledge, the anatomical parallels in these two systems are striking.

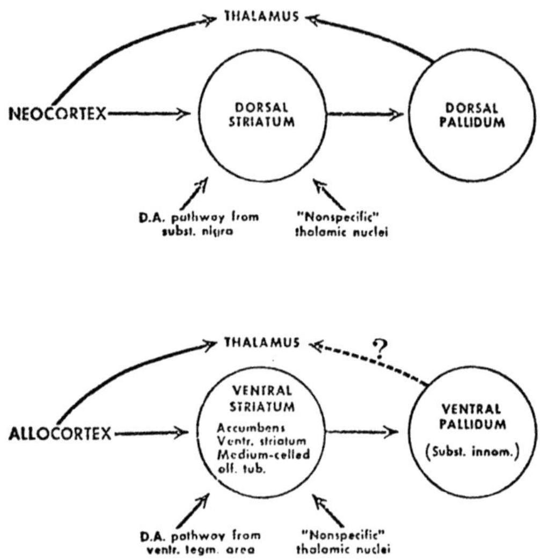

FIG. 6. Summary diagram from Heimer and Wilson (1975) illustrating the parallel efferent organization of dorsal and ventral striatum.

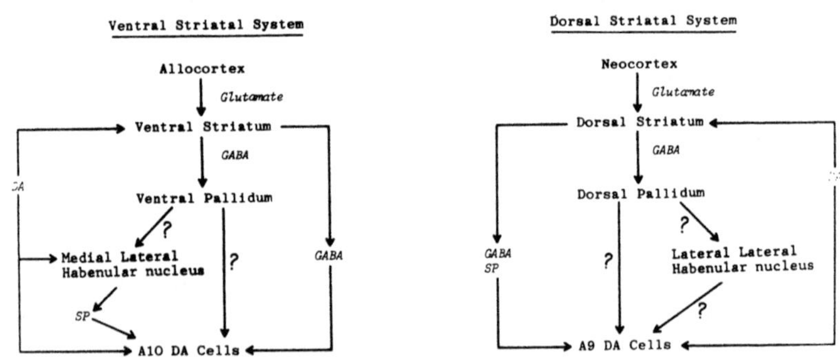

FIG. 7. Chemical coding of the ascending and descending anatomical links of the ventral (*left*) and dorsal (*right*) striatal complex (abstracted from a figure kindly supplied to SDI by Anders Bjorklund).

What Are the Functions of the Dorsal Striatal System?

With the discovery that patients dying of Parkinson's disease have degeneration of the nigrostriatal DA neurons, considerations of the role of the striatum have focused on motor functions. Parkinson's disease is characterized by akinesia, rigidity, and tremor, considered to reflect the unbalancing of extrapyramidal motor circuitries consequent upon the loss of the ascending DA innveration. But, although frank in its motor symptomology, is the disease purely one of motor dysfunction? It has been suggested that a deficiency of sensorimotor integration provides a more parsimonious explanation of the range of deficits seen in these patients. If sensory input is enhanced in the Parkinsonian patient, motor performance is improved; parallel lines drawn on the floor enhanced walking patterns, markers on a walking aid facilitate the initiation of stepping movements, and sight of an approaching bus elicits rapid movement. The thesis is that the DA innervation of the striatum is an enabling one, facilitating the integration of the sensory flow via cortex with motor responses. In support of this view are observations of the rat after unilateral degeneration of the nigrostriatal DA system. *Total* contralateral, multimodal, sensory neglect is observed (Marshall and Teitelbaum, 1974) and, as is more widely known, when the animal is activated to move, motor rotation occurs away from the side of the lesion or towards the side with intact sensory motor integration.

The dynamic balance of the striatal system is not solely dependent on the DA pathways. A striatal-nigral pathway involving non-dopaminergic cells of the SN zona reticulata and their output to the thalamus (di Chiara et al., 1978) also contributes to balanced motor control.

Bilateral lesions in the nigro-striatal DA system result in a total lack of behavior, including feeding and drinking, in rats. Ungerstedt (1971) described this effect originally, and pointed out that many years before, Teitelbaum and Epstein (1962) had reported similar deficits after bilateral, lateral hypothalamic lesions. It is now thought that their results were due to transection of the nigro-striatal pathway as it projects through the lateral hypothalamus. Ranje and Ungerstedt (1977) have studied the behavior of these severely handicapped rats in learning situations. Although spontaneous behavior is lacking, responding is possible when the animals are placed in demanding (one might say stressful) environments, such as a water maze, in which the rat is submerged in the start box and must swim to the open end of the maze. Animals with massive DA loss swim in this apparatus, but are unable to learn a visual discrimination in order to find the open arm of the maze and escape reliably.

Severe loss of DA from the striatum also modifies drug-induced behavior, in particular, the stereotyped response to large doses of amphetamine. Unlike the arousal seen after 1.5 mg/kg amphetamine, a dose of 5.0 mg/kg in the rat results in highly abnormal repetition of motor behavior; response elements from the normal behavioral repertoire occur with an abnormally high frequency. Lyon and Robbins (1975) have discussed this phenomenon and suggested that one response is not finished before the next is initiated.

Progressively, this leads to more frequent occurrence of responses which become increasingly truncated; the result is fractionated responses, and only elements of behavior which are normally completed in a short time can eventually be recognized. As a corollary, it is clear that behaviors such as grooming or social contact, which normally involve long sequences of complex responses, are the first to disappear as behavior disintegrates. Finally, the animal is repeating the shortest elements of behavior. If stereotypy is a consequence of overstimulation of the striatum by the drug-induced release of DA, this suggests that tonic release of DA is essential for the normal initiation and temporal sequencing of response patterns (Iversen, 1977, 1979).

A perusal of the experimental literature which predates the discovery of forebrain DA reveals that lesions to the body of the striatum (involving DA terminals and all other neuronal elements) result in deficits which are not obviously of a simple sensory-motor nature. Divac (1979) has continued to emphasize the disorders on delayed alternation and delayed response tasks after caudate lesions in the monkey. Rats with caudate lesions are also impaired on delayed alternation and spatial reversal. The DA innervation of the striatum is one feature of a complex neuronal architecture which includes several other chemically coded inputs and at least six different types of intrinsic neurons. Clearly, it is important to understand the role of DA, but equally its role must be viewed within the context of the overall functional organization of striatum. Perhaps in DA-induced stereotypy we are studying an artificially isolated feature of striatal function. Certainly, Divac (1979) considers that any general theory of striatal function should be couched in terms of *cognition* rather than simple motor function, and the existence of highly *organized* input from cortex to striatum reinforces this view. This has been demonstrated both in the monkey and rat; specific areas of cortex project to specific areas of caudate/putamen. What is more interesting is that these striatal foci receive overlapping projections from their afference inputs (Iversen, 1979). Two notable examples of this form of anatomical organization have been described recently.

In monkey, Yeterian and van Hoesen (1978) have defined an area of posterior neocortex having reciprocal connections with an area of anterior cortex in the arcuate sulcus; both these cortical areas project independently to the caudate nucleus, and the two projections overlap in this specified area of caudate. More recently, Beckstead (1979) has described another form of anatomical overlap. A group of DA cells in the SN were found to project to a specific region of medial caudate nucleus; the same DA cells innervate a focal area of frontal cortex in the pregenual area, which in turn was found to project to the identical area of striatum receiving the DA input. The importance of such topography and the role of cortico-striatal projections deserve experimental attention. It is difficult to know where to begin when faced with a structure of the neuronal complexity seen in the striatum. One approach we are pursuing involves the study of a variety of lesion types at a given site to see if any of the selective chemical lesions within the focus produce the same deficit as electrolytic removal of the whole striatal focus.

Local injections of 6OHDA can be used with desmethylimipramine (DMI) pretreatment to selectively removed DA terminals and, similarly, 5,7-dihydroxytryptamine can be used on 5HT terminals. A localized cortical lesion will destroy the corticostriate projection using glutamate as its transmitter, and a local injection of kainic acid into striatum destroys intrinsic neurons of striatum with relatively little loss of chemical transmitter terminals. Alternatively, local injection of the transmitters themselves may be used to activate particular components of the striatum. Neill (1976) has capitalized on this technique to manipulate cholinergic components of the striatum and has, in this way, produced behavioral deficits.

In view of the structural reappraisal of the dorsal striatum and its anatomical parallels with the ventral striatal complex, it is a matter of pressing urgency to discover more of its functional role in behavior.

Functional Relationships between the Ventral and Dorsal Striatal Systems

A number of hypotheses can be entertained concerning the dynamic interaction of the two forebrain striatal systems. One is that the VS and DS system have similar processing properties, but operate on different kinds of information. In this view, the VS is concerned with stimuli closely associated with meaningful or affective events, e.g., the presentation of reinforcers, novel stimuli, or aversive events which involve, as a major component, interoreceptive stimuli. By contrast, the DS is concerned with exteroreceptive stimuli processed by cortex. A second hypothesis is that the VS and DS are components of a sequential processing system. We may consider that a number of decisions have to be made between the receipt of a stimulus and the initiation of a response:

(a) What is this stimulus?
(b) What do I think about this stimulus?
(c) What shall I do in response to this stimulus?

These could occur in parallel, with the VS involved in (b) at the same time the DS is involved in (c). Alternatively, one can conceive of a system in which decision (b) is made before decision (c) and the latter does not proceed until triggered by (b). In such a system VS would need to communicate with DS. Do anatomical connections exist that would enable such cross-talk between the systems? Connections exist from the nucleus accumbens to the zona reticulata of SN. Furthermore, both systems project through globus pallidus, the habenular complex, the SN, and the brainstem tegmentum. Thus, on anatomical grounds, integration between the two systems is possible. But it will be difficult to devise experiments to distinguish these kinds of operational models of the striatal complex.

The processes of stimulus evaluation and response selection are both attentional in nature and are essential components of the associative learning mechanism (irrespective of the particular theoretical view of associative learning). Learning may reflect a correlation between activity in these two focusing mechanisms of striatum, which becomes increasingly probable with repetition of a particular stimulus and response.

If we turn to the animal learning theory literature, the terms *motivation* and *reinforcement* are those which most clearly relate to the dopamine-mediated arousal mechanisms discussed so far. Traditionally, there has been a fruitful marriage between learning theory and physiology in approaches to the study of motivation and reinforcement. Indeed, some of the methods used to unravel the neural substrates involved in reinforcement and motivation have generated results that highlight theoretical controversies and, in some areas, resolve them. Electrically-induced motivational states, intracranial self-stimulation (ICSS), and tail-pinch-induced behavior illustrate this point. It is now appreciated that the dopamine pathways are an integral part of the neural substrate of motivation, and it is inevitable that this new pharmacological approach to the study of motivation will find itself inextricably linked to the development of theoretical ideas. For this reason, we have included a section that illustrates the theoretical approach to motivation and the way in which physiological data underpins theoretical developments in this area.

THEORETICALLY ORIENTED APPROACHES TO THE STUDY OF MOTIVATION AND REINFORCEMENT

The most direct way of investigating the neural mechanisms of motivation is to study the behavior elicited by electrical stimulation of the brain (ESB). Stimulation of various areas, most notably the lateral hypothalamus, elicits a variety of consummatory acts in a wide range of species. Eating, drinking, licking, gnawing, and sexual behavior are most commonly found. Also, the same stimulation can be a powerful reinforcer. For instance, rats will typically make 100 responses per minute to receive exactly the same stimulation that produces eating. These findings have led to the suggestion that the lateral hypothalamus, in particular, might be concerned with motivation and reward mechanisms. In this section, the nature of these mechanisms will be examined and the role of the catecholamines in the mediation of electrically induced behavior will be considered.

Electrical Brain Stimulation

Following the discovery of eating deficits after lateral hypothalamic lesions, most of the work on behavior elicited by ESB has been concerned with eating during stimulation of the lateral hypothalamus. The stimulation could be producing eating for a variety of reasons other than activating a central mechanism that normally responds only when the animal is hungry. For instance, it could be generating the peripheral sensations by which the animal recognizes that it is hungry. Similarly, the stimulation might simply be eliciting the motor responses of jaw movements by activating a motor pathway. This last possibility appears not to be the case since in the absence of appropriate goal-objects, animals respond by exploring the environment, sniffing and biting at parts of the apparatus. A genuine motivational role is supported by observations that the stimulation will interact with external sensory factors; for instance, quinine inhibits the elicited eating (Tennen & Miller, 1964) and preferred tastes facilitate it (Smith, 1972).

A critical property of a motivational state is that it is capable of bringing about the learning of a response which leads to an appropriate goal. If ESB is to be regarded as motivational, it, too, must be shown to support new learning. Mendelson & Chorover (1965) showed that rats would learn a T-maze for food during ESB, and there have been similar demonstrations of learning mazes for the opportunity to gnaw on wood or to attack a prey. Coons et al. (1965) found that rats would respond selectively during ESB on whichever one of two levers produced food. They went on to show that the rats would continue to press on the most recently reinforced lever when they were transferred to food-deprivation in the absence of stimulation. Miller (1957) reported a similar transfer of a learned response when rats were switched from deprivation to ESB. These studies provide strong evidence that ESB is functionally equivalent to hunger.

However, while it is tempting to conclude that the ESB is activating a "hunger system," this conclusion may be backward. Rather, the stimulation could be acting non-specifically to arouse the animal, and evidence of transfer may indicate that hunger-motivation itself may be largely non-specific. Valenstein et al. (1970) have produced evidence that ESB is acting non-specifically. Rats given a choice of eating, drinking, or gnawing wood during ESB were observed to have a preference for one activity over the others, usually eating. When the preferred goal-object was removed, a second response would emerge, and re-introduction of the preferred goal-object resulted in the occurrence of both behaviors. Naive animals required considerable experience before they exhibited reliable consummatory behavior, and the threshold decreased with time, suggesting that they learned to eat in response to the stimulation. This is further supported by the demonstration by Valenstein that an eating response which developed slowly during experience of stimulation of one side of the brain occurred immediately when the other side of the brain was stimulated for the first time. These learning phenomena would not be expected if the stimulation were activating a specific eating mechanism.

An alternative interpretation of these data is that, in the lateral hypothalamus, many discrete motivational systems exist that are interdigitated to such an extent that it would never be possible to stimulate one system alone. Thus, the stimulated animal is faced with a multitude of conflicting desires, one of which is predominant. This idea is supported by the rigidity and compulsiveness of the behavior seen during ESB; once an animal has chosen a gold-object, it tends to stay with it. If the stimulation were really non-specific it might be predicated that the animals should shift between several goal-objects and never show a strong preference. Moreover, preference studies have revealed some unexpected properties of ESB not wholly consistent with the idea that the animals learn to eat. For instance, rats that have established a preference for food pellets over the same food in powdered form or water switched to the water, rather than the powdered food, when the food pellets were removed.

Wise and Erdmann (1973) have suggested an explanation for the rigidity of the behavior in terms of mixed effects of the stimulation. They adopt Kent and Grossman's (1969) proposal that the stimulation has an aversive component, which might make the annimals emotional, in addition to an appetitive component, which might make them hungry. They compared two groups of rats, one group well-habituated to the apparatus and well-handled, and the other non-habituated and unhandled, in a food preference test. The handled, habituated rats switched readily from food to food, in contrast to the unhandled, non-habituated rats which chose a single food and stayed with it. Thus, manipulations which were calculated to increase emotionality produced the rigidity of behavior characteristic of that elicited by ESB. Furthermore, the "emotional" rats exhibited similar, unusual changes of preference when exposed to the same preference tests as Valenstein's rats. Therefore, the rigidity of the behavior seems to be produced by very high levels of arousal or emotion. In most of the experiments of Valenstein et al., the rats preferred to indulge in behavior involving an intense licking or biting response, even when this meant changing to a novel goal-object. This rigid desire to bite something may be a reflection of the high state of arousal produced by the stimulation, an idea that is supported by the finding that the tranquilizer diazepam (Valium) increases ESB-elicited eating. The tranquilizer presumably reduces the aversive effects of the stimulation, allowing the appetitive affects to be unmasked. Nevertheless, it seems that it is probably impossible to distinguish satisfactorily between the non-specific arousal account of brain stimulation and an explanation in terms of simultaneous activation of many discrete systems. What is required is independent evidence that non-specific activating stimuli are sufficient to produce the motivational effects of ESB. Robbins and Fray (1980) have recently reviewed non-specific effects on eating, and there is no shortage of evidence. Electric shock, loud noises, handling, irrelevant drives (sex and aggression), novelty, social isolation *and* increased social interaction, and a variety of drugs have all been shown to increase eating under certain circumstances. Sexual and aggressive responses can also be elicited by electric shock (Barfield & Sachs, 1968; Caggiula & Eibergen, 1969).

Tail-pinch (a mild, sustained application of pressure to the tail with a hemostat, cuff, or paper-clip) has recently been studied in detail in order to assess the extent to which a non-specific arousing stimulus can be regarded as motivational. Antelman & Szechtman (1975) first demonstrated that tail-pinch would elicit eating, gnawing, and licking in nearly every rat tested. In the same way that ESB was shown to interact with natural motivational influences, Antelman et al. (1976) found that preloading the stomach with milk reduced tail-pinch-induced milk-drinking; isotonic saline was ineffective. A taste-aversion to saccharine-flavored pellets could be induced with lithium, with no effect on consumption of unflavored pellets. Diazepam facilitated a switch to a novel food, suggesting mixed effects of the pinch, which is supported by the finding of Robbins et al. (1977) that chlordiazepoxide (Librium) increased tail-pinch-induced eating at doses that have no effect on eating during control tests with no pinch.

Koob et al. (1976) found that the eating behavior takes some time to appear. During the first application of the pinch, not much eating is seen; instead, the rats run around and bite and lick at the apparatus and their tails. With repeated experience, the eating response strengthens until it is performed almost exclusively. As with ESB, it seems that the rats have to learn to eat.

It is important to demonstrate that tail-pinch would support new learning, and Koob et al. (1976) proceeded to show that rats with their tails pinched would learn a T-maze for the opportunity to gnaw on wood. Similar T-maze learning has been demonstrated for food. At first sight, it seems that the pinch is a purely aversive stimulus, and the animals ran the maze simply to escape it; perhaps they chose to run to the wood or food because gnawing afforded some relief from the discomfort of the pinch. This displacement activity interpretation of tail-pinch-induced behavior seems unlikely in the light of *increased* eating produced by tranquilizers. If the eating is maintained purely by the aversiveness of the pinch, a tranquilizer, which should reduce the aversiveness of the situation, should also reduce the eating. In the Koob et al. (1976) experiment, the pinch was applied throughout the maze; if the rats reached either goal-box they were confined there for 30 seconds; only one goal-box contained wood. Fray et al. (submitted) continued testing these rats with the wood switched to the opposite goal-box and the pinch was removed when the rats reached either goal-box. The rats were then replaced in the goal-box of their choice for 30 seconds. Rather than maintaining the previously learned habit, they actually preferred to *reverse* this habit in order to stay with wood after removal of the pinch, even though they did not gnaw it. In fact, the wood had acquired positive reinforcing properties as a result of the previous gnawing experience. Naive rats tested under these conditions (the pinch removed in both goal-boxes) did not learn to run the maze at all. These rats, in fact, started out running the maze, but wih experience preferred to remain in the start box and lick the floor, reaching a criterion of *not* running the maze in about the same number of trials as the experienced rats took to learn it. These rats actually chose to subject themselves to tail-pinch rather than escape it. Therefore the pinch cannot be purely aversive; in the absence of pairing wood and tail-pinch, it was more reinforcing to lick the floor than to have the clip removed. This forms a preliminary demonstration of the self-administration of tail-pinch. Obviously, a more rigorous demonstration is required, since, if tail-pinch is a genuine parallel to ESB, it should be possible to find the tail-pinch equivalent of ICSS.

The most compelling evidence of a functional similarity of two motivational states can be provided by the transfer of learning from one state to the other. Such transfer is difficult to demonstrate convincingly. For instance, rats trained to criterion to turn one way in a T-maze under food deprivation could be satiated and tested in the maze under tail-pinch. However, transfer might not be perfect and the rats might take some time to come back to criterion. Thus, a control group is required with which to compare the experimental animals in order to demonstrate that transfer has occurred. On the one hand, it is essential that the control group have the same experimental training as the experimental group; otherwise any difference between them might not reflect savings on the part of the experimental group, but poor performance by the controls. On the other hand, if the control group does not differ from the experimental group in its training, it cannot be distinguished from the experimental group. One way out of this dilemma is to train one large group of hungry rats in the maze, and then satiate them and divide them into two groups; both sub-groups are given transfer tests under tail-pinch, but one half continues with the same discrimination under tail-pinch and the other half is reversed. If the animals remember nothing about hunger, both sub-groups will have to learn about the maze as if new and will not be different. If, however, the rats continuing with the same discrimination reach criterion before the reversal rats, then clearly learning has transferred. This experiment has recently been carried out in our laboratory, and there is a clear difference between the two subgroups.

Thus, the evidence is as strong for a functional equivalence between tail-pinch and food deprivation as it is for ESB and food-deprivation. Rather than suggesting that tail-pinch actually makes rats hungry, as has been suggested for ESB, it is suggested that not only does ESB have its effects in a non-specific way, but so too does food-deprivation itself. Hunger itself may be a response that the organism has learned by a lifetime of association with food and eating behavior. Motivation, then, may be largely activation or arousal; the specificity of the motivational state is dictated by the particular internal and external stimuli producing the arousal, about which the organism has to learn or has learned previously (Fray et al., 1978).

Whether the arousal is rewarding or punishing may depend principally on context as well. Electric shock is traditionally thought of as a punisher, but it is now clearly established that animals can be trained to work for electric shocks as well as to avoid and escape them (Morse and Kelleher, 1977). Symmetrically, hungry rats and squirrel monkeys will work to *postpone* food presentation (Smith and Clark, 1972; Clark and Smith, 1977). Since a stimulus cannot be classified as intrinsically rewarding or punishing, its affective value can only be assessed by reference to the animal behavior. Thus, a stimulus is *defined* as a reward if the organism works for it or approaches it, and *defined* as a punisher if it works to avoid it or escape from it. It is circular to say that an animal is working for a stimulus *because* it finds it rewarding, since that state of reward can only be inferred from the fact that the animal is actively working for the stimulus (i.e., it is rewarding because he *works* for it). Therefore, reward and punishment may be the way we label the subjective feelings associated with approach and avoidance behavior, but they cannot explain that behavior. In fact, a pure reward or a pure punisher is indefinable. Rewards and punishers are particular stimuli in particular contexts, associated with particular behavior. Therefore, the effective valence of any particular arousing state may be dictated entirely by the context. Arousal is usually heralded by a pattern of sympathetic responses. Schachter (1966) has shown that adrenaline-induced arousal can generate either elation or anger in human subjects, depending on context and information the subject is given about the expected effects of the adrenaline.

A popular formation of arousal theory is that low levels are rewarding and high levels aversive (see Berlyne, 1967). This inverted U-shaped function along an arousal continuum (Fig. 1) is appealing, but since arousal is hard to define, and different measures of arousal often do not agree, it warrants careful investigation. Suffice it to say that the foregoing argument seriously calls into question the rationale not only for hard-wired motivational mechanisms, but also hard-wired reward mechanisms. Since logically such mechanisms cannot provide an explanation of behavior, they are therefore not required. The sterility of this approach is highlighted by the finding that a rat will work for the same stimulation in the absence of food that produces eating in the presence of food. That is, if eating in response to stimulation indicates that the stimulation is activating a hunger system and the observed self-stimulation indicates that it is also activating a reward mechanism, the rat must be pressing the lever to make itself extremely hungry. Since this hunger is not gratified with food, it is unclear why the rat finds it so rewarding. An account of motivation in terms of arousal does not have this problem; if the animal works for the stimulation, it must, by definition, be rewarding since reward is the manifestation of approach behavior.

Catecholamines and ICSS

The principal rationale for the search for the critical neural substrate of ICSS has been to discover the reward mechanism. We accept that ICSS is rewarding by definition, but it is suggested that this is a reflection of arousal, and the critical neural substrate will turn out to be an element of the arousal mechanism. Many sites in the brain support ICSS, and the ramifications of the catecholamine system, both NE and DA have been implicated. Reliable ICSS can be obtained from the region of the A9 and A10 DA cell bodies and the NE cell bodies of the locus coeruleus (Crow, 1972). The ventral noradrenergic bundle also passes near the A9 and A10 cell bodies. All these pathways come together in the medial forebrain bundle, which is the most common site for self-stimulation studies, notably at the level of the lateral hypothalamus.

Early evidence favored an important role for NE (Stein, 1968), but the manipulations used to interfere with the NE system in order to demonstrate this role mostly affected the DA system too. For instance, α-methyl-p-tyrosine (α-MPT), which inhibits synthesis of NE and DA, reduces ICSS, and monoamine oxidase inhibitors, which reduces metabolism of both NE and DA, increase it. In an attempt to distinguish the roles of DA and NE, Wise and Stein (1969) treated rats with the dopamine-β-hydroxylase (DBH) inhibitor, disulfiram, which depletes brain NE, but not DA. Self-stimulation was reduced, and was subsequently restored, by NE. However, Roll (1970) showed that the reduction in self-stimulation was largely due to sedation, and may not have been a reflection of a reduction in the rewarding value of the stimulation. Lippa et al. (1973) used the DBH inhibitor FLA-63, which does not produce sedation; it had no effect on self-stimulation.

Results of lesion experiments have caused the specific role of NE to be questioned, and have confirmed a principal role for DA. Cooper et al.

(1974) examined the effect of intracisternal injections of 6-OHDA on hypothalamic self-stimulation. Pargyline pretreatment, causing DA and NE depletion, produced a chronic deficit in self-stimulation. DMI pretreatment, resulting in selective DA depletion, produced a deficit from which the animals recovered. No pretreatment, resulting in a selective NE deplection, produced no deficit in self-stimulation. The first two groups (DA depletion) were highly disrupted by α-MPT, whereas the last group (NE depletion) was not. Lippa et al. (1973) found that self-stimulation rates recovered within seven days of intraventricular administration of 6-OHDA. Further administration of the NE-receptor blocker, phentolamine, had no effect, but the DA-receptor blocker, haloperidol, induced a 50 percent decline in self-stimulation rate.

Further evidence against a role for NE in ICSS comes from more specific lesion studies. Clavier et al. (1976) found that lesions of the dorsal nonadrenergic bundle did not reduce ICSS from the locus coeruleus, which gives rise directly to the fibers of the dorsal bundle. Similarly, Koob et al. (1976) showed that lesion of the locus coeruleus actually increased ICSS from the posterior hypothalamus. Calvier and Routtenberg (1976) found that lesions of the locus coeruleus or ventral nonadrenergic bundle did not affect brainstem ICSS.

Although the evidence favored DA rather than NE, the precise nature of DA's role was dubious. Antagonism of the DA system produces motor impairments, and rather than affecting motivation or reward, pharmacological and neurotoxic manipulations might simply be affecting the ability to move rather than the capacity to be rewarded. The problem of motor impairment produced by DA antagonism has been investigated by Rolls et al. (1974a). The DA blocker, spiroperidol, caused almost complete inhibition of self-stimulation at a dose that had only a small effect on locomotor activity and spontaneous rearing. In contast, phentolamine severely attenuated all three measures of behavior. In another experiment (Rolls et al. 1974b), spiroperidol produced a dose-dependent decrease in self-stimulation in the nucleus accumbens, septum, anterior hypothalamus, and ventral tegmentum. Spiroperidol caused a decrement in self-stimulation that was greater than the decrement in eating, which itself was greater that the decrement in drinking, at any one dose; thus, the drug may affect complex motor responses more than simple ones. When the rats were required to bar-press for food and water, they were equally sensitive to spiroperidol, and as sensitive as they had been when self-stimulating.

Thus, the effect on self-stimulation of DA blockade seems to be an impairment of the ability to make complex responses, rather than an effect on reward. Alternatively, it could induce an impairment of operant-learned behavior, which requires reward. Rolls et al. (1976b) suggested that the role of DA, then, could be in the high-level organization of motor responses, as illustrated by Wauquier and Niemegeers (1972), who showed that the selective DA receptor blocker, pimozide, disrupted many types of avoidance behavior and rewarded behavior to the same extent.

This problem was circumvented by employing a unilateral lesion technique, the rationale being that if the stimulation is processed in the same side of the brain to which it is applied, it can be predicted that a lesion of the critical system on the same side as the electrode would markedly reduce ICSS, but a lesion on the opposite side would have little effect. A pure motor impairment would produce a decrement regardless of the relative location of electrode and lesion. Koob et al. (1978) demonstrated that selective unilateral lesions of both the A9 and A10 systems markedly reduced ICSS from ipsilateral electrodes in the lateral hypothalamus, leaving ICSS from contralateral electrodes unaffected. Phillips et al. (1976) had previously shown that ICSS in the caudate nucleus was similarly affected. Here, the stimulation was applied anterior to the DA system so that the information had to travel down from the caudate to be fed into the DA system. Results with the electrodes in the substantia nigra are unclear. One study showed a similar result after unilateral DA lesions (Clavier et al., 1976), and another showed no differences between the ipsilateral and the contralateral lesion groups (Clavier and Fibiger, 1977). However, in the latter study, ICSS from the SN may have been complicated by motor effects of the stimulation. The contralateral group did not recover well after the lesion, making interpretation difficult. Phillips et al. (1976) have recently shown that ICSS from the ventral tegmental area, the region of the A10 cell bodies, and from the medial prefrontal cortex is reduced by an ipsilateral DA lesion. ICSS from the nucleus accumbens was reduced to a smaller extent. Koob et al. (1978) showed that ICSS from the locus coeruleus was also reduced by ipsilateral but not by contralateral lesions. Thus, it appears that even ICSS from a NE site depends not on NE for its mediation but on DA. This result demonstrates that ICSS is not necessarily maintained by the neurons at the electrode tip, as has previously been suggested (German and Bowden, 1974).

These experiments demonstrate a role for dopamine other than in the control of motor movements. However, the nature of the deficit produced by a dopamine lesion is by no means clear. It is possible that lesioned rats cannot feel the stimulation, or that it has lost its significance, or that the rats cannot associate it with a particular response. A simple reduction in rate of self-stimulation will not distinguish these possibilities; a more sophisticated procedure is required.

Relative Preference as a Measure of Reward

It has generally been assumed that high rates of ICSS reflect a high level of reward, and low rates reflect a lower level of reward; this is not necessarily the case. An animal might respond rapidly because the stimulation only affords a low level of reward, and rapid responding might be required in order to obtain sufficient stimulation. Equally, low rates could reflect a high level of reward, in which each stimulation provides a reward that can be savored for a period of time. Preference tests provide the only clear way of establishing the reactive rewarding value of two stimuli. These show that rats choose to work for stimulation of a brain site for which they respond at a low rate, in preference to stimulating from another site, for which they respond at a high rate (Hodos and Valenstein, 1962).

However, these measures only provide a qualitative measure of preference. The slightest difference between reinforcing value of the stimuli will induce a rat to spend virtually all its time with the preferred stimulus. An appropriate technique for quantifying relative preference for two reinforcing stimuli has been developed by Herrnstein (1961). He arranges food presentation for pigeons on two concurrently running variable interval (VI) schedules. The birds are assumed to be spending time on one schedule while they are pecking on one key, and, as soon as they change to the other key, they are assumed to be spending time on the other schedule. Since pecks are reinforced at random intervals on both keys independently, the pigeons must change over at fairly frequent intervals to earn the reinforcers as they become available. Within limits, they can vary the proportion of time they spend on the two schedules and still collect all the reinforcers due to them. The relative number of reinforcers set up on the two schedules can be varied by changing the average length of the two variable intervals such that, within a single session, a bird might earn one, two, four, or eight times as many reinforcers on one schedule as on the other. Herrnstein (1961) found that under these circumstances, pigeons would matche the relative number of responses on the two schedules to the relative number of reinforcers they earned in the session. In other words, if the left key provided *n* times as many reinforcers as the right key, the pigeons, after several sessions of training, would respond *n* times as often on the left key, even though this "matching" was not required for all the reinforcers to be earned. Herrnstein expressed this relationship in the following form, known as the matching relation:

$$\frac{R_1}{R_1 + R_2} = \frac{r_1}{r_1 + r_2} \qquad [1]$$

where R_1 and R_2 are the number of responses on the left and right keys, and r_1 and r_2 are the number of reinforcements earned on the left and right keys, respectively. It soon became apparent that pigeons were also matching the amount of time they spent on the two schedules as well, and so the following equation can be written:

$$\frac{T_1}{T_1 + T_2} = \frac{R_1}{R_1 + R_2} = \frac{r_1}{r_1 + r_2} \qquad [2]$$

where T_1 and T_2 are the time spent responding on the left and right keys, respectively. An alternative way of writing euqation [1] is:

$$\frac{R_1}{R_2} = \frac{r_1}{r_2} \qquad [3]$$

Baum (1974) has pointed out that this is, in fact, a special form of the equation

$$\frac{R_1}{R_2} = a\left[\frac{r_1}{r_2}\right]^b \qquad [4]$$

with *a* and *b* equal to 1.
Taking logs:

$$\log\,[R_1/R_2] = \log a + b \log\,[r_1/r_2] \qquad [5]$$

Baum has shown that apparent deviations from equation [1] are often due to a value of the parameter *a* which is not equal to one. This parameter gives a measure of an animal's non-specific bias to one key or the other. It also appears that the parameter *b* is often less than 1. In fact, this may be the rule rather than the exception (Lobb and Davison, 1975; Myers and Myers, 1977.)

Equation [4] can be seen as a form of Stevens' (1957) power law for relating the physical intensity of a stimulus (analogous to r_1/r_2) to its subjective intensity (analogous to R_1/R_2). Here, we are asking the animal to give an account of the relative reinforcing value of two levels of reinforcement. Stevens' experiments with a variety of sensory stimuli often produced an exponent of less than one, and this may be the case for animals, too. Other explanations for this "undermatching" are possible, but the parallel between Stevens' law and the matching relation is compelling if the two reinforcers to be compared are two intensities of brain stimulation. It is to this end that we have recently applied the matching relation to ICSS.

If rats could be induced to work on concurrent VI shedules for brain stimulation, a function could be established for each rat, defining the relationship between relative amount of reinforcement and relative responding on two levers. Then relative reinforcement could be varied, not by changing the VI schedules, but by manipulating the relative current intensity available on the two levers. With reference to the rat's own function, the relative rewarding value of a particular pair of current intensities could be evaluated.

Five rats were trained using the matching procedure. Two retractable levers were presented with independent VI schedules running on each. When a reinforcement was earned on either lever, both levers were retracted, and the rat could make several panel-push responses to obtain a train of lateral hypothalamic stimulation for each response. Both schedules were frozen during the collection of reinforcers. When the programmed number of stimulation trains had been collected the levers were presented again and the schedules proceeded. Several different pairs of VI schedules were given to the rats, and the results are plotted in Fig. 8. It can be seen that the data fit the equation [4] remarkably well. All rats undermatched, but the agreement between the exponent for responses and time is extremely good.

Relative reward is now being manipulated by changing the current intensities on the two levers, keeping both schedules at VI 60 seconds. Preliminary results indicate that the rats will indeed match their responses to the absolute ratio of the current intensities employed. The data points fall on the same regression lines when the axis represents relative current intensity. That is to say, within limits, 50 μA is twice as reinforcing as 25 μA.

Also, we have held both the VI schedules and the current intensities constant while varying the relative number of stimulation trains that can be earned for each reinforcement opportunity in order to test the hypothesis that, otherwise stated, 8 trains is twice as reinforcing as 4 trains. Again, the rats appeared to match relative responses to relative reinforcement in this way. These data confirm an earlier suggestive finding by Pliskoff and Hawkins (1967). Further, Coleman and Berger (1978) have recently reported suggestive evidence that rats will also match their responses to the relative length of the stimulation train. Thus, it appears that the rats actually match their responses and time to the relative amount of stimulation available on the two schedules regardless of how it is made up. If this is true, then it should be possible to compensate for a long VI schedule with a high current, or a large number of stimulation trains. Suitable substitution tests have yet to be carried out to confirm this.

We propose that the matching relation provides a powerful tool for the investigation of the neural substrate of ICSS. A quantitative increase of the rewarding value of the stimulation can be obtained, and changes in this value can be assessed after lesions or treatment with drugs. Since the effect of a manipulation is measured in terms of the relative rate of responding and relative time allocation, non-specific effects on overall rate of responding

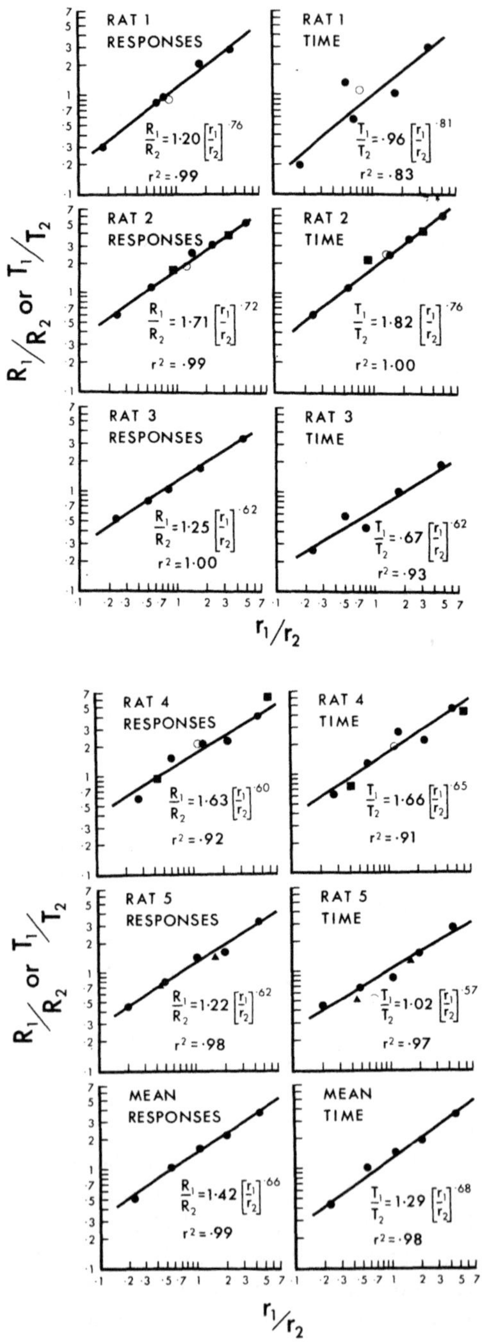

FIG. 8. Data of five rats responding on a series of concurrent VI/VI schedules reinforced by electrical stimulation of the lateral hypothalamus. Number of responses on the left lever divided by number of responses on the right lever (R_1/R_2), and time spent responding on the left lever divided by time spent on the right lever (T_1/T_2) are plotted as a function of the number of reinforcements earned on the left lever (r_1/r_2). Each point for individual rats is the median of seven consecutive determinations, taken when performance was judged stable. The last panel depicts the means of the points derived from the five rats. The VI schedules were arranged so that approximately the following total numbers of reinforcements were delivered each session: • = 60; ■ = 120; ▲ = 30; 0 = return to 60 after either 120 or 30. Equations were fitted by the method of least squares, using the filled-circle data only; r^2 indicates the proportion of the variance accounted for. The data indicate that the distribution of responses and time between the two schedules are determined by the relative number of reinforcers earned on the two concurrently running schedules, regardless of the total amount of reinforcement available in the session.

will have no effect. The exciting possibility exists of producing changes in the exponent and the bias of the equation independently. A change in bias would simply reflect a change in preference for the aspects of the situation unrelated to the programmed reinforcers on the two schedules. A change in exponent however, would indicate an actual change in the animal's expression of the relative value of the programmed reinforcers. Behavioral methods of this sophistication possess the analytic potential for advancing both the theoretical and physiological understanding of motivation.

MODELS OF THE MESOLIMBOCORTICAL DA SYSTEM IN RELATION TO MENTAL ILLNESS

Over the last ten years, an interesting body of multidisciplinary research on DA systems has accrued. The impetus for much of this work has been the belief that certain forms of mental illness in man are related to dysfunction of chemical transmitter systems of brain. We shall address ourselves particularly to the hypothesis that DA dysfunction in forebrain is a corollary of the major psychotic illness, schizophrenia. Hypotheses of this generality in biological psychiatry are dangerous and not unreasonably so; many people feel uncomfortable in embracing theories which they intuitively feel are too simple-minded. It may well prove to be the case that DA dysfunction is not primary to psychosis, but a relationship of some form cannot be denied. In the absence of other hypotheses, it remains worthwhile to continue exploring this relationship. In so doing, at least the normal role of DA in behavioral control should become clear and, at best, in studying the dysfunction of the DA system correlated with psychosis, other contributing factors will be revealed to yield a more complete explanation.

DA Models of Psychosis

The rationale for such models rests on several lines of investigation that have been reviewed many times in recent years and need only be referenced in this paper (Snyder, 1972). Briefly, these are:

(i) The drugs that control the florid symptoms of schizophrenia have, as their major CNS action, the ability to block catecholamine receptors in brain. Some of the most potent ones developed in recent years block DA receptors specifically, reinforcing the view that DA systems may be more involved in psychosis than NE systems.

(ii) Biochemical assay of post-mortem material from patients diagnosed as schizophrenic show raised levels of DA in certain forebrain limbic areas.

(iii) Amphetamine, a drug which releases DA and NE in brain, produces a form of psychosis in man similar to paranoid schizophrenia, when taken in large doses. Superficially one might question the details of this comparison. For example, in the chronic schizophrenic, blunted affect and thought disorder are cardinal symptoms. In amphetamine psychosis (AP), they are rarely, although sometimes, seen. Equally, visual hallucinations and prominant stereotypies are frequently seen in AP, but are less common in schizophrenia. It would thus appear that AP and schizophrenia share a wide range of symptoms, although their frequency in the two conditions may differ. It is thus reasonable to view this form of amphetamine-induced behavior as a model of psychosis.

(iv) In experimental animals, the acute behavioral effects induced by amphetamine are abolished by lesions of the forebrain DA pathways, but not of the NE pathways.

In view of these lines of evidence, animal preparations with heightened DA function would be potentially useful models of psychosis. These models, described in the following sections, include stereotypy induced by drugs which release DA from the CNS (e.g., sympathomimetic amines, such as amphetamine), behavioral effects induced by sustained stimulation with amphetamine (as released from implanted drug pellets), and the effects of priming activation of DA pathways on the subsequent response to DA-releasing drugs.

Acute Amphetamine and Stereotyped Behavior

Large, acute doses of amphetamine induce pronounced stereotyped behavior in all species studied. Stereotypy is abnormal behavior in which response elements from the normal behavioral repertoire are repeated with increasing frequency. Because of the physical limitations of the animal and the constraints of time, this results in a rapid fragmentation of behavior. Long sequences of responses can never be completed and quickly disappear, whereas short elements of behavior have a higher probability of completion. Eventually, brief fragments of the normal behavior remain and are repeated at a high frequency. Amphetamine-release of DA in the striatum underlies this behavioral response. Presumably, behavior is disrupted because of the abnormally high release of DA. Stereotypy appears autonomous but can be influenced by the external environment. If a particular response is highly probable before the drug is given, it is likely to be enhanced under the drug. For example, if rats are rewarded for making a particular response, e.g., lever-press, stereotyped lever pressing is seen following amphetamine, even though the animal does not retrieve the earned food reinforcements. Amphetamine addicts demonstrate dramatic sterotyped behavior in which patterns of thought are often repeated, and the nature of the stereotyped activities are determined by individual differences and favored activities.

Mechanically-minded people dismantle and reassemble complex machines such as cars or clocks, houseproud women clean endlessly, and tidy people sort their possessions. The blockade of drug-induced stereotyped behavior has provided one of the most valuable tools for identifying and ranking antischizophrenic drugs.

Behavioral Effects of Sustained Amphetamine Exposure

Schizophrenia and amphetamine psychosis are conditions associated with chronic states, whereas stereotypy is caused by acute drug dosage. Ellison et al. (1978) have suggested that a more appropriate animal model would involve sustained dopaminergic overactivity and, to this end, he devised a slow releasing depot injection of amphetamine which is implanted subcutaneously in the animal. Biochemical work has shown that 87 percent of the amphetamine is released continuously over 10 days. Brain levels of amphetamine are initially slightly lower than those seen after a systemic injection of 2 mg/kg amphetamine and they decrease linearly from this level. The behavior of the drugged rats changes over the six-day observation period. On day 1 and 2, the typical locomotor stimulation and stereotypy are observed in the arena. On day 3 the amphetamine-treated animals withdraw from the social colony (18 rats) and spend more time in the burrows during the next 24 hours. Gradually they re-emerge to indulge in abnormal social behavior with each other and with undrugged members of the colony. This takes the form of aggressive encounters with long bouts of "stand and box" behavior, persistently initiated by the drugged animals with the control rats. In view of the fact the brain levels of amphetamine are relatively low, the profound behavioral effect must be attributed to the sustained stimulation by amphetamine.

We have performed similar experiments in the monkey. A 175-mg pellet induced a number of behaviors, but most impressive and interesting are the hallucinatory-like episodes seen from about day 5 onward. In the absence of real-world stimuli, the amphetamine animal showed clear orientation, startle, and fleeing from apparently imaginary stimuli. At this stage, the monkey was divorced from the real world and barely responded to observers, even when threatened by them. Although repeated acute injections of amphetamine result in heightened behavioral responsiveness to DA-agonist drugs, surprisingly, after the chronic pellet treatment with amphetamine, no evidence of enhanced DA receptor sensitivity has been found. Such results confirm the impression that activity of the DA neurons and the state of the postsynaptic receptors are not causally related in a simple manner (Iversen et al., 1980).

In fact, the DA synapse is under the influence of a complex set of control mechanisms that include the DA level in the neuron and DA turnover, the state of DA autoreceptors on the terminals, and the state of the postsynaptic DA receptor. All of these mechanisms are susceptible to modification, but they are difficult to study in isolation, and we do not fully understand their role and contribution to the responsiveness of the DA synapse (Schwartz et al., 1978). Use or disuse may result in hypo- or hypersensitivity of the DA response, and it is clear that the DA neuron is a very highly tuned and sensitive neuronal system.

DA sensitivity, measured by receptor binding in post mortem material, is raised in schizophrenic brain. However, this may well be a reflection of chronic receptor blocking drugs used in treatment rather than a reflection of the state of the dopamine synapse. Indeed, if DA levels are raised in the schizophrenic, this is the exact opposite of the condition which commonly results in an increase in receptor sensitivity. Lowered levels of dopamine after lesions or chronic blockade of DA transmission with antagonist drugs are the most common manipulations which produce marked DA receptor supersensitivity.

Methods for Sensitizing the Response of Dopamine Neurons

Antelman and his colleagues have described a number of procedures which alter the subsequent responsiveness of the DA neurons to drugs and enhance the occurrence of unconditioned behavior thought to involve DA in their normal expression. Antelman became aware of the importance of the DA system in processes of behavioral arousal through the studies discussed in the previous section. Blockers of DA pathways prevent tail-pinch-induced arousal, as they do amphetamine responses. It has been shown that rats exposed to repeated, mild tail-pinch subsequently show greatly enhanced responses to amphetamine. Other stimuli that result in similar sensitization include pretreatment with amphetamine and electrical self-stimulation of the NAS or medial frontal cortex (Eichler and Antelman, 1979). Thus, it has been suggested that such stimuli act as mild stressors to increase the functional capacity of the DA neurons. This kind of responsiveness to the environment would be of obvious biological value, and thus a reasonable amount of stress may not be harmful. He went on to reason that excessive stress would clearly be disadvantageous and raises the possibility that schizophrenia and its associated DA hyperactivity may reflect an inherent tendency to over-respond to stress.

For a number of years, Stevens has been investigating the responsiveness of certain forebrain sites to repeated chemical or electrical stimulation in experiments modeled on the classical kindling procedure of Goddard et al. (1969). In particular, she has focused on the mesolimbic dopamine pathway and has found that local injection of the GABA antagonist, bicuculline, into the VTA produced marked changes in the behavior of cats, including intense arousal, hypervigilance, orientating, side-to-side looking behavior, slinking, and crouching (Stevens et al., 1974). This behavior was associated with abnormal electrical spike activity in the NAS. It is reasonable to assume that inhibition of the normal inhibitory action of GABA on the VTA dopamine neurons resulted in increased dopaminergic activity and the associated behavioral arousal. Electrical stimulation of the VTA produced similar results in some animals. Stevens has coined the term "behavioral kindling" for the phenomenon and has shown a decreased threshold for electrically-induced kindling at the injection or stimulation site (Stevens and Livermore, 1978). Abnormal spike activity has been noted in the limbic areas of schizophrenic patients (Heath, 1962) and it has been suggested that this may arise as a result of a chronic disorder of the normal inhibitory influences on the DA neurons of the VTA. Pursuing such reasoning, it has been proposed that kindling of these inhibitory pathways to DA neurons may be able to compensate for the dopaminergic dysfunction.

Which DA System Is Principally Involved In Schizophrenia?

The forebrain DA is contained in three different terminal areas: striatum, limbic structures, and cortex, albeit cortex strongly linked functionally with the limbic system. Are all of these DA systems involved in schizophrenia, and do neuroleptics control the florid symptoms of the disease by blocking receptors at all these sites? We do not have definitive answers to either of these questions. First, it would not be surprising to find widespread forebrain dysfunction in an illness with symptoms ranging from hallucinations, through affect, to motor stereotypy. Second, from a large number of biochemical studies investigating the interaction between neuroleptic drugs and DA neurons, it is fair to say that all DA receptors respond to such drugs. Differences have emerged, but most of these have been of a *quantitative* rather than a *qualitative* nature. The biochemical response to neuroleptics of mesolimbic DA neurons is said to be greater than that of nigro-striatal neurons; differential tolerance to the biochemical effects of neuroleptics on DA metabolism have been reported, with mesolimbic areas showing less tolerance. Two further lines of evidence suggest a particularly important role of the mesolimbocortical system in relation to psychosis. The atypical neuroleptics such as thioridazine and clozapine, which have muscarinic activity, are thought to be without functional blocking capacity in the striatum, where cholinergic interneurons are in functional balance with the DA terminals. In line with this observation, chronic clozapine and the thioridazine do not induce extrapyramidal side effects, particularly tardive dyskinesia, to the same extent as those neuroleptics with strong antidopaminergic and weak anticholinergic activity. Yet, these atypical neuroleptics control psychotic systems, suggesting that sites outside the striatum play a major role in the expression of psychotic behavior. Finally, in experiments investigating environmental factors which modify the activity of DA neurons, limbic and cortical areas are found to be more sensitive than striatum and, within the former group of structures, Thierry et al. (1978) have reported the mesofrontal cortex to be especially sensitive to stress-induced changes in DA turnover.

However, despite these clues, the contribution of the various forebrain DA sites to schizophrenia and its control remain to be defined.

Interaction Of DA With Other Chemically Coded Forebrain Systems

It would be misleading to conclude this review without reference to the functional importance of interaction between DA neurons and other forebrain circuits, some of which are also chemically coded. These interactions are of two kind: first, those concerned with the local control of activity within dopaminergic systems neurons, and, second, those between DA neuron systems and the other forebrain modulatory systems.

The local control of activity within dopaminergic neuron systems exerted by direct projections of non-dopaminergic neurons has been most extensively studied in the nigro-striatal system. Several central interactions, including those with ACh interneurons of striatum, enkephalin interneurons of striatum, descending striato-nigral GABA neuron system to globus pallidus and SN, descending Substance P pathway to SN, and a non-dopaminergic striato-nigral-thalamic output system have been identified. In the non-striatal system, ACh interactions do not appear to be as important as in the striatum. However, in the non-striatal systems, evidence of GABA, SP and enkephalin interactions in the VTA has been found. In both the SN and the VTA, local manipulations of GABA (Mogenson et al. 1979), SP (Kelley et al., 1979), and enkephalin (Kelley et al., 1980) have been found to produce behavioral and biochemical changes consistent with altered activity of the DA neurons. In most cases, the fine structure of these chemical interactions remains to be demonstrated with appropriate anatomical techniques. With respect to interactions extrinsic to the DA neurons, both NE and 5HT play modulatory roles at forebrain sites innervated by the DA neurons. Lesions to one part of such a balanced system result, not unexpectedly, in changes in spontaneous and drug-induced behavior. These results have been admirably reviewed by Antelman and Caggiula (1977).

CONCLUDING STATEMENT

Considerations of balance provide an appropriate concluding point for this review. In seeking to understand the role of chemically coded pathways in brain, we are the captive of the available techniques and of the traditional ways of viewing brain structure in relation to function. Current research strategies employ techniques to interfere with a pathway or structure in order to study the subsequent effects on behavior. The change in behavior inevitably reflects not only the loss of a specific contribution made by the lesioned system to forebrain integration, but also reflects disruption of a finely balanced circuitry associated with the DA neurons and extending far beyond. It is very difficult to tease these two effects apart. The lesion technique is inadequate when used in isolation. The value of results obtained with this method must rely heavily on parallel anatomical, biochemical, and electrophysiological studues of the DA neurons in the normally functioning brain. The chemical coded circuits of brain may not serve specific information processing functions in the sense that primary visual cortex does; rather they may serve enabling functions essential for the integration of the various forms of neural processing achieved by the forebrain. In this sense, the non-striatal DA system is not involved in sensory coding or the initiation of specific responses. Rather, DA systems appear to serve an arousal process which allows the animal to focus on biologically relevant stimuli in the environment, and is thus essential for organized motivational and emotional behavior.

REFERENCES

Angrist, B.M., and Gershon, S. The phenomenology of experimentally induced amphetamine psychosis — preliminary observations. *Biol. Psychiat.* 2, 95–107 (1970).

Antelman, S.M., and Caggiula, A.R. Norepinephrine—dopamine interactions and behaviour. *Science* 195, 646–653 (1977).

Antelman, S.M., Rowland, N.E., and Fisher, A.E. Stimulation bound ingestive behavior: A view from the tail. *Physiol. Behav.* 17, 743–748 (1976).

Antelman, S.M., and Szechtman, H. Tail pinch induces eating in sated rats which appears to depend on nigrostriatal dopamine. *Science* 189, 731–733 (1975).

Barfield, R.J., and Sachs, B.D. Sexual behavior: Stimulation by painful electric shock to skin in male rats. *Science* 161, 392–393 (1968).

Baum, W.M. On two types of deviation from the matching law: Bias and undermatching. *J.Exp. Anal. Behav.* 22, 231–242 (1974).

Beckstead, R.M. Convergent prefrontal and nigral projections to the striatum of the rat. *Neurosci. Letters* 12, 59–64 (1979).

Berlyne, D.E. Arousal and reinforcement, in *Symposium on Motivation*, Vol. 15. D. Levine, ed. University of Nebraska Press, Lincoln, Nebraska (1967), pp. 1–110.

Caggiula, A.R., and Eibergen, R. Copulation of virgin male rats evoked by painful peripheral stimulation. *J. Comp. Physiol. Psychol.* 69, 414–419 (1969).

Clark, F.C., and Smith, J.B. Schedules of food postponement. II. Maintenance of behavior by food postponement and effects of the schedule parameter. *J. Exp. Anal. Behav.* 28, 253–269 (1977).

Clavier, R.M., and Fibiger, H.C. On the role of ascending catecholaminergic projections in intracranial self-stimulation of the substantia nigra. *Brain Res.* 131, 271–286 (1977).

Clavier, R.M., Fibiger, H.C., and Phillips, A.G. Evidence that self-stimulation of the region of the locus coeruleus in rats does not depend upon noradrenergic projections to telencephalon. *Brain Res.* 113, 71–81 (1976).

Clavier, R.M. Phillips, A.G., and Fibiger, H.C. Effects of unilateral nigrostriatal bundle lesions with 6-hydroxydopamine on self-stimulation from the A9 dopamine cell group. *Neurosci. Abs.* 1, 479 (1975).

Clavier, R.M. and Routtenberg, A. Brain stem self-stimulation attenuated by lesions of medial forebrain bundle, but not by lesions of locus coeruleus or caudal ventral norepinephrine bundle. *Brain Res.* 101, 251–271 (1976).

Coleman, W.R., and Berger, L.H. Utility scaling of intracranial reinforcement duration. *Physiol. Behav.* 21, 485–490 (1978).

Coons, E.E., Levak, M., and Miller, N.E. Lateral hypothalamus: Learning of food-seeking response motivated by electrical stimulation. *Science* 150, 1320–1321 (1965).

Cooper, B.R., Cott, J.M., and Breese, G.R. Effects of catecholamine-depleting drugs and amphetamine on self-stimulation of the brain, following various 6-hydroxydopamine treatments. *Psychopharmacologia (Berl.)* 37, 235–248 (1974).

Creese, I., and Iversen, S.D. The role of dopamine systems in amphetamine induced stereotyped behaviour in the rat. *Psychopharmacologia (Berl.)* 39, 345–357 (1974).

Crow, T.J. Catecholamine-containing neurones and electrical self-stimulation: A review of some data. *Psychol. Med.* 2, 414–421 (1972).

Darwin, C. *The Expression of the Emotions in Man and Animals.* Reprinted University of Chicago Press (1965).

DiChiara, G., Porceddu, M.L., Morelli, M., Mulas, M.L., and Gessa, G.L. Strio-nigral and nigro-thalamic GABA-ergic neurons as output pathways for striatal responses, in *GABA-Neurotransmitters.* Alfred Benzon Symposium, (1978), pp. 465–481.

Divac, I. Current conceptions of neostriatal functions, in *History and Evaluation in the Neostriatum.* I. Divac and R.G.E. Oberg, eds. Pergamon Press, Oxford and New York (1979), pp. 215–230.

Eichler, A.J. and Antelman, S.M. Sensitization to amphetamine and stress may involve nucleus accumbens and medial frontal cortex. *Brain Res.* 176, 412–416 (1979).

Ellinwood, E.H., Jr., Sudilovsky, A., and Nelson, L. Evolving behaviors in the clinical and experimental amphetamine (model) psychosis. *Am. J. Psychiat.* 29, 1088–1092 (1973).

Ellison, G., Eison, M.S., and Huberman, H.S. Stages of constant amphetamine intoxication: Delayed appearance of abnormal social behavior in rat colonies. *Psychopharmacologia* 56, 293–299 (1978).

Fallon, J.H., and Moore, R.Y. Catecholamine innervation of the basal forebrain. IV. Topography of the dopamine projection to the basal forebrain and neostraiatum. *J. Comp. Neurol.* 180, 545–580 (1978).

Fallon, J.H., Riley, J.N., and Moore, R.Y. Substantia nigra dopamine neurons: Separate population project to neostriatum and allocortex. *Neurosci, Letters* 7, 157–162 (1978).

Fray, P.J., Koob, G.F., and Iversen, S.D. Tail pinch versus brain stimulation: Problems of comparison (reply). *Science* 201, 841–842 (1978).

Fray, P.J., Koob, G.F., and Iversen, S.D. Tail-pinch elicited behaviour in rats: preference, plasticity and learning. Submitted.

German, D.C., and Bowden, D.M. Catecholamine systems as the neural substrate of intracranial self-stimulation. *Brain Res.* 73, 381–419 (1974).

Goddard, G.V., McIntyre, D.C., and Leech, C.K. A permanent change in brain function resulting from daily electrical stimulation. *Exper. Neurol.* 25, 296–330 (1969).

Heath, R.G. Common characteristics of epilepsy and schizophrenia: clinical observation and depth electrode studies. *Am. J. Psychiat.* 118, 1013–1026 (1962).

Heimer, L., and Wilson, R.D. Perspectives in neurobiology, in *The Golgi Centennial Symposium.* M.M. Santini, ed. Raven Press, New York (1975), pp. 177–193.

Herrnstein, R.J. Relative and absolute strength of response as a function of frequency of reinforcement. *J. Exp. Anal. Behav.* 4, 267–272 (1961).

Hodos, W., and Valenstein, E.S. An evaluation of response rate as a measure of rewarding intracranial stimulation. *J. Comp. Physiol. Psychol.* 55, 80–84 (1962).

Iversen, S.D. Behaviour after neostriatal lesions in animals, in *The Neostriatum.* I. Divac and R.G.E. Oberg, eds. Pergamon Press, Elmsford (1979), p. 195–212.

Iversen, S.D. Striatal Function and Behaviour, in *Psychobiology of the Striatum.* A. Cools, ed. Elsevier, New York (1977), pp. 99–118.

Iversen, S.D., and Iversen, L.L. *Behavioural Pharmacology.* Oxford Press, New York (1975), Chapter 5.

Iversen, S.D., Howells, R.B., and Hughes, R.P. Behavioural consequences of long-term treatment with neuroleptic drugs, in *Long-Term Effects of Neuroleptics.*, Adv. Biochem. Psychopharmacol., Vol. 22. Cattaberi et al., eds. Raven Press, New York (1980), in press.

Kelley, A.E., Stinus, L., and Iversen, S.D. Behavioural activation induced in the rat by substance P infusion into ventral tegmental area: Implication of dopaminergic A10 neurones. *Neurosci. Letters* 11, 335–339 (1979).

Kelley, A.E., Stinus, L., and Iversen, S.D. Interactions between d-ala-met-enkephalin, A10 dopaminergic neurones, and spontaneous behaviour in the rat. *Behav. Brain Res.* 1, 3–24 (1980).

Kelly, P. Drug-induced motor behaviour, in *Handbook of Psychopharmacology,* Vol. 8, Chapter 7. S.D. Iversen, L.L. Iversen, and S. Snyder, eds. Plenum Press, New York/London (1978), pp. 295—331.

Kent, E., and Grossman, S.P. Evidence for a conflict interpretation of anomalous effects of rewarding stimulation. *J. Comp. Physiol. Psychol.* 69, 381–390 (1969).

Koob, G.F., Fray, P.J., and Iversen, S.D. Tail-pinch stimulation: Sufficient motivation for learning. *Science* 194, 637–639 (1976).

Koob, G.F., Fray, P.J. and Iversen, S.D. Self-stimulation at the lateral hypothalamus and locus coeruleus after specific uniliteral lesions of the dopamine system. *Brain Res.* 146, 123–140 (1978).

Lippa, A.S., Antelman, S.M., Fisher, A.E., and Canfield, D.R. Neurochemical mediation of reward: A significant role for dopamine? *Pharmacol. Biochem. Behav.* 1, 23–28 (1973).

Lobb, B., and Davison, M.C. Performance in concurrent interval schedules: A systematic replication. *J. Exp. Anal. Behav.* 24, 191–197 (1975).

Lyon, M., and Robbins, T.W. The action of central nervous system stimulant drugs: a general theory concerning amphetamine effects, in *Current Developments in Psychopharmacology.* W. Essman and L. Valzelli, eds. Spectrum Publications, New York (1975), Vol. 2, pp. 79–163.

Marshall, J.F., and Teitelbaum, P. Further analyses of sensory inattention following lateral hypothalamic damage in rats. *J. Comp. Physiol. Psychol.* 86, 375–395 (1974).

Mendelson, J., and Chorover, S.L. Lateral hypothalamic stimulation in satiated rats: T-maze. Learning for food. *Science* 149, 559–561 (1965).

Meyers, D.L., and Myers, L.E. Undermatching: A reappraisal of performance on concurrent variable-interval schedules of reinforcement. *J. Exp. Anal. Behav.* 25, 203–214 (1977).

Millenson, J.R. *Principles of Behavioral Analysis.* Macmillan, New York (1967).

Miller, N.E. Experiments on motivation. *Science* 126, 1271–1278 (1957).

Mogenson, G.J., Wu, M., and Manchanela, S.K. Locomotor activity initiated by microinfusions of picrotoxin in the ventral tegmental area. *Brain Res.* 161, 311–319 (1979).

Moore, K.E. Amphetamines: Biochemical and behavioral actions in animals, in *Handbook of Psychopharmacology*. L.L. Iversen, S.D. Iversen, and S.H. Snyder, eds. Plenum Press, New York and London (1978), Vol. II, pp. 41–98.

Morse, W.H., and Kelleher, R.T. Determinants of reinforcement and punishment, in *Handbook of Operant Behavior.*. W.K. Honig and J.E. Staddon, eds. Prentice-Hall, Englewood Cliffs, New Jersey (1977), pp. 174–200.

Nauta, W.J.H., and Domesick, V.B. Crossroads of limbic and striatal circuitry: Hypothalamonigral connections in limbic mechanisms, in *Limbic Mechanism,* K.E. Livingstone and O. Hornykiewicz, eds. Plenum Press, New York and London (1978), pp. 75–93.

Nauta, W.J.H., Smith, G.P., Faull, R.L.M., and Domesick, V.B. Efferent connection and nigral afferents of the nucleus accumbens septi in the rat. *Neuroscience* 3, 385–401 (1978).

Neill, D.B. Fronto-striatal control of behavioral inhibition in the rat. *Brain Res.* 105, 89–103 (1976).

Phillips, A.G., Carter, D.A., and Fibiger, H.C. Dopaminergic substrates of intracranial self-stimulation in the caudate-putamen. *Brain Res.* 104, 222–232 (1976).

Phillips, A.G., and Fibiger, H.C. The role of dopamine in maintaining intracranial self-stimulation in the ventral tegmentum, nucleus accumbens, and medial prefrontal cortex. *Canad. J. Psychol.* 32, 58–66 (1978).

Pliskoff, S.S., and Hawkins, T.D. A method of increasing the reinforcement magnitude of intracranial stimulation. *J. Exp. Anal. Behav.* 10, 281–289 (1967).

Ranje, C., and Ungerstedt, U. Lack of acquisition in dopamine denervated animals tested in an underwater Y-maze. *Brain Res.* 134, 95–111 (1977).

Robbins, T.W., and Fray, P.J. Stress-induced eating: fact, fiction or misunderstanding? *Appetite* 1, 103–133 (1980).

Robbins, T.W. Phillips, A.G., and Sahakian, B.J. Effects of chlordiazepoxide on tail-pinch induced eating in rats. *Pharmacol. Biochem. Behav.* 6, 297–302 (1977).

Roll, S.K. Intracranial self-stimulation and wakefulness: effect of manipulating ambient brain catecholamine. *Science* 168, 1370–1372 (1970).

Rolls, E.T., Kelly, P.H., and Shaw, S.G. Noradrenaline, dopamine and brain-stimulation reward. *Pharmacol. Biochem. Behav.* 2, 735–740 (1974).

Rolls, E.T., Rolls, B.J., Kelly, P.H., Shaw, S.G., Wood, K.J., and Dale, R. The relative attenuation of self-stimulation, eating and drinking produced by dopamine-receptor blackade. *Psychopharmacologia (Berl.)* 38, 219–230 (1974b).

Rylander, G. Chemical and medico-criminological aspects of addictions to ventral stimulating drugs, in *Abuse of Central Stimulants.* F. Sjoquist and M. Tottil, eds. Raven Press, New York (1969), pp. 251–273.

Schachter, S. The interaction of cognitive and physiological determinants of emotional state, in *Anxiety and Behavior.* C.D. Spielberger, ed. Academic Press, New York and London (1966), pp. 193–224.

Schwartz, J.C., Costenin, J., Martres, M.P., Protais, P., and Baudry, M. Modulation of receptor mechanisms in the CNS: Hyper- and hyposensitivity to catecholamines. *Neuropharmacology* 17, 665–685 (1978).

Smith, D.A. Incentive as a factor in the behaviors of rats given lateral hypothalamic stimulation. *Physiol. Behav.* 8, 1077–1086 (1972).

Smith, J.B., and Clark, F.C. Two temporal parameters of food postponement. *J. Exp. Anal. Behav.* 18, 1–12 (1972).

Snyder, S.H. Catecholamines in the brain as mediators of amphetamine psychosis. *Arch. Gen. Psychiat.* 27, 169–179 (1972).

Stein, L. Chemistry of reward and punishment, in *Psychopharmacology, a Reveiw of Progress: 1957–1967.* D.H. Efron, ed. U.S. Government Printing Office, Washington, D.C. (1968), pp. 105–123.

Stevens, J.R., and Livermore, A. Kindling of the mesolimbic dopamine system: animal model of psychosis. *Neurology* 28, 36–46 (1978).

Stevens, J., Wilson, K., and Foote, W. GABA blockade, dopamine and schizophrenia: experimental studies in the cat. *Psychopharmacologia* 39, 105–119 (1974).

Stevens, S.S. On the psychophysical law. *Psychol. Rev.* 64, 153–181 (1957).

Stinus, L., Gaffori, O., Simon, H., and LeMoal, M. Disappearance of hoarding and disorganization of eating behavior after ventral mesencephalic tegmentum lesion in rats. *J. Comp. Physiol. Psychol.* 92, 289–296 (1978).

Teitelbaum, P., and Epstein, A.N. The lateral hypothalamic syndrome: recovery of feeding and drinking after lateral hypothalamic lesions. *Physiol. Rev.* 69, 74–90 (1962).

Tennen, S.S., and Miller, N.E. Strength of electrical stimulation of lateral hypothalamus. Food deprivation and tolerance for quinine in food. *J. Comp. Physiol. Psychol.* 58, 55–62 (1964).

Thierry, A.M., Tassin, J.P., Blanc, G., and Glowinski, J. Studies on mesocortical dopamine systems, in *Advances in Biochemical Psychopharmacology,* Vol. 19, Raven Press, New York (1978), pp. 205–216.

Tourtellotte, W.W., Farley, I.J., and Hornykiewicz, O. Binding of ^{3}H-neuroleptics and ^{3}H-apomorphine in schizophrenic brains. *Nature* 274, 897–900 (1978).

Ungerstedt, U. Is interruption of the nigro-striatal system producing the "lateral hypothalamus syndrome"*Acta Physiol. Scand.* 80, 35A–36A (1970).

Ungerstedt, U. On the anatomy, pharmacology and function of the nigro-striatal dopamine system. *Acta Physiol. Scand.* Suppl. 367 (1971).

Valenstein, E.S., Cox, V.C., and Kakolewski, J.W. Re-examination of the role of the hypothalamus in motivation. *Psychol. Rev.* 77, 16–31 (1970).

Wauquier, A., and Niemegeers, C.J.E. Intracranial self-stimulation in rats as a function of various stimuli parameters II. Influence of haloperidol, pimozide and pipamperone. *Psychopharmacologia (Berl.)* 27, 191–202 (1972).

Wise, R.A., and Erdmann, E. Emotionality, hunger and normal eating: implications for the interpretation of electrically-induced behavior. *Behav. Biol.* 8, 519–531 (1973).

Wise, C.D., and Stein, L. Facilitation of brain self-stimulation by central administration of norepinephrine. *Science* 163, 299–301 (1969).

Yeterian, E.H., and van Hoesen, G.W. Cortico-striate projections in the rhesus monkey: the organization of certain cortico-caudate connections. *Brain Res.* 139, 43–63 (1978).

PART IV

Pain

Copyright © 1982, Spectrum Publications, Inc.
The Neural Basis of Behavior

13

Neural Mechanisms in Pain and Analgesia: An Overview

Kenneth L. Casey

Acute pain is an adaptive warning of impending or actual tissue damage. It interrupts ongoing behavior, directs attention to the site of injury, and motivates behavior to escape from the offending stimulus. Chronic, intractable pain is an equally compelling, but typically maladaptive, state often associated with profound affective disturbances in patients. These descriptions emphasize two major features of pain which must be considered in attempting to understand the underlying neural mechanisms. First, pain is a somatic or visceral sensation which can be localized in time, space, and along a continuum of intensities; like other sensations, pain has discriminative features. Second, pain is unpleasant; unlike most other sensations, it has an affective dimension which is a necessary component of the experience. A neurophysiology of pain must ultimately account for both the discriminative and affective features of pain.

A complete understanding of pain mechanisms would provide a satisfactory explanation for the many pain phenomena seen in everyday life and in medical practice. How can the athlete sustain a serious injury without realizing it until the action is over? How does hypnosis prevent the pain of childbirth? Why are some neuropathies painful? What is the mechanism of phantom limb pain? Why do some lesions of the central nervous system produce pain, and why does pain return after neurosurgical operations to relieve pain? How do analgesics work? These are among the many questions which will remain unanswered until we have a more complete understanding of the normal anatomy, physiology and biochemistry of pain mechanisms. Recent advances in all these areas, however, indicate that continued research will eventually lead, not only to a better understanding of pain, but to exciting and fruitful insights into many other areas of nervous system function.

PERIPHERAL MECHANISMS

It is now well established that receptors which are uniquely sensitive to painful stimuli are found in skin, muscle, and deeper tissues (Burgess and Perl, 1973; Mense and Schmidt, 1974). These *nociceptors* excite afferent discharges in finely myelinated (Aδ) or unmyelinated (C) sensory fibers. Morphological studies have yet to reveal distinctive structural features that clearly distinguish nociceptors from all other somatic or visceral sensory endings, but they appear to be among the group of undifferentiated terminals that lack a specialized structure or transducing apparatus. The mechanism by which noxious stimuli activate nociceptors is not known, but various investigators have presented evidence that chemical events are probably important links between the receptor and the surrounding stimulated tissue (Lim, 1970). Stimuli which are potentially or frankly tissue-damaging may release ions, such as potassium, or organic substances (histamine or specific peptides) which bind specifically with receptors on the terminal membrane, triggering the depolarization that leads to the generation of action potentials in the afferent fiber. This "chemoreceptor" hypothesis would help explain why some nociceptors (called "polymodal") respond to any stimulus, thermal, mechanical or chemical, which threatens tissue integrity. There are other nociceptors, however, that respond only to intense mechanical or thermal stimuli; the basis for this selectivity if not known and is not easily explained by chemoreceptor mechanisms.

Nociceptors have been studied by recording from Aδ and C fiber sensory afferents in experimental animals and humans (Torebjork, 1974). These investigations have shown that some commonly experienced features of pain may be at least partially explained by the physiological properties of nociceptor afferents. A sudden, brief, noxious stimulus, for example, typically elicits two distinct types of pain: a sharp, stinging sensation (first pain) followed by a longer duration pain which often has a burning quality (second pain). These distinct sensations can be attributed to the fact that many Aδ afferents conduct impulses at an average velocity of 15 m/sec and respond with relatively brief discharges to noxious mechanical or thermal stimuli, while the C fiber afferents conduct impulses much more slowly (1 m/sec) and have a prolonged discharge which outlasts the stimulus. Direct recordings from single sensory afferents in humans support this explanation of the "double pain" phenomenon: sharp, pricking sensations are associated with Aδ fiber activity while C fiber discharges are accompanied by more prolonged burning sensations. Another common experience is that previously damaged tissue, such as sunburned skin, is more sensitive to noxious stimuli. The experimental counterpart of this phenomenon has been demonstrated in animal experiments (Perl, 1976). It has been shown that both Aδ and C fiber nociceptive afferents have markedly lower discharge thresholds for hours following a noxious thermal stimulus. Observations such as these, plus clinical-neuropathological studies of disturbances of pain sensation in humans, leave little doubt that nerve impuses giving rise to pain are transmitted to the central nervous system along specific nociceptive afferents included among the Aδ and C sensory fibers.

Since the time of Bell and Magendie, there has been general acceptance of the theory that all sensory information from the body and viscera entered the central nervous system via fibers in the dorsal spinal roots or their counterparts in the cranial nerves of the brainstem. This theory, long considered a bedrock of neurologic fact, has now been challenged by recent anatomical and physiological studies (Coggeshall et al., 1975). Approximately 20 to 30 percent of the ventral root fibers in cat and man are unmyelinated; animal experiments have shown that about one-half of these C fibers are sensory afferents which respond to noxious cutaneous or deep stimuli similar to those activating polymodal nociceptors. The cell bodies of these ventral root nociceptive afferents are in the dorsal root ganglion, but the central connections of their axons are not yet established. The finding of nociceptive afferents in ventral roots may explain the frequent failure of dorsal rhizotomy to relieve pain in man.

CENTRAL CONNECTIONS OF NOCICEPTIVE AFFERENTS

Two anatomically and physiologically distinct types of neurons receive input from nociceptive afferents and send axons toward the brain via the contralateral spinothalamic tract (Kerr, 1975a). Many of the cells capping the dorsal margin of the substantia gelatinosa (marginal cells of Waldeyer) respond exclusively to noxious stimuli and transmit impulses to substantia gelatinosa (SG) cells in neighboring segments and to the contralateral thalamus. Deeper in the dorsal horn are larger neurons with dendrites extending into the substantia gelatinosa. These cells have a wide dynamic range of response; they are excited by large-diameter myelinated touch-pressure afferents and respond with increasing frequency as stimulus intensity is brought into the noxious range. Axons of the deeper cells project to the reticular formation of the brainstem as well as to the contralateral thalamus. The major features of this description apply also to the caudal portion of the trigeminal sensory nucleus, which receives nociceptive input from the face.

There is anatomical and physiological evidence for extensive interaction and cross-modulation among neural elements at the initial stage of processing input from nociceptive afferents (Kerr, 1975b). Consequently, neither the dorsal horn of the spinal cord nor the caudal portion of the trigeminal sensory nucleus can be thought of as simple relay stations. Much of the interactive modulation is mediated by small, short-axon SG interneurons which are excited directly by somatic afferents. Some excitatory SG interneurons may mediate input from tactile and nociceptive afferents onto the deep dorsal horn neurons. On the basis of current evidence, however, it is reasonable to suggest that many, perhaps most, SG interneurons exert an inhibitory influence. The inhibitory effect of SG interneurons may be produced by presynaptic inhibition of sensory afferents or by postsynaptic inhibition of spinothalamic tract neurons. In presynaptic inhibition, it is hypothesized that there is a reduction in the amount of neurotransmitter (possibly a peptide such as substance P) released by impulses in nociceptive afferent fibers. There is evidence that presynaptic inhibition can be elicited by input from both tactile and nociceptive afferents, thus producing a type of negative feedback control on the input itself. In addition, both excitatory and inhibitory influences on somatic and visceral sensory input are produced by the axons of neurons located in supraspinal structures; these descending systems will be discussed later.

It is apparent that the output of spinal or trigeminal neurons projecting to the brain is not simply determined by the intensity of nociceptive afferent discharge. Some sensory inputs may exert a predominant inhibitory influence on nociceptive transmission. Perhaps this is why rubbing, vibratory stimulation, or, in some cases, innocuous electrical stimulation relieves pain to a moderate degree. In contrast, removal of the inhibitory input, such as might occur with partial deafferentation or in the case of some peripheral neuropathies, could produce a hyperpathic state with an increased sensitivity to noxious or even innocuous somatic stimuli.

ASCENDING CENTRAL PATHWAYS

Since pain is an experience which has discriminative and affective dimensions, and includes autonomic and somamotor responses, it is not surprising that this diversity is reflected by the underlying anatomy (Mehler et al., 1960) and physiology (Casey, 1978). The diagram in Fig. 1 shows the major features of the ascending systems now thought to be important in mediating pain and pain-related behavior.

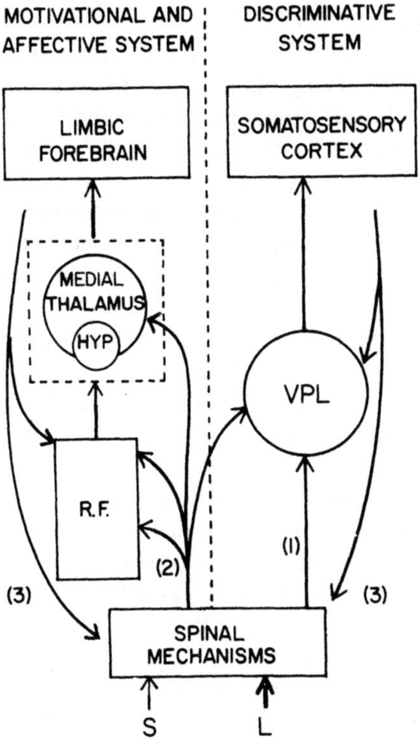

FIG. 1. Diagram of neural systems important in pain and pain modulation. Small diameter nociceptive afferents (S) and larger diameter non-nociceptive fibers (L) activate spinal mechanisms leading to the generation of impulses ascending to higher centers. Neurons in the ventrobasal thalamus (ventralis posterolateralis shown here: VPL) receive input from fibers of the dorsal column-medial lemniscal system (1) and from that portion of ventrolateral spinal cord (2) forming the spinothalamic tract. Projection of these neurons to the somatosensory cortex provides the basis for the discriminative aspects of somesthesis, possibly including pain. Other fibers ascending from the ventrolateral spinal cord (2) send projections into the brainstem reticular formation (RF) and to the medial thalamus. Ascending reticular formation fibers also project to the medial thalamus and hypothalamus where they may influence limbic forebrain mechanisms subserving the motivational and affective components of pain. Both discriminative and motivational-affective systems are modulated by descending pathways (3) acting at thalamic, brainstem, and spinal levels. Some of these modulating influences may be mediated by endogenous opiate-like compounds.

The spinothalamic tract (STT) neurons comprise the classical pain pathway projecting directly to the posterior lateral thalamus. The trigeminal counterpart is the trigeminothalamic tract. The responses of these dorsal horn or caudal trigeminal nucleus neurons to noxious stimuli suggest that there should be a substantial population of posterior lateral thalamic neurons which are exclusively or differentially responsive to nociceptor input. It is rather surprising, then, that recordings of neural activity in animals have generally failed to confirm this expectation, possibly because of the anesthetics often used in such experiments or because certain neurons have been missed by sampling errors (Poggio and Mountcastle, 1963). However, the posterolateral thalamus has been electrically stimulated or destroyed in humans and in animal experiments, and the results also suggest that other pathways and structures must play an equally important and necessary role in pain mechanisms. In the human, for example, reports of pain accompanying postero-lateral thalamic stimulation are surprisingly rare—and lesions in this area may result in a "thalamic syndrome" in which normally innocuous stimuli have an unpleasant or even severely painful quality (White and Sweet, 1969). Furthermore, there is little clinical and experimental evidence to indicate that the cortical projections of posterolateral thalamic neurons are critical for pain perception; surgical extirpation of this cortical tissue has been notably unsuccessful in relieving clinical pain (White and Sweet, 1969). Neurophysiological and clinical observations have, however, established that nociceptive information is transmitted to the posterolateral thalamus and associated cortex, and there is general agreement that the neurons of this system mediate the discriminative aspects of somesthesis. On the evidence at hand, it is reasonable to suggest that the direct STT system subserves the discriminative aspects of pain, permitting the organism to recognize that potential or actual tissue damage has occurred, to localize it in space and time, and perhaps to recognize the physical nature of the stimulus (thermal, mechanical, chemical).

Dorsal horn neurons projecting to the medullary or mesencephalic reticular formation form the spinoreticular tract (SRT). A comparable system originates from the caudal portion of the trigeminal nucleus. Neurophysiological experiments performed in several different laboratories have shown that a substantial proportion of brainstem reticular formation neurons respond either differentially or exclusively to noxious stimuli. (Casey, 1978). Most often, the response of these neurons resembles that of the deeper dorsal horn cells with a wide dynamic range; there is a relatively weak response to innocuous stimuli but a longer and more intense discharge when noxious stimuli are applied. Similar responses have been recorded from neurons of the medial thalamus which receive input via reticulo-thalamic projections; some of these medial thalamic neurons may also receive input from STT neurons. Localized lesion and electrical stimulation experiments in animals have also indicated that the reticular formation and medial thalamus are an essential part of CNS pain mechanisms (Casey, 1978). Medial thalamic lesions, for example, have been used for some time to relieve intractable pain in cancer sufferers (White and Sweet, 1969).

The above evidence notwithstanding, the medial spinoreticulothalamic (SRTT) system cannot be considered an exclusive, specific pain pathway. Many of these reticular and medial thalamic neurons respond to innocuous somatic stimuli, and some are activated by visual and auditory input. Furthermore, reticular formation neurons typically respond to stimulation anywhere within an extensive area of the body surface. It is unlikely that such cells could encode the spatial information necessary to localize pain. The output of reticular neurons is similarly extensive. Many, if not most, of these cells have multifocal axonal projections to the thalamus, spinal cord, and within the brain stem. Many experiments have shown that the reticular formation is not simply a sensory pathway; reticular neurons undoubtedly mediate motor and autonomic responses to the various inputs they receive.

If the SRTT is not an exclusive pathway mediating all aspects of the pain experience, what functions might this system subserve? There is currently insufficient evidence to answer this question, but the available data suggest that neurons in the reticular formation are important determinants of non-discriminative aspects of pain experience and response. There is no doubt that reticular neurons which respond differentially to noxious stimuli, and that project to bulbar and spinal outflow systems, can help establish the basic somatomotor and autonomic responses to tissue damage. These and other reticular neurons with ascending projections forming the SRTT may also mediate the affective and motivational dimension of the pain experience (Melzack and Casey, 1968). The medial thalamus and hypothalamus, which receive SRTT input, both project to limbic system forebrain structures, such as the cingulate gyrus and hippocampal formation, which are known to play an important role in motivational and affective mechanisms. Selective lesions within limbic forebrain structures of humans and animals, for example, have been shown to markedly attenuate the aversive quality of noxious stimuli without interfering with the discriminative aspects of somesthesis. There is also evidence that the narcotic analgesics act on reticular formation neurons to modulate SRTT activity (Pert and Yaksh, 1974), perhaps accounting, in part, for the reduction of suffering in clinical pain while preserving much of the discriminative ability to recognize noxious stimuli.

The neural system mediating motivational and affective mechanisms is not, of course, a specialized pain pathway. Many other inputs are important determinants of affective state and can motivate behavior. Pain, however, is an especially compelling experience, so it is reasonable to expect that nociceptive afferents would be among the major inputs to a system which may provide the essential affective-motivational component of the pain experience.

MODULATION OF PAIN

One of the major findings of modern neurophysiology is that the central nervous system (CNS) regulates sensory input. Sensory experience is thus determined not only by ongoing afferent activity but by the activity of sensory control systems in the CNS. The sensitivity of muscle stretch receptors, for example, is directly controlled by CNS efferent fibers (gamma motoneurons), and the central effect of cutaneous afferent discharge is determined by dorsal horn interneurons described earlier in this chapter. Recent research has begun to reveal more about the mechanisms of action of CNS pathways which are probably important in the modulation of pain (Mayer and Price, 1976).

In animal experiments, it has been shown that electrical stimulation within certain parts of the CNS can produce an analgesia which typically outlasts the duration of stimulation, sometimes for several minutes. This stimulation-produced analgesia (SPA) has been most consistently demonstrated by stimulation within the midline raphe nuclei of the brainstem, a group of serotonin-containing neurons extending from the mesencephalon through the medulla.

There is substantial evidence that the axons of medullary raphe cells descend in the dorsolateral fasciculus (DLF) to terminate in the dorsal horn where they markedly attenuate the response of spinothalamic and other dorsal horn cells to noxious stimuli. Surgical section of the DLF eliminates this suppressive effect and prevents the analgesic affect of medullary raphe stimulation. Additional experiments have indicated that this descending pain-attenuation mechanism can also be activated by midbrain raphe neurons and by stimulation within the periventricular gray substance of the diencephalon. Some experiments have suggested that the cerebral cortex may also participate in this system.

The mechanisms underlying SPA appear closely related to the analgesia produced by morphine in experimental animals (Mayer and Price, 1976). Raphe system lesions, DLF lesions, and blockage of the synthesis of serotonin within raphe neurons all reduce the analgesic effect of morphine and SPA. Furthermore, naloxone reverses the analgesia of both morphine and SPA and repeated exposure to SPA or morphine results in the development of tolerance to either agent. Some neurophysiological experiments have also shown that there are neurons within the raphe system which increase their frequency of discharge following systemic or local intracerebral injections of morphine. These responses are also blocked by the specific narcotic antagonist, naloxone.

The above findings suggest the presence of endogenous opiate-like substances and receptors in the brain that are important for the normal, physiological operation of pain modulation systems. Recent research has, in fact, supported this hypothesis and has opened up new and exciting frontiers in brain research. Radioactive labeling of opiate agonists reveals the presence of opiate receptors in the brain; the receptor binding of the labeled opiate is specifically blocked by naloxone (Pert et al., 1975). The opiate receptors are found at several CNS sites, but the binding with opiate agonists is most dense in portions of the limbic system, medial thalamus, and the periaqueductal gray of the midbrain. Some neurons in these regions are thought to be important in mediating the affective dimension of pain. Neurons within the periaqueductal gray are also part of the proposed pain suppression system. In the spinal cord, opiate receptors are found in the substantia gelatinosa of the dorsal horn where a significant proportion appear to be located on the membranes of primary afferent terminals.

The discovery of opiate receptors in the CNS was soon followed by the finding that the mammalian brain synthesizes small peptides with opiate-like pharmacologic properties (Hughes, 1975; Hughes et al., 1975). Of particular importance to pain mechanisms are two pentapeptides, met-enkephalin and leu-enkephalin, which have a CNS distribution similar to that of the opiate receptors.

There is evidence that the enkephalins are released from the terminals of short-axon interneurons to act as neuro-modulators or perhaps as neurotransmitters to modulate synaptic transmission between neurons mediating pain (Iversen et al., 1978). Both met-enkephalin and leu-enkephalin are released from brain slices and from isolated synaptic endings (synaptosomes) by potassium ions, veratridine, and electrical stimulation; this release is enhanced by calcium and is blocked by lack of calcium and by tetrodotoxin, consistent with the expected effects on normal synaptic release mechanisms. In the brain, enkephalin-containing nerve processes and endings have been identified by immunohistochemical methods. The release of enkephalin from these endings is likely to have powerful effects on synaptic transmission since, like morphine, met-enkephalin has been shown to inhibit cholinergic, adrenergic and dopaminergic transmission. Additional experiments have indicated that the enkephalins may inhibit the release of another peptide, substance P, which is found in the terminals of sensory afferents in the dorsal horn of the spinal cord and in the trigeminal nucleus. The available evidence, then, strongly supports the hypothesis that, whatever additional functions they may subserve, endogenously synthesized opioid peptides in the CNS are important mediators of pain modulation.

A major problem for further research is to demonstrate both the normal physiological mechanisms of activation of the proposed pain-suppression system and the behavioral states in which such activation occurs. There is little evidence, for example, that the administration of the opiate antagonist naloxone has any effect on the pain threshold of normal humans or experimental animals. This may indicate that the enkephalinergic pain attenuation mechanisms are not tonically active, but are brought into play only under special circumstances. Some recent experiments have suggested that certain forms of stress in experimental animals and the placebo reaction in humans are conditions in which moderate degrees of analgesia may be mediated by an enkephalinergic system. If future research reveals more about the normal activation of enkephalin-mediated pain suppression, perhaps we will be able to develop more effective means of controlling pain where current methods are unsatisfactory.

SUMMARY

Pain is a complex phenomenon, involving the activation of specific somesthetic discriminative mechanisms and neural systems subserving motivation and affective experience (Fig. 1). The pluridimensional nature of pain is reflected in the central organization of neurons which respond exclusively or differentially to noxious stimuli. Recent research has begun to reveal physiological and biochemical mechanisms by which pain may be suppressed by drugs, brain stimulation, or by normal physiological processes. The continued investigation of the neural mechanisms of pain and analgesia is likely to provide further fruitful insights not only into clinical problems of pain but into many other areas relating neural function to behavior.

ACKNOWLEDGEMENTS

Supported by grants NS12015 and NS12581 from the National Institute of Health (USPHS).

REFERENCES

Burgess, P.R., and Perl, F.R. Cutaneous mechanoreceptors and nociceptors, in *Handbook of Sensory Physiology, Vol. II, Somatosensory System*. A. Iggo, ed. Springer Verlag, New York (1973), pp. 29–78.

Casey, K.L. Neural mechanisms of pain, in *Handbook of Perception*, Vol. VIB. E.C. Carterette, and M.P. Friedman, eds. Academic Press, Inc., New York (1978), pp. 183–230.

Coggeshall, R.E., Applebaum, M.L., Fazen, M., Stubbs, T.B., and Sykes, M.T.. Unmyelinated axons in human ventral roots, a possible explanation for the failure of dorsal rhizotomy to relieve pain. *Brain* 98, 157–166 (1975).

Hughes, J. Isolation of an endogenous compound from the brain with pharmacological properties similar to morphine. *Brain Res.* 88, 295–308 (1975).

Hughes, J., Smith, T.W., Kosterlitz, H.W., Fothergill, L.A., Morgan, B.A., and Morris, H.R. Identification of two related pentapeptides from the brain with potent opiate agonist activity. *Nature* 258, 577–579 (1975).

Iversen, L.L., Nicoll, R.A., and Vale, W.W. Neurobiology of peptides. *Neurosci. Res. Prog. Bull.* 16(2), 211–370 (1978).

Kerr, F.W.L. Neuroanatomical substrates of nociception in the spinal cord. *Pain* 1, 325–356 (1975a).

Kerr, F.W.L. Pain: A central inhibitory balance theory. *Mayo Clin. Proc.* 50, 685–690 (1975b).

Lim, R.K.S. Pain. *Ann. Rev. Physiol.* 32, 269–288 (1970).

Mayer, D.J., and Price, D.D. Central nervous system mechanisms of analgesia. *Pain* 2, 379–404 (1976).

Mehler, W.R., Feferman, M.E., and Nauta, W.J.H. Ascending axon degeneration following anterolateral cordotomy. An experimental study in the monkey. *Brain* 83, 718–750 (1960).

Melzack, R., and Casey, K.L. Sensory, motivational, and central control determinants of pain, in *The Skin Senses*. D.R. Kenshalo, ed. C.C. Thomas, Springfield, Illinois (1968), pp. 423–443.

Mense, S., and Schmidt, R.F. Activation of group IV afferent units from muscle by analgesic agents. *Brain Res*. 72, 305–310 (1974).

Perl, E.R. Sensitization of nociceptors and its relation to sensation, in *Advances in Pain Research and Therapy, Vol. I* (Proceedings of the First World Congress on Pain). J.J. Bonica and D.G. Albe-Fessard, eds. Raven Press, New York (1976), pp. 17–28.

Pert, A., and Yaksh, T. Sites of morphine-induced analgesia in the primate brain: relation to pain pathways. *Brain Res*. 80, 135–140 (1974).

Pert, C.B., Kuhar, M.J., and Snyder, S.H. Autoradiographic localization of the opiate receptor in rat brain. *Life Sci*. 16, 1849–1854 (1975).

Poggio, G.F., and Mountcastle, V.B. The functional properties of ventrobasal thalamic neurons studied in unanesthetized monkeys. *J. Neurophysiol*. 26, 775–806 (1963).

Torebjork, H.E. Afferent C units responding to mechanical, thermal and chemical stimuli in human non-glabrous skin. *Acta Physiol. Scand*. 92, 374–390 (1974).

White, J.C., and Sweet, W.H. *Pain and the Neurosurgeon: A Forty-Year Experience*. C.C. Thomas, Springfield, Illinois (1969).

Copyright © 1982, Spectrum Publications, Inc.
The Neural Basis of Behavior

14

Opiate Receptors

Eric J. Simon

INTRODUCTION

Morphine and related analgesics have aroused the curiosity of scientists longer than perhaps any other drugs. While there has always been much interest in the way these drugs produce analgesia, it must be admitted that their tendency to induce addiction and the great problems this creates for the individual and for society was undoubtedly a major impetus for the great research effort in this area. The search for a non-addictive analgesic, however, did not yield to an empirical approach, but seemed to demand an understanding of the mode of action of analgesic drugs. It is therefore not surprising that research on opiates has led to advances that seem at the present time to have greater relevance to our understanding of pain and analgesia than of the addictive process. This knowledge should prove beneficial since there are many more people who suffer severe, chronic pain than there are narcotic addicts. Research on pain is only now beginning to receive the attention and support that it should have received long ago.

This chapter will be largely restricted to the opiate receptor, since separate discussions of the opioid peptides (the putative endogenous ligands of the receptor) and the involvement of the opiate receptor-endorphin system in pain modulation will be provided by Hans Kosterlitz and Huda Akil.

DISCOVERY OF OPIATE RECEPTORS

Pharmacological evidence for the concept that opiates must bind to specific sites in the CNS (and other target tissues) in order to produce their pharmacological effects has been available for several decades. It was based on the high degree of steric and structural specificity exhibited by analgesia and most other responses to opiates. Thus, for a large number of synthetic opiates studied, only the levorotatory enantiomer is active while the dextrorotatory isomer shows little or no analgesic activity. The most interesting structural change is the substitution of the N-methyl group by a larger alkyl group, such as allyl or cycloproplylmethyl, which for most opiates results in molecules with potent, specific antagonistic activity against morphine-like analgesics. Both "pure" antagonists (e.g., naloxone and naltrexone) and mixed agonist-antagonist drugs (e.g., nalorphine, cyclazocine) have been produced. All of the observed specificities are most readily explicable by the existence of binding sites that exhibit complementary specificity. These binding sites together with a transducing element that permits the binding to trigger appropriate biochemical or biophysical events resulting in the observed responses have been called opiate receptors, in analogy to hormone receptors.

Biochemical identification of opiate receptors proved difficult. Van Praag and Simon (1966) were the first to utilize brain homogenate in the search for receptor binding. It proved easy to demonstrate binding but far more difficult to distinguish between specific and non-specific binding. This was attempted by determining the proportion of binding that was sensitive to displacement by the opiate antagonist nalorphine, but this approach was not successful at that time.

Ingoglia and Dole (1970) first used the principle of stereospecificity in the search for opiate receptors. They injected l- and d-methadone into the lateral ventricle of rats but found no difference in the rate of diffusion of the enantiomers into brain tissue.

Goldstein et al. (1971) used stereospecificity as the criterion of receptor binding in brain homogenates. They incubated mouse brain homogenates with [^{3}H]levorphanol in the presence of a large excess of unlabeled levorphanol or of its inactive enantiomer dextrorphan. Since dextrorphan has neither agonist nor antagonist activity it is presumed not to be recognized by the receptor. Stereospecific binding was, therefore, defined as that portion of the binding of the labeled drug which is prevented by levorphanol but not by dextrorphan. In their experiments, Goldstein's group found only about 2 percent of the total binding to be stereospecific. However, in 1973, three laboratories (Simon et al., 1973; Terenius, 1973a; Pert and Snyder, 1973), each using similar modifications of the Goldstein procedure, independently and simultaneously reported the observation of stereospecific opiate binding in rat brain homogenate which represented the major portion of total binding. The modifications involved the use of very low concentrations of labeled ligand, made possible by high specific activity, and the washing of homogenates after incubation and centrifugation or filtration with cold buffer to remove contaminating unbound and loosely bound radioactivity. Since that time, these results have been confirmed in many laboratories, and much evidence has accumulated suggesting that these stereospecific binding sites indeed represent receptors to which opiates must bind in order to produce their pharmacological responses. They have been found in man (Hiller et al., 1973) and in all vertebrates so far studied, but not in invertebrates (Pert et al., 1974a).

PROPERTIES OF OPIATE BINDING SITES

The stereospecific binding sites are found in the central nervous system and in the innervation of certain smooth muscle systems such as the myenteric plexus of the guinea pig ileum. They are tightly associated with membrane fractions of tissue homogenates and have been reported to be most concentrated in the synaptosomal cell fraction (Hitzeman et al., 1974; Pert et al., 1974b), suggesting a location in the vicinity of synapses.

Stereospecific opiate binding is saturable, and binding at saturation amounts to about 0.35 pmol per mg of rat brain protein in a crude brain membrane preparation. Both agonists and antagonists bind with high affinity. Dissociation constants range from 0.025 nM for certain potent derivatives of fentanyl (Stahl et al., 1977) to low or undetectable affinity for drugs that possess little or no opiate-like activity. The striking discrimination between stereoisomers is best exemplified by levorphanol and dextrorphan which differ by four orders of magnitude in their affinities (Simon et al., 1973; Pert and Snyder, 1973).

The pH optimum for opiate binding is in the physiological range, between 6.5 and 8. The addition of various salts to the incubation medium tends to reduce binding. Sodium represents an exception which will be dealt with in some detail in a later section (see *Conformation Changes in Opiate Receptors*).

The inhibition of stereospecific opiate binding by proteolytic enzymes (Simon et al., 1973; Pasternak and Snyder, 1973) and a wide variety of protein reagents, including sulfhydryl reagents (Simon et al., 1973; Terenius 1973b), strongly suggests that one or more proteins are involved in opiate binding. The role of lipids is less clear since binding is inhibited by treatment with phospholipase A from some sources but is virtually unaffected by phospholipase C (Simon et al., 1973; Pasternak and Snyder, 1973). Ribonuclease, deoxyribonuclease, and neuraminidase are without effect.

The most convincing evidence indicating that the observed binding sites represent pharmacological receptors comes from the close correlation between binding affinities and pharmacological potencies observed for a large number of drugs in several studies. Thus, good correlation was found for a homologous series of ketobemidones differing only in the length of their alkyl substitution on the nitrogen (Wilson et al., 1975). Creese and Snyder (1975) found excellent correlation between binding of a series of opiate agonists and antagonists to receptors in the guinea pig ileum and their pharmacological potency in this system.

Stahl et al. (1977) studied a series of 26 coded drugs from the repertory of Janssen Pharmaceutica. The binding affinities of these drugs were assessed by competition with labeled naltrexone for stereospecific binding. These affinities were compared to analgesic potencies measured in Belgium by the tail withdrawal reaction following intravenous administration of drug. In this series, in which the drugs varied in pharmacological potencies over six orders of magnitude, a rank correlation coefficient of 0.9 was found.

The drugs studied included a number of neuroleptics, such as haloperidol and droperidol, which were found able to compete with labeled opiates for binding in the micromolar range, in agreement with reports by others (Clay and Brougham, 1975; Creese et al., 1976).

The stereospecificity, saturability, and high affinity of the opiate binding sites and, above all, the excellent correlation between pharmacological potency and binding affinity for a large number of opiates and antagonists support the hypothesis that these sites represent the binding portion of pharmacologically relevant receptors.

REGIONAL DISTRIBUTION OF OPIATE RECEPTORS IN THE CNS

The precise regional distribution of opiate receptors in human and animal brain has been determined in considerable detail. In earlier studies, human brain obtained at autopsy (Hiller et al., 1973) and animal brain (Kuhar et al., 1973) were dissected, and binding of tritiated opiates was measured in homogenates of specific brain regions. More recently these results have been confirmed and extended by autoradiography (Atweh and Kuhar, 1977a; 1977b; 1977c) in rat CNS.

These studies can be summarized by stating that opiate receptors are widely distributed in the CNS, but not randomly. Areas of high opiate binding are largely areas that had previously been suspected by investigators, using very different approaches, to be sites of opiate action. In particular, opiate binding was shown to be high in the limbic system and in all regions that have been implicated in pain conduction and modulation, such as the substantia gelatinosa of the dorsal spinal cord, the nucleus raphe magnus, the periventricular and periaqueductal gray areas and the thalamus. The limbic system has long been held responsible for the ability of morphine to ameliorate the affective aspects of pain perception.

The distribution of opiate receptors is well correlated with the distribution of the enkephalins, though there are exceptions. The most striking such exception is the globus pallidus which contains the highest levels of both met- and leu-enkephalin but exhibits relatively low opiate binding. The reason for this discrepancy is not understood. Brain β-endorphin, which may also have a role in endogenous pain modulation, is restricted to a single cell group in the arcuate nucleus of the hypothalamus. From here it radiates by axonal transport to various other regions including the preoptic area, the septal nuclei, the periaqueductal region of the midbrain, the dorsal raphe and the locus coeruleus. Figure 1 depicts the striking difference in distribution between enkephalins (and opiate receptors) and β-endorphin.

The question of whether opiate receptors are located pre- or postsynaptically has received a good deal of attention. After dorsal rhizotomy in monkeys, Lamotte et al. (1976) observed a 50 percent reduction of opiate receptors in the dorsal horn of the spinal cord, suggesting a presynaptic location. However, as pointed out by the authors, a transsynaptic effect on receptors localized on postsynaptic cord neurons could not be excluded. The

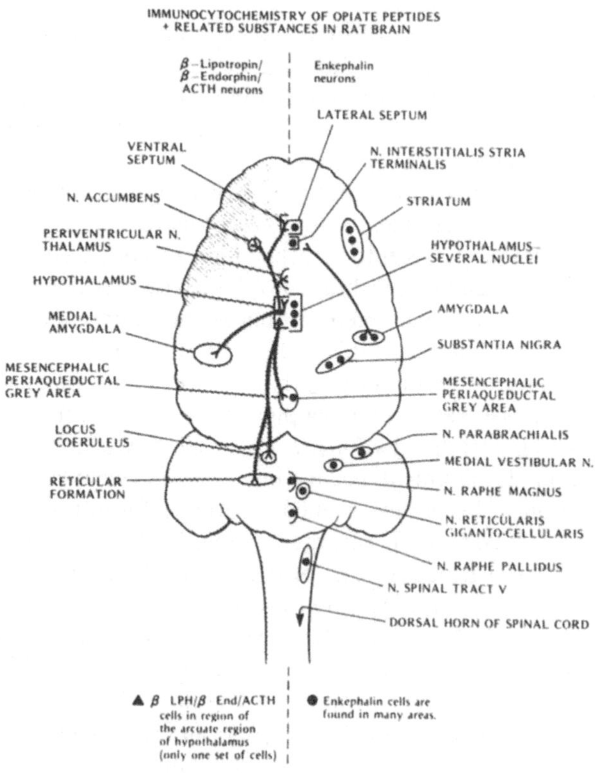

FIG. 1. Localization of the enkephalins and of β-endorphin in rat brain. From Barchas et al. (1978). Reprinted by permission. Courtesy of A.A.A.S.

most direct evidence for presynaptic opiate receptors comes from studies in tissue culture. A high level of opiate receptors was found in the neuritic outgrowth from dorsal root ganglia explanted from 14-day mouse embryos by Hiller et al. (1978). Since opiate receptors were present even when the ganglia were cultured in the absence of spinal cord, they appear to be located on nerve fibers which are destined to provide presynaptic afferent input into the dorsal spinal cord. Not all published results point to a presynaptic site of opiate action. Thus, electrophysiological experiments by Zieglgansberger and Fry (1976) showed that opiates and endorphins exert inhibitory effects on electrical stimulation due to glutamate, which is known to act postsynaptically. It is therefore very likely that opiate receptors are located pre- as well as postsynaptically, a conclusion reached recently for dopamine receptors.

ONTOGENY OF THE OPIATE RECEPTOR

The ontogenetic development of opiate receptors in the brain of rat and guinea pig was investigated by Clendeninn et al. (1976). In the rat, the rate of increase of opiate binding is greatest between the midfetal stage and three weeks postpartum (three- to fourfold). Thereafter, until adulthood (10–20 weeks) the rise is more gradual (about twofold). Scatchard analysis of saturation curves for naltrexone binding in rat brain from one day after birth to the age of ten weeks has shown that the increase in binding is due to an increase in number of receptors rather than to enhanced affinity.

Opiate binding to guinea pig brain homogenates has demonstrated no significant difference in either receptor number or binding affinity between late fetal life and adulthood in this species. Binding in brain homogenate from a midterm fetus is about one half that oberved late in pregnancy and in adult guinea pigs. The fact that guinea pigs are born with a full complement of receptors is well correlated with previous reports that in the guinea pig almost full brain development occurs before birth, whereas in the rat a significant portion of brain development continues for at least three weeks after birth. In rat brain, the percentage increase of opiate receptors from newborn to adult in various regions of the brain differs widely (Coyle and Pert, 1976). For example, receptor binding in the hippocampus and parietal cortex increases by 830 percent and 690 percent, respectively, but in the medulla, pons and corpus striatum by only 270 percent and 300 percent.

A very close association was found by Garcin and Coyle (1976) in rat brain between development of opiate receptors and level of enkephalin. This is consistent with the notion that these are components of a developing neurotransmitter or neuromodulator system.

CONFORMATIONAL CHANGES IN OPIATE RECEPTORS

The studies discussed so far do not permit distinction between a potent agonist and an equally potent antagonist by a receptor binding assay. Both types of drugs compete with each other for the same receptor and show identical binding characteristics. A method which permits the distinction between agonists and antagonists by their binding characteristics arose from what appeared to be an experimental discrepancy between two laboratories. Pert and Snyder (1973) reported that the addition of salt had little effect on binding, while Simon et al. (1973) reported profound inhibition. Since the NYU group was using the potent agonist etorphine and the Hopkins group was using the "pure" antagonist naloxone, Simon et al. suggested that the apparent discrepancy might represent a general difference in the manner in which agonists and antagonists bind to the receptor. It was indeed found that the binding of all agonists examined was inhibited by salt while the binding of antagonists was enhanced. It was also shown (Pert and Snyder, 1974) that this ability to "discriminate" between agonists and antagonists was not a general effect of salts, but a very unique property of the cation Na^+. The effect is not shown by the other alkali metals K^+, Rb^+, and Cs^+, while Li^+ does exhibit this action but to a much smaller degree. No other inorganic cations nor a series of organic cations studied (Simon et al., 1975a) were found to exhibit this property. This ability of sodium ions to "distinguish" between such closely related molecules as an opiate and its corresponding antagonist (allyl or cyclopropylmethyl analogue) is of considerable interest, especially in light of the uniqueness of Na^+ in this respect. The effect of sodium reaches its maximum at 100 mM and is completely reversible upon removal of sodium from the incubation mixture.

Manganese and magnesium salts have been reported to enhance agonist binding while they depress antagonist binding (Pasternak et al., 1975). This effect is observed most clearly when sodium is also present and may represent a reversal of the sodium effect by the divalent cations.

Studies of the mechanism of the sodium effect were carried out. The first question raised was whether the differences in binding represented changes in the number of sites or in the affinity of binding. Pert and Snyder (1974) reported that sodium caused an increase in the number of high affinity binding sites for naloxone and a decrease of binding sites for dihydromorphine. Simon et al. (1975b), on the other hand, found that sodium increased the affinity of naltrexone for the receptor and other antagonists while reducing the affinity of agonists. No change in the number of binding sites was noted. These results were consistent with a model involving a conformational change of the opiate receptor in the presence of sodium ions. The experimental discrepancies have never been completely resolved. However, studies carried out in both laboratories, involving competition experiments, favor the changes in affinity. When a relatively pure antagonist is allowed to compete for binding with a labeled antagonist, there is little or no change in the IC_{50} of the competitor when sodium is added to the incubation mixture. When an unlabeled agonist is allowed to compete with a labeled antagonist, the IC_{50} for the agonist is increased drastically in the presence of sodium (10- to 60-fold). Such a shift in IC_{50} reflects a change in affinity but not in the number of binding sites.

The best evidence for an alteration in receptor conformation by sodium ions came unexpectedly from a study of the kinetics of receptor inactivation by the sulfhydryl alkylating reagent, N-ethylmaleimide (NEM) by Simon and Groth (1975). When a membrane fraction from rat brain was incubated with NEM for various periods, followed by inactivation or removal of unreacted NEM, there was a progressive decrease in the ability of the membranes to bind opiates stereospecifically. The rate of receptor inactivation follows pseudo-first-order kinetics, consistent with the existence of one SH-group per receptor essential for binding. Protection against inactivation was achieved by the addition of low concentrations of opiates or antagonists during the preincubation with NEM, suggesting that the SH-group is located near the opiate binding site of the receptor.

Considerable protection was observed (half time of inactivation was increased to 30 minutes from 8 minutes) when inactivation was carried out in the presence of 100 mM NaCl. Since sodium salts were without effect on the alkylation of model SH-compounds, such as cysteine or glutathione, this suggested that the SH-groups were made less accessible to NEM by a conformational change in the receptor protein. The fact that this protection exhibited a) the same ion specificity (Na^+ protects, Li^+ protects partially, K^+, Rb^+, or Cs^+ not at all) and b) the same dose-response to Na^+ as the differential changes in ligand affinities, suggests that the conformational change

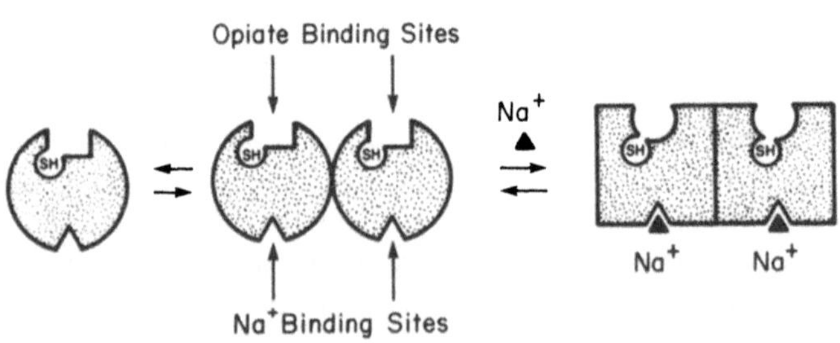

FIG. 2. Model for the allosteric effect of sodium ions on the conformation of the opiate receptor.

which masks SH-groups is the same as that which results in increased affinity of antagonists and decreased affinity of agonists.

The simple model for the allosteric effect of sodium ions on opiate receptors shown in Fig. 2 encompasses the various changes in receptor properties discussed. The reason for representing the receptor as a dimer is the existence of evidence, not discussed here, for cooperativity of binding.

These studies illustrate that opiate receptors possess a certain plasticity that could play a role in the events subsequent to opiate binding. The change in conformation of a protein by sodium is not without precedent since a number of enzymes are known that are specifically activated by sodium ions. Moreover, conformational changes in synaptic proteins during membrane depolarization have also been reported (Clark and Strickholm, 1971).

THE ROLE OF LIPIDS IN OPIATE BINDING

The possible role of lipids in the binding of opiates to their receptors has been the subject of considerable investigation. H.H. Loh and his collaborators have published extensively on the ability of cerebroside sulfate to bind opiates stereospecifically and have provided evidence that cerebroside sulfate may be a component of opiate receptors (Loh et al., 1978).

The work of Abood and his collaborators (Abood and Takeda, 1976; Hoss et al., 1977) suggests a role for phospholipids, especially phosphatidylserine in receptor binding. Further evidence comes from the exquisite sensitivity of opiate receptors to certain phospholipases. Phospholipase A from bee venom or from the venom of *V. russelli* inhibits binding at concentrations in the nanogram per ml range (Pasternak and Snyder, 1973), whereas phospholipase A from *Crotalus adamanteus* and various preparations of phospholipase C have little effect on opiate binding (Simon et al., 1973).

We have recently reported the observation (Lin and Simon, 1978) that inhibition of opiate receptors by phospholipase A from *V. russelli* was dramatically reversed by incubation with bovine serum albumin (BSA) subsequent to treatment with and removal of the enzyme (by centrifugation). As shown in Table 1, incubation with phospholipase A reduced binding of etorphine, naltrexone and met-enkephalin to 10 percent of that observed in untreated membranes. However, after treatment with BSA binding of all three ligands was restored to 80–85 percent of control values. Other serum albumins including human, porcine, chicken, and rabbit were also effective. Curiously, egg albumin was the only albumin tested that did not restore binding activity.

Table 1. Effect of bovine serum albumin on phospholipase A-treated rat brain membranes

Ligand	*Phospho-lipase A*	*1% BSA*	*Stereospecific binding (fmoles/mg protein)*	*% of individual control*
	–	–	136.7	100
	+	–	11.8	8.6
^{3}H-etorphine	–	+	126.3	100
	+	+	104.6	82.8
	–	–	139.2	100
	+	–	7.9	5.7
^{3}H-naltrexone	–	+	134.2	100
	+	+	116.5	86.8
	–	–	61.2	100
	+	–	3.9	6.4
^{3}H-enkephalin	–	+	78.9	100
	+	+	62.0	78.6

Membrane fractions derived from rat brain were treated with phospholipase A from *Vipera russelli* (11 units/mg protein, Sigma Co.) and incubated with or without BSA (Pentex, Fraction V) as described in text. Opiate receptor stereospecific binding was assayed by incubation of the phospholipase A-treated and control membranes with 1.1 nM ^{3}H-etorphine (16.5 Ci/nmole) or 1.8 nM ^{3}H-naltrexone (10.6 Ci/mmole) with or without 1 μM unlabeled levallorphan at 37° for 15 minutes. Samples were placed in an ice bath for 10 minutes before filtration through GF/B filters. ^{3}H-Met-enkephalin (15.9 Ci/mmole) was used at a concentration of 4.6 nM and incubation was carried out at 4° for 1.5 hours with or without 20 μM unlabeled enkephalin. (Reprinted from Lin and Simon, 1978, by permission from MacMillan Journals, Ltd).

The simplest explanation of these findings is that end products of phospholipolysis inhibit opiate receptor binding and that BSA is effective in removing these products. However, attempts to reverse inhibition of binding by fatty acids (linoleic acid) or lysophosphatides (lysolecithin) with BSA have so far not been successful. It may be, though, that inhibitory effects of fatty acids and lysocompounds produced *in situ* occur at much lower concentrations than those observed when such materials are added as crude sonicated suspensions.

At present, there are two possible explanations for the inhibition of opiate receptor binding by phospholipase A. One is a direct toxicity by fatty acids and/or lysophospholipids, generated by phospholipase, on the receptor. The second is the possibility that membrane phospholipids hold the opiate receptor in its active conformation. The generation of hydrolysis products in the vicinity of the receptor may perturb its conformation, and removal of these products by BSA may restore the appropriate phospholipid environment for receptor activity. The ability to assess the effects of phospholipolysis products directly on a solubilized receptor molecule would be helpful in the ultimate resolution of the mechanism of this phenomenon.

BIOCHEMICAL EVENTS FOLLOWING OPIATE BINDING

The nature of the events that are triggered by opiate or endorphin binding to their receptors, and which result in the observed pharmacological or physiological changes, is still obscure. However, some efforts to penetrate this "black box" will be described.

The results suggesting that the opiate receptor can exist in alternative conformations make it attractive to postulate that such changes could mediate opiate effects by causing modifications in the neighboring synaptic membrane. To date, the evidence that such alterations are involved in either acute or chronic actions of opiate is scant. However, this hypothesis is, in the author's view, well worth pursuing.

Cyclic nucleotides have been shown to act as "second messengers" in a number of hormonally controlled phenomena. A considerable literature is accumulating describing attempts to implicate cyclic AMP or GMP in the action of opiates.

Collier and Roy (1974) reported the inhibition by opiates of prostaglandin E-stimulated adenylate cyclase in brain homogenates. This effect was stereospecific, reversible by opiate antagonists, and well correlated with analgesic potency. Collier's group also reported that the administration of large doses of phosphodiesterase inhibitors (e.g., theophylline) produced behavior patterns in naive rats that resembled the opiate-withdrawal syndrome. They termed this a quasimorphine-withdrawal syndrome (QMWS) and assumed that it resulted from an increase in brain cyclic AMP.

Bonnet (1975) has reported that systemic injections of morphine produced dose-dependent increases in the level of cAMP and adenylate cyclase in the striatum and thalamus of rat brain, whereas in the substantia nigra and the periventricular gray area the level of cAMP was found to be reduced. More recently, Bonnet and Gusik (1976) have demonstrated that the increases in thalamic adenylate cyclase were reversible by naloxone, suggesting the involvement of opiate receptors in this effect. They also found that the level of Ca^{2+} (up to 1.3 mM) tended to enhance the opiate stimulation of adenylate cyclase in the thalamus while high levels of Ca^{2+} tended to suppress it.

Similar findings to those of Collier and Roy have been reported in the mouse neuroblastoma × rat glioma hybrid cell line (NG-108-15) found by

Klee and Nirenberg (1974) to contain high levels of opiate receptors. Levels of cAMP (Traber et al., 1974) and adenylate cyclase (Sharma et al., 1975a) were found to be reduced by opiates in a stereospecific, antagonist-reversible manner. This effect, unlike the findings in brain homogenates, were not restricted to PGE-stimulated cyclase but were also observed for adenosine stimulation and for basal enzyme activity. The opiate-specific nature of this inhibition received support from the finding that in various cell lines the extent of inhibition was correlated with the level of opiate receptors.

An interesting biochemical effect of chronic treatment with opiates, thought to be related to tolerance and dependence, has been observed in cell culture (Sharma et al., 1975b; Traber et al., 1975). When neuroblastoma × glioma hybrid cells are cultured in the presence of morphine for 4 days there is a gradual rise in both basal and PGE_1-stimulated adenylate cyclase (measured after removal of morphine). After 2–3 days of growth in morphine, both basal and PGE_1-stimulated adenylate cyclase, measured in the presence of morphine, were about the same as in control cells (preincubated in the absence of morphine) assayed in the absence of morphine. The authors suggest that this is the cells' equivalent to tolerance in animals and man. The cells also exhibit dependence on opiates, in the sense that adenylate cyclase is abnormally high in pretreated cells unless opiates are present during the assay. Dependence is demonstrated dramatically when cAMP levels are measured in cells exposed briefly to the antagonist naloxone after pretreatment with morphine for several days. Such cells show as much as a fivefold increase in cAMP levels, a phenomenon suggested as analogous to precipitated withdrawal in animals and man. Adenylate cyclase levels were shown to return to normal within 24 hr after withdrawal of morphine from the culture medium.

It will be of great interest to learn to what extent these findings in cell culture apply to the action of opiates in the central nervous system.

A TISSUE CULTURE MODEL FOR THE STUDY OF OPIATE RECEPTORS

The complexity of the mammalian brain has led investigators to seek simpler models. The guinea pig ileum has been a useful model for a number of years, but it is not CNS tissue, and basic differences in opiate action are possible. Neuroblastoma × glioma hybrid cell lines have been very valuable, but they are tumor cell lines with the attendant disadvantages and, to date, are unable to form functional synapses with other neurons.

In collaboration with Stanley M. Crain, we have developed a model system which, in our view, possesses exciting potential for the study of opiate action. The system consists of a cross section of spinal cord with attached dorsal root ganglia (DRG) explanted from 14-day fetal mice. These cultures are maintained on collagen-covered coverslips in Maximow depression-slide chambers in suitable nutrient medium containing nerve growth factor. There is abundant outgrowth of neurites from the DRG, which increases with time in culture during the first 2–3 weeks. After 1–2 weeks in culture, focal stimulation of DRG and extracellular recording in the spinal cord cross section gives rise to complex, negative slow wave potentials, restricted to the dorsal region of the cord, that resemble primary and secondary sensory-evoked synaptic network responses in dorsal spinal cord *in situ*. This represents strong evidence for the formation of functional synapses between DRG neurites and dorsal cord (Crain and Peterson, 1974).

Introduction of morphine sulfate into the culture bath at concentrations of 10^{-7}–10^{-6} M led to marked depression of the DRG-evoked negative slow wave response in the dorsal cord (Crain et al., 1977). Etorphine exerted a similar effect at even lower concentrations (10^{-8}–10^{-7} M). Levorphanol was active at 10^{-7} M while its enantiomer, dextrorphan, was ineffective at 10^{-6} M. Introduction of the opiate antagonist, naloxone, at low concentrations (10^{-8}–10^{-6} M) restored cord responses within minutes, while restoration of response by return of cultures to opiate-free medium required 30–60 minutes. It was of special interest that naloxone added to cultures not previously exposed to opiates elicited in most cases increases in both amplitude and duration of the sensory-evoked negative slow wave potentials. This suggests the presence of enkephalinergic networks in the isolated cord-DRG cultures. It was also noted that the explants develop marked tolerance after chronic exposure to opiates.

More recently, we have shown that the electrical response of the dorsal cord is also inhibited by a variety of enkephalins, enkephalin analogues, and longer-chain endorphins, and that the inhibitory effectiveness correlates well with their analgesic potencies in rodents (Crain et al., 1978).

The electrophysiological effectiveness of opiates and endorphins caused us to study opiate receptor levels and localization in these cultures (Hiller et al., 1978). Receptor binding was assayed using the potent opiate antagonist [^{3}H]diprenorphine labeled at high specific activity (22.3 Ci/nmole). It was observed that opiate receptors are present in cord-DRG cultures and that similar levels can be found in the simpler cultures in which DRG's are explained in the absence of spinal cord. Fresh explants had little or no opiate binding, but receptor levels increased with time in culture and reached maximum levels at 11 to 14 days after explantation. When the neuritic outgrowth was assayed separately from the original DRG explants, most of the receptor binding was consistently found in the outgrowth.

As stated earlier, this represents the most clearcut evidence for a presynaptic location of opiate receptors, evidence that is difficult to explain in alternative ways.

This organotypic culture system has already proved very useful, and we hope that a great deal can be learned from it about the mode of action of opiates and endorphins.

HETEROGENEITY OF OPIATE RECEPTORS

The idea that there may be multiple opiate receptors derives from the many pharmacological effects elicited by opiates and endorphins and from the knowledge that receptors for other neurotransmitters almost invariably exist in two or more forms. Thus multiple receptors have been found for acetylcholine, norepinephrine, dopamine, and serotonin.

The earliest evidence that this may also be true for opiate receptors came from experiments of Martin and co-workers (Martin et al., 1976; Gilbert and Martin, 1976) in chronic spinal dogs. Striking differences in pharmacological responses to different types of narcotic analgesics and their inability to substitute for each other in the suppression of withdrawal symptoms in addicted animals led to the postulate of three types of receptors in the CNS of the dog. These were named for the prototype drugs that gave rise to the distinction: μ(morphine), κ(ketocyclazocine) and σ(SKF 10047).

Kosterlitz' group has published convincing data suggesting that the receptors in the mouse vas deferens are different from those present in the guinea pig ileum. This group has also reported evidence based on binding studies for heterogeneity of opiate receptors in rat brain (Lord et al., 1977). We have repeated very similar experiments, and the results shown in Table 2 confirm the results of Lord et al. These data may indeed reflect two separate kinds of receptor sites, but it is difficult to rule out the possibility that enkephalins and opiate alkaloids bind to the same receptor in a somewhat different manner. The concept of different types of receptors has received additional support from recent results in our laboratory (Groth et al., 1979). Binding competition studies were carried out in different brain areas. IC_{50} values in certain regions, e.g., the caudate nucleus and the periventricular gray, were similar to those observed in the whole brain. However, a reproducible and significant difference was found in the thalamus. Here, naloxone is able to compete equally well with [^{3}H]leu-enkephalin as with [^{3}H]naloxone (IC_{50} = 3 nM for each), while, as shown in Table 2, in whole brain its IC_{50} for displacement of leu-enkephalin is 12. This result suggests that the thalamus contains a predominance of "morphine" receptors, while the PVG and caudate contain a mixture of "morphine" and "enkephalin"

Table 2. Competition for opiate receptor binding

Compound	*[³]naloxone*	*[³H]D-ala²-met-enkephalinamide*	*[³H]leu-enkephalin*
Naloxone	2	4	12
Morphine	13	10	150
Etorphine	1	1	2.5
Met-enkephalin	30	5	3
Met-enkephalin amide	14	4	7
D-ala²-met-enkephalin	20	2	0.5
D-ala²-met-enkephalinamide	2	3	3
Leu-enkephalin	80	10	8
D-ala²-leu-enkephalin	19	4	3

The numbers listed are IC_{50} values. All binding experiments were carried out at 0° for 150 minutes in the presence and absence of a large excess of unlabeled ligand corresponding to the tritiated ligand used. [^{3}H]naloxone and [^{3}]leu-enkephalin were used at 1 nM, D-ala^2-met-enkephalinamide at 0.5 nM. The results are the average of at least three closely similar experiments.

receptors similar to that present in whole brain. Such a regional difference is probably the strongest evidence for the existence of multiple opiate receptors.

PROGRESS IN RECEPTOR SOLUBILIZATION AND PURIFICATION

Progress in research aimed at obtaining a soluble opiate receptor purified to homogeneity has been slow. This has been due to the absence of an electric fish or similar organism rich in opiate receptors, the unavailability of highly specific affinity-labeling compounds, and above all, to the remarkable sensitivity of opiate receptors to even small concentrations of most ionic and even non-ionic detergents.

There has been some progress in modestly enriching (three- to fivefold) small (sonicated) membrane fragments that carry opiate receptors (Lin and Simon, unpublished results). The use of a number of affinity chromatography columns prepared in our laboratory (Simon et al., 1972; Simon, 1974) for further purification of receptor-bearing membrane fragments has been surprisingly unsuccessful, especially in view of their effectiveness in the purification of morphine antibodies (Walker and Simon, 1977).

The most promising advance has been the solubilization of an etorphine-bound macromolecule that has properties suggesting that it is an etorphine-receptor complex (Simon et al., 1975a). This solubilization was achieved by the use of the non-ionic detergent Brij 36T and the use of columns of Amberlite XAD-2 for the separation of free and bound [^{3}H]etorphine. As much as 25–30 percent of prebound (in the presence of dextrorphan) radioactivity present in the supernatant from ultracentrifugation at 100,000 × g appeared in the void volume of the XAD column as bound etorphine. When binding was carried out in the presence of excess unlabeled levorphanol or etorphine, virtually no bound radioactivity appeared in the solubilized protein fraction, providing evidence for the stereospecificity of the solubilized macromolecular complex. The bound etorphine was released by proteolytic enzymes, heat, and sulfhydryl reagents, suggesting the participation of protein in binding. The molecular weight of the solubilized complex determined on a calibrated Sepharose 6B column was about 400,000. All the evidence so far obtained is consistent with the notion that this solubilized material is an etorphine-receptor complex.

This work has recently been repeated with identical results and extended by Zukin and Kream (1979). They found that an enkephalin-receptor complex can be solubilized by the use of the same detergent and procedure utilized by us for solubilization of the etorphine complex. They then proceeded to show that it was possible to cross-link prebound enkephalin to the solubilized receptor by treatment with the cross-linking reagent dimethyl suberimidate.

Zukin and Kream have been able to detect a labeled band of molecular weight 35,000 by electrophoresis on SDS-polyacrylamide gel. This cross-linking procedure may prove useful for the purification of a receptor- or receptor-subunit-enkephalin complex.

CONCLUDING COMMENTS

This section has dealt in considerable detail with opiate receptors. The relationship of the work discussed here to pain mechanisms is, perhaps, not immediately evident. However, it should be remembered that pain relief produced by the opiates clearly requires their interaction with the receptors, and that these receptors, or at least one or more sub-classes, seem to be also the receptors for the endogenous opioid peptides. The evidence for the involvement of endorphins and their receptors in endogenous pain modulation is increasingly impressive. Moreover, recent evidence regarding other receptors strongly suggests that it is the receptor rather than the ligand that carries the important information for physiological function. In the case of the insulin receptor, binding of specific antibodies to the receptor results in insulin-like activity in the total absence of insulin. Thus, the excitement about the endorphins should not obscure the importance of the receptors.

The evidence for a presynaptic location of opiate receptors and the well-known ability of opiates and endorphins to inhibit neurotransmitter release has led to the postulate that the enkephalins (and perhaps brain β-endorphin) may be neuromodulators. Thus, it is thought that activation of a descending pain modulating system that originates in the periventricular gray area results in the release of enkephalins from interneurons in the dorsal spinal cord which react with presynaptic receptors on nociceptive primary afferent nerve fibers to reduce the release of neurotransmitter and thereby block the pain impulse. There is evidence that suggests that the neurotransmitter involved in the conduction of pain impulses in the spinal cord may be the peptide substance P. Figure 3 shows a schematic model of how enkephalins are thought to exert their analgesic effects.

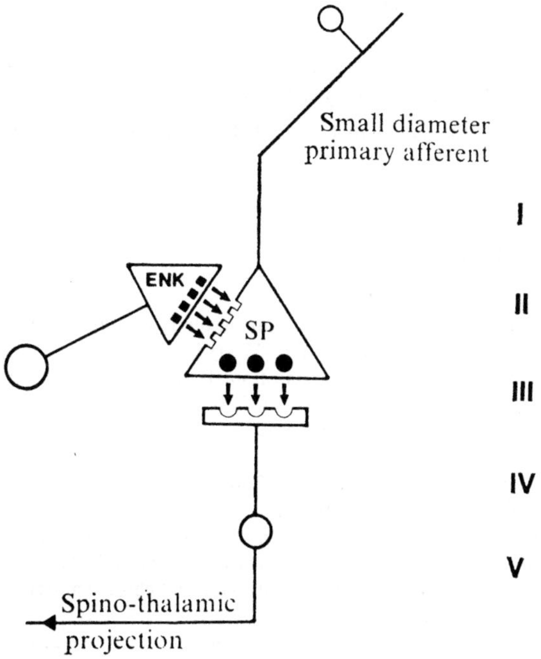

FIG. 3. Schematic representation of a possible mechanism for opiate-induced suppression of substance P (SP) release. SP is shown localized within the terminal of a small diameter afferent fiber which forms an excitatory axodendritic synapse with the process of a spinal cord neuron originating in lamina IV or V and projecting rostrally. A local enkephalin-containing inhibitory interneuron (ENK), confined to laminae II and III, forms a presynaptic contact on the terminal of the primary afferent. Opiate receptor sites are depicted presynaptically. Roman numerals on the right refer to the laminae of Rexed. From Jessel and Iverson (1977). Reprinted by permission. Courtesy of Macmillan Journals, Ltd.

There has been great progress in this field during the last six years, but there is much left to be learned. The events that occur between endorphin or opiate binding and analgesia represent a great challenge. The questions of which endogenous peptides have physiological functions and what are these functions are ones that we hope will be answered within the next few years.

Many of the structural and functional properties of the opiate receptors will be understood only when an active receptor is solubilized and purified. This is a difficult technical problem, the solution of which holds the key to many important pieces of this puzzle.

Finallly, it should be pointed out that the strategy that proved so successful in the opiate field is being generalized to other drugs. Thus, evidence has recently been obtained in several laboratories for the existence of specific binding sites for benzodiazepine tranquilizers. An active search is in progress in numerous laboratories for one or more endogenous ligands for this receptor. So far, none of the known neurochemicals have been found to bind to the benzodiazepine receptor with high affinity, and the possibility is being explored that the endogenous ligands are as yet unknown compounds that represent the body's own tranquilizing neurotransmitters.

ACKNOWLEDGEMENT

The author's research was supported by grant DA-00017 from the National Institute on Drug Abuse. We also gratefully acknowledge financial assistance from Hoffman-LaRoche, Inc., and E.I. DuPont de Nemours and Company.

REFERENCES

Abood, L.G., and Takeda, F. Enhancement of stereospecific opiate binding to neural membranes by phosphatidyl serine. *Eur. J. Pharmacol.* 39, 71–77 (1976).

Atweh, S.F., and Kuhar, M.J. Autoradiographic localization of opiate receptors in rat brain. I. Spinal cord and lower medulla. *Brain Res.* 124, 53–67 (1977a).

Atweh, S.F., and Kuhar, M.J. Autoradiographic localization of opiate receptors in rat brain. II. The brainstem. *Brain Res.* 129, 1–12 (1977b).

Atweh, S.F., and Kuhar, M.J. Autoradiographic localization of opiate receptors in rat brain. III. The telencephalon. *Brain Res.* 134, 393–406 (1977c).

Barchas, J.A., Akil, H., Elliot, G.R., Holman, R.B., and Watson, S.J. Behavioral neurochemistry: neuroregulators and behavioral states. *Science* 200, 964–972 (1978).

Bonnet, K.A. Regional alterations in cyclic nucleotide levels with acute and chronic morphine treatment. *Life Sci.* 16, 1877–1882 (1975).

Bonnet, K.A., and Gusik, S. Endorphin or morphine alter brain adenylate cyclase activity depending on calcium ion levels. *Soc. Neurosic. Abs.* 2, 849 (1976).

Clark, H.R., and Strickholm, A. Evidence for a conformational change in nerve membrane with depolarization. *Nature* 234, 470–471 (1971).

Clay, G.A., and Brougham, L.R. Haloperidol binding to an opiate receptor site. *Biochem. Pharmacol.* 24, 1363–1367 (1975).

Clendeninn, N.J., Petraitis, M., and Simon, E.J. Ontological development of opiate receptors in rodent brain. *Brain Res.* 118, 157–160 (1976).

Collier, H.O.J., and Roy, A.C. Hypothesis: Inhibition of E-prostaglandin-sensitive adenyl cyclase as the mechanism of morphine analgesia. *Prostaglandins* 7, 361–376 (1974).

Coyle, J.T., and Pert, C.B. Ontogenetic development of [^{3}H]naloxone binding in rat brain. *Neuropharmacol.* 15, 555–560 (1976).

Crain, S.M., and Peterson, E.R. Enhanced afferent synaptic function in fetal mouse spinal cord-sensory ganglion explants following NGF-induced ganglion hypertrophy. *Brain Res.* 79, 145–152 (1974).

Crain, S.M., Peterson, E.R., Crain, B., and Simon, E.J. Selective opiate depression of sensory-evoked synaptic networks in dorsal horn regions of spinal cord cultures. *Brain Res.* 133, 162–166 (1977).

Crain, S.M., Crain, B., Peterson, E.R., and Simon, E.J. Selective depression by opioid peptides of sensory-evoked dorsal-horn network responses in organized spinal cord cultures. *Brain Res.* 157, 196–201 (1978).

Creese, I., Feinberg, A.P., and Snyder, S.H. Butyrophenone influences on the opiate receptor. *Eur. J. Pharmacol.* 36, 231–235 (1976).

Creese, I., and Snyder, S.H. Receptor binding and pharmacological activity of opiates in the guinea pig intestine. *J. Pharmacol. Exp. Ther.* 194, 205–219 (1975).

Garcin, F., and Coyle, J.T. Ontogenetic development of [^{3}H]naloxone binding and endogenous morphine-like factor in rat brain, in *Opiates and Endogenous Opioid Peptides*. H.W. Kosterlitz, ed. Elsevier/North-Holland Biomedical Press, Amsterdam (1976) pp. 267–273.

Gilbert, P.E., and Martin, W.R. The effects of morphine- and nalorphine-like drugs in the non-dependent, morphine-dependent and cyclazocine-dependent chronic spinal dog. *J. Pharmacol. Exp. Ther.* 198, 66–82 (1976).

Goldstein, A., Lowney, L.I., and Pal, B.K. Stereospecific and nonspecific interactions of the morphine congener levorphanol in subcellular fractions of mouse brain. *Proc. Natl. Acad. Sci. USA* 68, 1742–1747 (1971).

Groth, J., Bonnet, K., Hiller, J.M., and Simon, E.J. Evidence for differential distribution of opiate receptor types in rat caudate nucleus and thalamus. Abs. for meeting of Int. Soc. Neurochem. Jerusalem, Israel, Sept. 1979.

Hiller, J.M., Pearson, J., and Simon, E.J. Distribution of stereospecific binding of the potent narcotic analgesic etorphine in the human brain: predominance in the limbic system. *Res. Commun. Chem. Pathol. Pharmacol.* 6, 1052–1062 (1973).

Hiller, J.M., Simon, E.J., Crain, S.M., and Peterson, E.R. Opiate receptors in cultures of fetal mouse dorsal root ganglia (DRG) and spinal cord: Predominance in DRG neurites. *Brain Res.* 145, 396–400 (1978).

Hitzeman, R.J., Hitzeman, B.A., and Loh, H.H. Binding of [^{3}H]naloxone in the mouse brain: Effect of ions and tolerance development. *Life Sci.* 14, 2393–2404 (1974).

Hoss, W., Abood, L.G., and Smiley, C. Enhancement of opiate binding to neural membranes with an ethyl glycolate ester of phosphatidyl serine. *Neurochem. Res.* 2, 303–309 (1977).

Ingoglia, N.A., and Dole, V.P. Localization of *d*- and *l*-methadone after intraventricular injection into rat brains. *J. Pharmacol. Exp. Ther.* 175, 84–87 (1970).

Jessel, T.M., and Iversen, L.L. Opiate analgesics inhibit substance P release from rat trigeminal nucleus. *Nature* 268, 549–551 (1977).

Klee, W.A., and Nirenberg, M. A neuroblastoma × glioma hybrid cell line with morphine receptors. *Proc. Natl. Acad. Sci. USA* 71, 3474–3477 (1974).

Kuhar, M.J., Pert, C.B., and Snyder, S.H. Regional distribution of opiate receptor binding in monkey and human brain. *Nature* 245, 447–450 (1973).

LaMotte, C., Pert, C.B., and Snyder, S.H. Opiate receptor binding in primate spinal cord: Distribution and changes after dorsal root section. *Brain Res.* 112, 407–412 (1976).

Lin, H.K., and Simon, E.J. Phospholipase A inhibition of opiate receptor binding can be reversed by albumin. *Nature* 271, 383–384 (1978).

Loh, H.H., Law, P.Y., Oswald, T., Cho, T.M., and Way, E.L. Possible involvement of cerebroside sulfate in opiate receptor binding. *Fed. Proc.* 37, 142–152 (1978).

Lord, J.A.H., Waterfield, A.A., Hughes, J., and Kosterlitz, H.W. Endogenous opioid peptides: Multiple agonists and receptors. *Nature* 267, 495–499 (1977).

Martin, W.R., Eades, C.G., Thompson, J.A., Hoppler, R.E., and Gilbert, P.E. The effects of morphine- and nalorphine-like drugs in the nondependent and morphine-dependent chronic spinal dog. *J. Pharmacol. Exp. Ther.* 197, 517–532 (1976).

Pasternak, G.W., Snowman, A.M., and Snyder, S.H. Selective enhancement of [^{3}H]opiate agonist binding by divalent cations. *Molec. Pharmacol.* 11, 735–744 (1975).

Pasternak, G.W., and Snyder, S.H. Opiate receptor binding: Effects of enzymatic treatment. *Molec. Pharmacol.* 10, 183–193 (1973).

Pert, C.B., Aposhian, D., and Snyder, S.H. Phylogenetic distribution of opiate receptor binding. *Brain Res.* 75, 356–361 (1974a).

Pert, C.B., Snowman, A.M., and Snyder, S.H. Localization of opiate receptor binding in synaptic membranes of rat brain. *Brain Res.* 70, 184–188 (1974b).

Pert, C.B., and Snyder, S.H. Opiate receptor: Demonstration in nervous tissue. *Science* 179, 1011–1014 (1973).

Pert, C.B., and Snyder, S.H. Opiate receptor binding of agonists and antagonists affected differentially by sodium. *Mol. Pharmacol.* 10, 868–879 (1974).

Sharma, S.K., Klee, W.A., and Nirenberg, M. Dual regulation of adenylate cyclase accounts for narcotic dependence and tolerance. *Proc. Natl. Acad. Sci. USA* 72, 3092–3096 (1975a).

Sharma, S.K., Nirenberg, M., and Klee, W.A. Morphine receptors as regulators of adenylate cyclase activity. *Proc. Natl. Acad. Sci. USA* 72, 590–594 (1975b).

Simon, E.J. Morphine and related drugs, in *Affinity Techniques, Methods in Enzymology*, Vol. 34B. W.B. Jacoby and M. Wilchek, eds. Academic Press, New York (1974), pp. 619–623.

Simon, E.J., Dole, W.P., and Hiller, J.M. Coupling of a new, active morphine derivative to Sepharose for affinity chromatography. *Proc. Natl. Acad. Sci. USA* 69, 1835–1837 (1972).

Simon, E.J., and Groth, J. Kinetics of opiate receptor inactivation by sulfhydryl reagents: evidence for conformational change in presence of sodium ions. *Proc. Natl. Acad. Sci. USA* 72, 2404–2407 (1975).

Simon, E.J., Hiller, J.M., and Edelman, I. Stereospecific binding of the potent narcotic analgesic [^{3}H]etorphine to rat brain homogenate. *Proc. Natl. Acad. Sci. USA* 70, 1947–1949 (1973).

Simon, E.J., Hiller, J.M., and Edelman, I. Solubilization of a stereospecific opiate-macromolecular complex from rat brain. *Science* 190, 389–390 (1975a).

Simon, E.J., Hiller, J.M., Groth, J., and Edelman, I. Further properties of stereospecific opiate binding sites in rat brain: on the nature of the sodium effect. *J. Pharmacol. Exp. Ther.* 192, 531–537 (1975b).

Stahl, K.D., van Bever, W., Janssen, P., and Simon, E.J. Receptor affinity and pharmacological potency of a series of narcotic analgesic, antidiarrheal and neuroleptic drugs. *Eur. J. Pharmacol.* 46, 199–205 (1977).

Terenius, L. Stereospecific interaction between narcotic analgesics and a synaptic plasma membrane fraction of rat cerebral cortex. *Acta Pharmacol. Toxicol.* 32, 317–320 (1973a).

Terenius, L. Characteristics of the "receptor" for narcotic analgesics in synaptic plasma membrane fraction from rat brain. *Acta Pharmacol. Toxicol.* 32, 377–384 (1973b).

Traber, J., Fischer, K., Latzin, S., and Hamprecht, B. Morphine antagonizes the action of prostaglandin in neuroblastoma cells but not of prostaglandin and noradrenaline in glioma and glioma × fibroblast hybrid cells. *FEBS Letters* 49, 260–263 (1974).

Traber, J., Gullis, R., and Hamprecht, B. Influence of opiate on the levels of adenosine 3′, 5′-cyclic monophosphate in neuroblastoma × glioma hybrid cells. *Life Sci.* 16, 1863–1868 (1975).

Wilson, R.S., Rogers, M.E., Pert, C.B., and Snyder, S.H. Homologous N-alkylnorketobemidones. Correlation of receptor binding with analgesic potency. *J. Med. Chem.* 18, 240–242 (1975).

Van Praag, D., and Simon, E.J. Studies on the intracellular distribution and tissue binding of dihydromorphine-7,8-[^{3}H] in the rat. *Proc. Soc. Exp. Biol. Med.* 122, 6–11 (1966).

Walker, M.C., and Simon, E.J. The purification of anti-morphine antibodies by affinity chromatography. *J. Pharmacol. Exp. Ther.* 203, 360–364 (1977).

Zieglgansberger, W., and Fry, J. Actions of enkephalin on cortical and striatal neurons of naive and morphine tolerant/dependent rats, in *Opiates and Endogenous Opioid Peptides.* H.W. Korsterlitz, ed. Elsevier/North Holland Biomedical Press, Amsterdam (1976), pp. 231–238.

Zukin, R.S., and Kream, R.M. Chemical crosslinking of a solubilized enkephalin macromolecular complex. *Proc. Natl. Acad. Sci. USA* 76, 1593–1597 (1979).

Copyright © 1982, Spectrum Publications, Inc.
The Neural Basis of Behavior

15

Enkephalins, Endorphins, and Their Receptors

H.W. Kosterlitz

One of the more important developments during recent years has been the increasing evidence for the view that peptides of relatively small weight play an important role not only in the regulation of endocrine function but in the control of certain pathways in the central and peripheral nervous systems. The discovery of the opioid peptides which mimic the actions of morphine and other opiates is of particular interest, since it may give a better understanding of the physiological modulation of the responses to painful experiences. We now know that there are at least three opioid peptides which occur naturally; first, two short-chain peptides, methionine-enkephalin and leucine-enkephalin (Hughes et al., 1975), which are widely but unevenly distributed throughout the nervous system (Elde et al., 1976; Hughes et al., 1977; Simantov et al., 1977), and second, the long-chain β-endorphin, which extends from the hypothalamic-pituitary axis at first rostrally and then caudally in the midline regions as far as the anterior pons (Bloom et al, 1978; Rossier et al., 1977; Watson and Barchas, 1979).

Evidence has accumulated that the receptor population with which these peptides interact is not homogeneous. There are at least two receptors. Peptides which interact with the δ-receptors are characterized by their high affinity to the leucine-enkephalin binding sites in the brain and their preferential pharmacological action on δ-receptors in the mouse vas deferens. In contrast, peptides which interact with the μ-receptors have a high affinity to the dihydromorphine binding sites in the brain, and they act preferentially on the μ-receptors in the guinea pig ileum. There is a certain amount of cross-reactivity between the two types of receptors. β-Endorphin has equal affinity to both receptors, leucine-enkephalin has a much higher affinity to the δ-binding site than to the μ-binding site, and finally, methionine-enkephalin has characteristics between the two extremes (Lord et al., 1977; Kosterlitz et al., 1980). From a comparison of the relative affinities with the antinociceptive potencies, the conclusion may be drawn that μ-receptors appear to be more important for antinociception than δ-receptors (Kosterlitz et al., 1980; Kosterlitz, 1978; Ronai and Berzetei, 1979).

Since the naturally occurring enkephalins are readily inactivated by enzymes, many analogues have been synthesized. It is important to examine to what extent the peptide molecules may be altered without changing their pharmacological patterns. Since this problem has been discussed recently in detail (Kosterlitz et al., 1980), no further consideration is necessary, except to state in general terms that many of the modifications decrease the enkephalin-like character with a concomitant change towards the properties of morphine-like drugs.

Since the distinction between μ- and δ-receptors is of fundamental importance, experiments were designed to demonstrate the specific protection of μ- and δ-receptors by their respective ligands (Robson and Kosterlitz, 1979). Phenoxybenzamine has been found to cause a long-lasting inactivation of opiate receptors in homogenates of guinea pig brain. Both μ- and δ-receptors are affected to the same extent. This effect is selectively prevented when, before the exposure to phenoxybenzamine, the homogenate is pre-incubated with ligands of high affinity to either the μ- or δ-receptor binding site: dihydromorphine for the former and D-Ala^2-D-Leu^5-enkephalin for the latter.

As far as the physiological functions of the opioid peptides are concerned, little is known in spite of the fact that our knowledge of their pharmacological effects is quite considerable. In this respect they mimic the actions of morphine, although there are certain differences. It would appear that pain control is only one of the many functions of opioid peptides. In general terms, it can be stated that the function of the enkephalins will depend on the neuronal circuits on which they act, either in the central or peripheral nervous system, including the hypothalamus, which is particularly important for the control of endocrine functions. Our knowledge of the function of β-endorphin is also limited. It is probably of particular importance in endocrine control but may also play an important role in pain control in the diencephalon. It is likely that all natural and synthetic opioid peptides are liable to produce tolerance and dependence. There is no evidence, however, that under physiological conditions animals or man are tolerant to, and dependent on, their endogenous opioid peptides. This situation is probably due to the sequestration of the peptides in subcellular structures and the rapid destruction, particularly of the short-chain enkephalins, after their release from the nerve endings. Thus, the exposure of the receptors to their ligands would be short enough to avoid the development of tolerance and dependence.

REFERENCES

Bloom, F., Battenberg, E., Rossier, J., Ling, N., and Guillemin, R. Neurons containing β-endorphin in rat brain exist separately from those containing enkephalin: immunocytochemical studies. *Proc. Natl. Acad. Sci. USA* 75, 1591–1595 (1978).

Elde, R., Hokfelt, T., Johansson, O., and Terenius, L. Immunohistochemical studies using antibodies to leucine-enkephalin: initial observations on the nervous system of the rat. *Neuroscience* 1, 349–351 (1976).

Hughes, J., Kosterlitz, H.W., and Smith, T.W. The distribution of methionine-enkephalin and leucine-enkephalin in the brain and peripheral tissues. *Brit. J. Pharmacol.* 61, 639–647 (1977).

Hughes, J., Smith, T.W., Kosterlitz, H.W., Fothergill, L.A., Morgan, B.A., and Morris, H.R. Identification of two related pentapeptides from the brain with potent opiate agonist activity. *Nature* London 258, 577–579 (1975).

Kosterlitz, H.W. Opioid peptides and their receptors, in *Endorphins '78*. L. Graf, M. Palkovits, and A.Z. Ronai, eds. Akademiai Kiado, Budapest (1978), pp. 205–216.

Kosterlitz, H.W., Lord, J.A.H., Paterson, S.J., and Waterfield, A.A. Effects of changes in the structure of enkephalins and narcotic analgesic drugs on their interactions with μ-receptors and δ-receptors. *Brit. J. Pharmacol.* 68, 333–342 (1980).

Lord, J.A.H., Waterfield, A.A., Hughes, J., and Kosterlitz, H.W. Endogenous opioid peptides: multiple agonists and receptors. *Nature* (London) 267, 495–499 (1977).

Robson, L.E., and Kosterlitz, H.W. Specific protection of the binding sites of D-Ala^2-D-Leu^5-enkephalin (δ-receptors) and dihydromorphine (μ-receptors). *Proc. Roy. Soc. Lond. B.* 205, 425–432 (1979).

Ronai, A.Z., and Berzetei, I. Similarities and differences of opioid receptors in different isolated organs, in *Endorphins '78*. L. Graf, M. Palkovits, A.Z. Ronai, eds. Akademiai Kiado, Budapest (1979), pp. 237–257.

Rossier, J., Vargo, T.M., Minick, S., Ling, N., Bloom, F.E., and Guillemin, R. Regional dissociation of β-endorphin and enkephalin contents in rat brain and pituitary. *Proc. Natl. Acad. Sci. USA* 74, 5162–5165 (1977).

Simantov, R., Kuhar, M.J., Uhl, G.R., and Snyder, S.H. Opioid peptide enkephalins: immunohistochemical mapping in the rat central nervous system. *Proc. Natl. Acad. Sci. USA* 74, 2167–2171 (1977).

Watson, S.J., and Barchas, J.D. Anatomy of the endogenous opioid peptides and related substances: The enkephalins, β-endorphin, β-lipotropin, and ACTH, in *Mechanisms of Pain and Analgesic Compounds*. R.F. Beers, Jr., and E.G. Bassett, eds. Raven Press, New York (1979), pp. 227–237.

Copyright © 1982, Spectrum Publications, Inc.
The Neural Basis of Behavior

16

On the Role of Endorphins in Pain Modulation

Huda Akil

It is well known that reactions to pain, particularly in man, are modifiable by many factors such as social environment, cultural values, the significance of the painful stimulus, and the individual's past history and biological predisposition. For example, some cultures encourage expression of discomfort while others favor a more stoic attitude. However, the differences in responsiveness to a painful stimulus appear to go beyond the level of expression. Certain states appear conducive to changes in pain sensation or perception. There are several striking examples of manipulations that lead to dramatic reduction in pain sensitiviy, such as hypnosis (Hadfield, 1917; Hilgard, 1967), acupuncture (Mau and Chen, 1972) or coping with a situation that threatens the survival of the organism. Among the most cited examples is a study by Beecher (1959) showing that soldiers who are injured at war appear to perceive their injuries as less painful, presumably because they signify the end of the war for these individuals.

Such factors affecting pain perception have often been termed "psychological," and by implication, removed from the realm of biology. However, in 1965, Melzack and Wall proposed their gate theory of pain transmission. Aside from its impact in hypothesizing a mechanism of pain transmission at the spinal level, this theory suggested that influences descending from the brain could modulate pain transmission at the very first synapse. These factors would presumably include cognitive and emotional variables which would alter more than pain processing, or pain responsiveness. They would, in fact, affect pain input and transmission at the lowest point of integration.

In the last twenty years, a great deal of evidence has accumulated to support this notion. In general, we have become more aware that pain is not merely a sensation. In fact, emotional responsiveness constitutes its core. A stimulus, no matter how intense, is not painful unless it is "upsetting." In fact, no theory that ignores the basic, limbic components of pain appreciation could ever describe adequately the underlying neural mechanisms of pain control. Neuroscience has begun to explore the neural mechanisms that can modulate both the emotional and the sensory components of pain appreciation. Analgesia, a state of little or no sensitivity to painful stimuli, can be conceived as an extreme case of pain modulation. It has been the subject of many studies both because of its theoretical implications and its potential for clinical applications.

The most potent pharmacological tools for producing analgesia are the opiate alkaloids. Morphine and its analogues are known to inhibit acute pain in animals, and to block clinical pain in man. It is conceivable that morphine could act in one of two ways. Opiates could be interrupting the transmission of noxious input along the neuraxis, in which case morphine injection would be akin to a transection anywhere along the pain pathways. Alternatively, opiates could activate a system in the brain that normally function to dampen pain without completely interrupting its transmission. There is evidence for the second mechanism in many studies that have demonstrated the active nature of opiate analgesia and its dependence on the integrity of various neurotransmitters, such as the monoamines, for full effectiveness (Proudfit and Anderson, 1974; Verri et al., 1968; Vogt, 1974). Further support for an active role of opiates has come from structure-activity studies that pointed to the presence of opiate receptors in the central nervous system (Goldstein et al., 1971) as well as in the periphery (Henderson et al., 1972). The existence of these opiate receptors (Pert and Snyder, 1973; Simon et al., 1973; Terenius, 1973) and of their endogenous ligands (Hughes et al., 1975; Li and Chung, 1976) are described elsewhere in this volume. These findings have had a major impact on the neurosciences. They have also suggested very strongly that the brain possesses a system potentially capable of blocking pain, and that morphine may act by activating this system.

Several years prior to the discovery of enkephalins, we (Mayer et al., 1971; Akil et al., 1972) had suggested the existence of such a system based on a somewhat different line of evidence. The work of Reynolds (1969) had shown that electrical stimulation of the periaqueductal grey produces a dramatic decrease in responsiveness to pain in the rat. Our group at U.C.L.A. (Drs. J. Liebeskind, D. Mayer, and myself) explored and characterized this phenomenon, termed stimulation-produced analgesia or SPA. There are several excellent reviews of this work (Liebeskind et at., 1976; Mayer and Price, 1976), and I will briefly summarize here the relevant findings. Stimulation-produced analgesia has been shown to occur in several species including rat, cat, monkey, and man (Mayer et al., 1971; Liebeskind et al., 1973; Richardson and Akil, 1977a,b) and consists of a selective loss in responsiveness to pain, with little or no loss in other sensations. It derives from stimulation of a mesial brain system, particularly aroung the fourth ventricle, the Aqueduct of Sylvius, and the third ventricle. Several lines of evidence led us to suggest that analgesia thus obtained was not due to the interruption of pain transmission. Rather, as is the case with morphine, it resulted from the activation of an endogenous pain inhibitory system. For example, SPA was dependent on the integrity of serotonin (Akil and Mayer, 1972), dopamine and norepinephrine (Akil and Liebeskind, 1975) for its effectiveness. Furthermore, electrolytic lesions, placed at the effective stimulation sites, did not result in analgesia (Kelly and Glusman, 1968; Liebman et al., 1970). There were also some striking parallels with morphine's action. Neuro-anatomical studies demonstrated a general correspondence between loci sensitive to morphine microinjection (Jacquet and Lajtha, 1973) and sites that yielded analgesia upon electrical stimulation. Naloxone, the specific opiate antagonist, was able to reverse SPA in some of our animals (Akil et al., 1972, 1976b). Finally, SPA appeared subject to cross-tolerance with morphine (Mayer and Hayes, 1975). Based on the several lines of evidence, we suggested that SPA was acting by releasing an endogenous factor akin to morphine (Akil et al., 1976b). Under this hypothesis, both morphine and SPA would be activating the same system, but in different ways. SPA would be releasing the endogenous ligands, whereas morphine would be binding directly to the opiate receptor. The merits and limitations of this hypothesis will be discussed below. It, nonetheless, focused attention on the possible existence of such a pain inhibitory system with opiate-like properties. At this point, it is necessary to describe our current knowledge of endogenous opioid systems in mammalian brain, before discussing their potential role in pain modulation.

MULTIPLE ENDOGENOUS OPIOID SYSTEMS

In the last few years, it has become clear that there are several endogenous opioid systems and that these may serve multiple and complex functions. Three opioid peptides have been shown to exist within brain neurons and pituitary cells. There are also several peptides awaiting final identification or anatomical mapping.

Hughes, Kosterlitz, and their co-workers (1975) first identified two closely related pentapeptides, methionine- and leucine-enkaphalin, differing by a single residue at the COOH terminal. These peptides were shown by numerous studies to possess opiate-like properties, including the ability to produce analgesia (Beluzzi et al., 1976), tolerance and dependence (Wei and Loh, 1976). However, their effects were short-lived, due to their rapid breakdown. Several laboratories raised antibodies to the two enkephalins in order to study their distributions, levels, and responses to environmental physiological changes. Elde, Hokfelt and their co-workers (1976) were the first to visualize the enkephalins in the CNS. They described a complex system with multiple cell groups and short pathways distributed throughout the neuraxis. Several groups have confirmed this distribution, employing a number of antisera directed against methionine- or leucine-enkephalin (Watson et al., 1977; Simantov et al., 1977). Although many of these sera had good specificity against one or the other of the enkephalins, the general pattern of distribution of both peptides is very similar. At this point, two possibilities exist: either methionine and leucine enkephalin occur in the same neurons, or they are localized in separate systems that exhibit very similar regional distribution.

The mammalian brain also contains a second well-identified opioid system with β-endorphin (β-END) as the putative transmitter. Hughes et al. (1975) first pointed to the existence of methionine enkephalin's structure within the sequence of β-lipotropin (β-LPH). This latter hormone had been identified and sequenced by Li et al. (1966), and was thought to be the prohormone of α-melanocyte-stimulating-hormone (α-MSH). Soon thereafter, two groups demonstrated that the 31 amino acid carboxy terminal residues of β-lipotropin (61-91) had potent opiate-like properties (Cox et al., 1976; Bradbury et al., 1976). While this peptide, termed β-endorphin, was primarily found in the pituitary, it appeared conceivable that it was the precursor of brain enkephalins. Alternatively, it was possible to conceive of enkephalins as neurotransmitters and of β-endorphin as a pituitary hormone. However, neither of these hypotheses appears to be entirely true. It is now clear that β-endorphin exists in brain as well as in pituitary, and that it does not function there merely as the enkephalin precursor. Our own work (Akil et al., 1978a; Watson et al., 1978a) as well as that of the group at the Salk Institute (Bloom et al., 1978) has demonstrated that β-endorphin exists as a separate system in brain. β-endorphin-like immunoreactivity can be found with a simple group of neurons located in the arcuate region of the hypothalamus and projecting via long axons to various limbic structures, traversing the medial thalamus, the central grey area, and terminating at the level of the major noradrenergic cell group—the locus coeruleus. There appears to be no overlap between the distribution of the enkephalins and that of β-endorphin. In fact, the notion that methionine-enkephalin is derived from β-endorphin has received little support. A recent report of a leucine-enkephalin-containing peptide, α-neo-endorphin, which does not resemble β-endorphin in structure (Kangawa et al., 1979), further points to a separate synthetic pathway for the enkephalins.

It is therefore clear that the mammalian brain contains at least three opioid systems: leucine-enkephalin, methionine-enkephalin, and β-endorphin. The β-endorphin system has some interesting properties. β-endorphin and β-lipotropin have been shown to coexist with adrenocorticotropin hormone (ACTH) in pituitary (Moon et al., 1973) and to be derived from a common precursor—31K or pro-opiocortin (Mains et al., 1977). This precursor contains a 16K fragment of unknown function, the full structure of $ACTH_{1\text{-}39}$, which includes α-MSH structure, and the full structure of β-lipotropin which includes α-MSH and β-endorphin structure. We and others (Watson et al., 1978b; Watson and Akil, 1979) have shown that the brain hypothalamic system which contains β-endorphin also demonstrates immunoreactivity against every fragment of the 31K precursor available for testing. Our most recent work suggest that pro-opiocortin in brain is processed to β-endorphin (from β-lipotropin) and α-MSH (from ACTH) (Watson and Akil, 1980). Whether both substances are simultaneously released, and their potential interaction, remains the subject of our studies.

In sum, the endogenous opioid systems in brain are far from simple. There are many identified to date, possibly with more to come. The enkephalins are short-acting and appear to be localized in interneurons. β-endorphin is much longer acting, is localized within a simple limbic system, and contains other neuroactive peptides, particularly ACTH and its fragments. Interestingly, enkephalins and β-endorphin appear to possess different pharmacological properties (Bloom et al., 1978), in spite of the fact that they can be all characterized as opioids. Most striking is the long duration of action seen with β-endorphin, which is occasionally difficult to reverse with naloxone. Our recent work with ^{3}H-β-endorphin binding (Akil et al., 1980) shows that this peptide tends to bind very tightly to the opiate receptor, dissociating with a slow rate, which correlates well with behavioral observation. The implications of this mode of action and the relative resistance to enzymatic breakdown of β-endorphin brings about interesting questions as to the mode of action in brain and to its potential role in modulating pain responsiveness.

ROLE OF ENDORPHINS IN PAIN CONTROL

The analgesic effects of morphine, enkephalins, and β-endorphin would naturally lead to the hypothesis that endogenous opioids play an important role in regulating pain. While this is both an obvious and attractive hypothesis, it faces a number of difficulties and requires several refinements.

The first refinement to be made is that analgesia is not a typical physiological state. Rather, it is an extreme of pain modulation, which results from pharmacological or other "unphysiological" manipulations. It is therefore unlikely that endogenous opioids are there to produce analgesia, any more than that dopamine's function is to produce motor stereotypy. However, these extremes do shed light on the nature of more subtle modulation which might occur in the behaving animal.

A second point to be remembered is that the "opiate receptor," when studied *in vitro*, recognizes all of the endogenous opioids. Therefore, when we administer a given endogenous opioid peptide, and it produces analgesia, we cannot conclude that pain control is its natural function. We can merely deduce that the peptide interacted with many opiate receptors, some of which are critically situated to produce pain inhibition. To date, it is not possible to determine which of the systems described above is most critical in pain control—nor is it possible to invoke a single circuit which is most important in modulation of pain appreciation.

Because of the above difficulties with pharmacological studies, it would be advantageous to have a model for studying endogenous opioid function without administering the peptides in question. The use of a specific antagonist would serve to block the receptor, preventing the endogenous opioids from being effective. Any sensory or behavioral descriptions resulting from such treatment could be construed as results of the blockade and reflections of the natural function of the opioids. This approach has been employed using the antagonist naloxone, which is known to bind to the opiate receptor to reverse the effects of both opiate alkaloids and opioid peptides.

Naloxone's Effect on Pain Responsiveness

Jacob and his co-workers (1974) were the first to show that naloxone administration produces hyperalgesia on the hot plate test. One interpretation of this finding is that pain responsiveness is under inhibitory control of endorphins, and that their blockade results in hypersensitivity to noxious input. If this is the case, then, other types of pain tests should be similarly affected. Yet, there are several negative reports using other tests in rat and man (Goldstein et al., 1976; Grevert and Goldstein, 1977). While there are some reports of naloxone affecting the tail flick test (Bernston and Walker, 1977), the effect tends to be small and elusive. In man, naloxone appears to have little effect on experimental pain (Grevert and Goldstein, 1977), although there are reports of naloxone effects in some experimental situations and in clinical pain, as well as reversal of placebo effects in man

(Buchsbaum et al., 1977; Levine et al., 1978, 1979). There is also a recent report showing that patients who are congenitally insensitive to pain show some pain responsiveness after naloxone injection (Dehen et al., 1978). The above findings are all new, require replication, and typically involve situations where pain responsiveness has been running away from homeostasis. However, naloxone is, generally speaking, relatively impotent in producing significant hyperalgesia in animals or in man.

Such negative evidence flies in the face of an hypothesis that would place endogenous opioids at a critical junction in circuits modulating pain responsiveness. One possible explanation is that the endogenous opioid modulation of pain sensation is not tonic; rather, opioids have to be activated first by some environmental or physiological stimulus before they exhibit their modulation of pain. Under this hypothesis, certain types of pain tests, such as the hot plate test employed by Jacob et al. (1974), would succeed in activating endogenous opioids which would result in naloxone-reversible increases in pain threshold. Other potential hypotheses that might account for the discrepant effects of naloxone on pain responsiveness would have to incorporate multiple pain inhibitory mechanisms with complex interactions. Such a model will be proposed and discussed below.

Opioids and Stimulation-Produced Analgesia

Before turning to a model, however, it would be useful to address the first hypothesis, and explore some of the possible ways that endogenous opioids can be activated, and whether they appear to produce naloxone-reversible analgesia. The most direct activation would result from direct stimulation of opioid pathways within the brain. This, of course, is far from physiological. However, our work on stimulation-produced analgesia in animals and man (Mayer et al., 1971; Richardson and Akil, 1977a and b; Akil et al., 1979) does point to the importance of endorphins in the control of pain. SPA has been employed to alleviate pain in over thirty human patients. The stimulation site is very medial, immediately adjacent to the ventricular system, at the junction of the third ventricle and the Aqueduct of Sylvius. The analogous sites in lower animals are extremely rich in endogenous opioids, particularly β-endorphin. We (Akil et al., 1979) and Hosobuchi et al. (1977) have reported that this analgesia can be reversed by the opiate antagonist, naloxone; this was congruent with our previous animal findings (Akil et al., 1972, 1976b) which had led us to suggest that SPA resulted from release of endogenous opioids.

We therefore undertook the study of the cerebrospinal fluid (CSF) from stimulated human patients to determine whether stimulation which results in pain relief is accompanied by release of endogenous opioids. In two separate studies, we examined levels of enkephalin-like material and of β-endorphin-like immunoreactivity before and after analgetic electrical stimulation in our patients (Akil et al., 1978a, b, d). The fluids were collected in the operating room during the implantation procedure. Enkephalin-like material was characterized on two chromatographic methods, which separated it from β-endorphin, and was measured with two bioassays which recognized opiate-like material, the opiate binding assay, and the vas-deferens bioassay. These strategies helped us determine that the material being measured was indeed an active endogenous opioid, which had several properties like enkephalin and unlike β-endorphin.

In the second study, we employed a radioimmunoassay which recognized β-endorphin but not methionine-enkephalin; detection of β-lipotropin was only ⅙th–¹/₁₀th as effective on a molar basis (Akil et al., 1978a). Both studies demonstrated a significant rise in opioid peptides throughout twenty minutes of stimulation. Enkephalin-like material was elevated by approximately 50%, whereas β-endorphin-like material was elevated several-fold (up to 20-30-fold). Hosobuchi et al. (1979) have also demonstrated a substantial rise in β-endorphin inmunoreactivity upon electrical stimulation in humans.

This correlation between analgesia and an increased release of opioids is necessary but not sufficient to prove a role of endorphins in modulating pain or producing analgesia. While the studies with SPA have been critical in pointing to the role of endogenous opioids in pain regulation, they also began to point to the complexities of pain modulation. Even the first studies of naloxone's effect on SPA in rat (1972–1976) showed that only a proportion of the animals exhibited naloxone-reversible analgesia. Other animals, which were not easily distinguishable by any other means, had full-blown analgesia which remained totally resistant to the effects of opioids. Other investigators could not produce reversal of SPA with naloxone (Akil et al., 1976a). However, recently we have begun to uncover some of the factors involved in this paradigm. A report at the 1978 Neuroscience meeting by Dr. Larry Stein suggested that naloxone-reversibility of SPA and self-stimulation were very much a function of current parameters. More recent work in the laboratory of Dr. John Liebeskind (Prieto et al., 1979) suggest that naloxone reversibility is site-specific. Stimulation of ventral central grey produces naloxone-reversible analgesia, whereas more dorsal sites appear resistant to naloxone's effect. It is possible that stimulation of sites presynaptic to an endorphinergic synapse would lead to naloxone-reversible analgesia, whereas stimulation of a post-synaptic site would produce naloxone-resistant analgesia. However, it is also possible that there are mechanisms of pain inhibition which do not involve opioids at all. That such do exist is further indicated by studies described below.

Stress-Induced Analgesia

If we entertain the hypothesis that endogenous opioid control over pain is tonically "silent," then it must be engaged by physiological or environmental stimuli. Stressful or painful situations are known to produce short-term or long-term changes in pain responsiveness. We and others (Akil et al., 1976a; Madden et al., 1977; Hayes et al., 1978) have shown that stress can bring about changes in pain responsiveness, including full-blown analgesia. We (Akil et al., 1976a; Madden et al., 1977) demonstrated that footshock stress resulted in a rise in endogenous opioid levels in brain, and that the analgesia was partially reversible by naloxone. Recently, Frederickson and co-workers (1978) have shown a rise in enkephalin immunoreactivity upon heat stress, and the changes exhibited a circadian rhythm congruent with that of naloxone's effect on pain reponsiveness in the hot plate test (1977). Stress is also known to release β-endorphin peripherally (Rossier et al., 1977), although the effect of this peripheral release on analgesia is not clear.

One can therefore construct a model whereby environmental stress would engage endogenous opioids in brain, altering their levels and turnover, and producing, under some conditions, analgesia which is susceptible to naloxone. The hot-plate test of Jacob and co-workers can be construed as constituting a type of stress, since the noxious stimulus builds up slowly (unlike the case in the tail-flick test). It might then raise the pain threshold via endorphin activation and be susceptible to the effect of naloxone.

While the above model of stress-induced activation of endorphin is attractive, it is too simplistic. Whereas naloxone is clearly capable of reversing the analgesic effects of stress in our hands (Akil et al., 1976a and unpublished data) and those of others (Bodnar et al., 1978a), the effect is at best partial, and other researchers using shorter stress do not see any naloxone effects (Hayes et al., 1978).

While stress-induced analgesia exhibits cross-tolerance with morphine in the hands of one group studying mice (Chesher and Chan, 1977), it does not exhibit cross-tolerance in our hands (Akil et al., 1978c) or those of Bodnar and co-workers (1978b). In fact, we have observed a dramatic increase in stress-induced analgesia in opiate-tolerant rats (Akil et al., 1978a), a paradoxical finding which has been recently replicated by others (J. VanRee, personal communication). Thus, the partial effects of naloxone and the paradoxical effects of tolerance to morphine on stress-induced analgesia also point to the need for a more complex model of pain regulation.

Other Modes of Indirect Analgesia and the Relation to Endorphins

As mentioned earlier, placbo analgesia has been reported to be naloxone reversible (Levine et al., 1979), whereas hypnotic analgesia does not appear to be (Goldstein and Hilgard, 1975). Mayer and co-workers (1977) were the first to report that acupuncture analgesia is naloxone reversible, a finding also elaborated in mice by Pomeranz and co-workers (1976).

Bodnar and his co-workers have studied several other methods of producing analgesia, including the use of insulin hypoglycemia, and shown that many of them can be partially or totally resistant to naloxone.

Among the above paradigms, however, few, if any, have directly correlated changes in endorphin levels with changes in pain responsiveness. In fact, the work studying pain responsiveness and endorphins directly consists merely of the above-reported studies on SPA and changes in endogenous opioids, and the pioneering work performed by Terenius and coworkers (Terenius and Wahlstrom, 1975; VonKnorring et al., 1978). These authors have demonstrated that opioids in the CSF, some of them still unidentified, appeared lower in some patients suffering from chronic pain. They have evolved a classification of pain types and a correlation between them and certain opioid-containing fractions in human CSF.

In sum, the evidence for a role of endorphins in pain modulation can be stated as follows:

1. Pharmacological administration of endogenous opioids produces analgesia.
2. Some chronic pain patients exhibit lowered levels of endorphins in CSF.
3. Analgesic electrical stimulation causes release of endorphins in CSF.
4. Naloxone produces complex effects partially or totally reversing SPA, stress-induced analgesia, acupuncture, and placebo analgesia, and altering threshold to clinical pain and to some animal tests. On the other hand, naloxone fails to reverse analgesia in some animals undergoing electrical stimulation at certain sites or responding to stress, fails to reverse hypnosis analgesia, and does not appear to alter experimental pain in man.
5. Cross-tolerance of some analgesias with morphine have only been tested in a few paradigms. Such cross-tolerance occurs with SPA, but shows paradoxical interaction with stress-induced analgesia.

The above summary points to a few features of this field. Most studies suggest that even if endorphins are involved in pain regulation, one must invoke non-endorphinergic mechanisms of analgesia as well (cf. Mayer and Price, 1976). Furthermore, many of the classifications appear to depend primarily on the use of naloxone, with little other evidence. While naloxone-reversibility might be construed as necessary, we will discuss below why it may not be sufficient to implicate endorphins in any given analgesic phenomenon. Furthermore, naloxone does not distinguish well enough between various opioid systems even though it may be differentially effective in reversing their action. The following section is aimed at suggesting a working model for pain inhibition and pointing to some of the pitfalls in researching the role of endorphins in pain.

A MODEL FOR PAIN MODULATION

The findings surveyed above raise a number of problems for a simplistic view that opioid peptides function exclusively to suppress pain. Two complexities are immediately apparent: opioids have numerous other functions—from affecting eating and drinking to being implicated in psychosis (cf. Watson et al., 1979)—and pain appears to be modulated by non-opiate mechanisms.

If we accept this last point, then we are clealy in need of defining criteria for calling an analgesic phenomenon opioid in nature. Is naloxone reversibility a necessary and sufficient condition? Can it, alone, be the basis for classifying analgesic phenomena as "opioid" and "non-opioid"? In order to address these issues, I am suggesting a model of pain modulation which takes into consideration the information we already possess, and hopes to integrate the apparent complexities many researchers have encountered.

It should be stated from the outset that this is merely a working model. We know much too little about many of the facets of this problem to have any certainty in assigning circuitry, directionality, or even determining the critical components in such a model. My main goal is to show the reader how a reasonable working hypothesis can be evolved which points to the pitfalls of using naloxone as a sole criterion for determining the opioid nature of an analgesic phenomenon. I hope to use the model to evolve reasonable criteria for dissecting opioid and non-opioid mechanisms, and for putting in perspective the role of endorphinergic mechanisms in pain control. I fully expect that future data will lead to the modification of this suggested hypothesis, most probably to the addition of many unforeseen interactions.

Any current model of pain modulation needs to address a number of broad issues that have arisen in the literature in the last few years. These can be summarized as follows:

1. Are there opioid and non-opioid mechanisms of analgesia? How do they relate to each other and how do their interactions affect pain transmission and perception?

2. Why does naloxone, which reverses opiate alkaloids readily, exhibit minimal effects on many baseline pain behaviors and partial, or variable effects on many analgesic phenomena?
3. How is it possible to have an analgesic phenomenon which is susceptible to naloxone but not to opiate tolerance?
4. What determines the activation on opioid vs. non-opioid mechanisms of analgesia?
5. Can we evolve criteria for teasing apart opioid from non-opioid mechanisms?

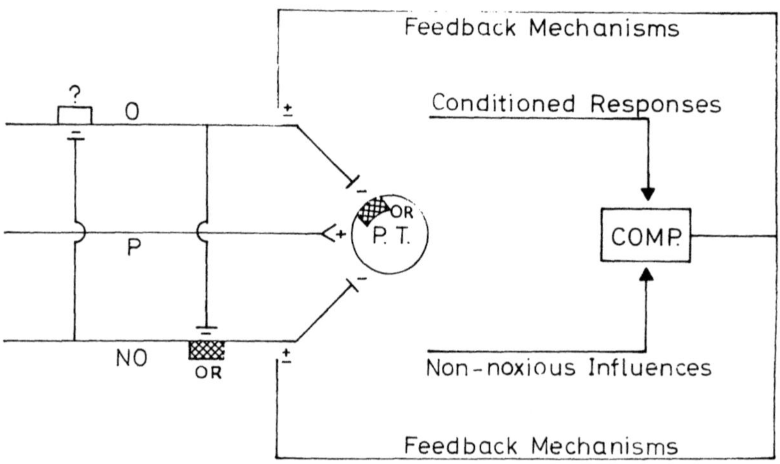

FIG. 1. A schematic diagram of the working model of endorphinergic and non-endorphinergic components of pain modulation (cf. text for more detail).

The circle in the middle of Fig. 1 labelled PT represents pain transmission. The model depicts PT as being determined by three major factors: P, or pain input; O, or an opioid pain inhibitory system; and NO, or a non-opioid pain inhibitory system. Obviously, pain input would facilitate pain transmission, whereas O and NO are analgesic mechanisms and would therefore inhibit pain transmission. This pain inhibition by the opiate system would be mediated via an opiate receptor (OR) depicted on PT. Moreover, O and NO are not likely to function in isolation. They are seen as being capable of interaction with each other, possibly by mutual inhibition, in order to prevent extreme and long-lasting analgesia and to maintain the organism's critical ability to respond to pain. Here again, the modulation of NO by O would be mediated via an opiate receptor (OR on NO). Pain transmission, in turn, can be integrated with other inputs, and via comparator mechanisms modulate both opioid and non-opioid systems, allowing them to become more or less active. The large arrows in the scheme point to some of the influences on the comparator circuit which affect its feedback onto O and NO. These include complex perceptual events, the subject's mood and drive state, non-noxious but possible stressful influences, and conditioned or anticipatory responses resulting from the organism's history with pain in general, and the noxious event in particular.

A number of points should be made clear before discussing the implications of the model. First, the modulation of pain in this manner is not necessarily localized in one site within the CNS. Rather, these complex interactions are likely to take place at several levels of the neuraxis, from the first synapse in the spinal cord (where the model is quite consistent with the gate control hypothesis of Melzack and Wall, 1965) to the midbrain, limbic structures, thalamus, and even cortex. Secondly, each of the components, such as P, O, NO, are not thought to involve a single connection or neurotransmitter. Rather, they represent multisynaptic systems, some of which involve opioids at a critical junction (O), while others do not (NO). It is quite likely that there are many opioid and non-opioid systems, with different connectivities at different sites. Remember, for instance, the existence of enkephalin in the spinal cord "at the gate," and the presence of both enkephalin and β-endorphin in central grey and in many limbic structures.

Finally, while this model does not address the controversy of "pain as a modality" versus "pain as a pattern of inputs," it obviously accepts the notion that pain transmission is a highly modifiable event. As such, it is consistent with the broader principles of the gate control theory (Melzack and Wall, 1965). Its main goal, however, is to specifically define the role of endorphinergic vs. non-endorphinergic mechanisms of pain control.

According to this working model, our sensitivity to pain is under tonic control by all three components (P, O, NO), which are regulated by peripheral and central influences. What can we expect, if we administer naloxone to an otherwise "normal" animal and test for pain responsiveness? While naloxone may block the opiate receptor on PT, thus decreasing the inhibitory effect of the O system, the opiate receptor on NO would also be blocked. This would release NO from inhibition, allowing it to be more active, and restoring an ideal balance at the level of PT. We may, therefore, detect little or no change in pain responsiveness. This does not mean that we never expect naloxone to affect pain threshold. There are states or behaviors where the relative importance of O in modulating PT is much greater, where non-opiate mechanisms may not compensate adequately, and where naloxone would have an effect. Many variables, such as the circadian rhythm, the general drive state of the animal, and the test being employed would determine the relative weights of O and NO in the final balance. Still, one would expect naloxone effects on baseline pain responsiveness to be subtle and task specific. What this would suggest is that a lack of naloxone effect on "baseline pain responsiveness" does not eliminate a role of opioids in pain control. It merely speaks to a well-balanced system striving toward homeostasis.

If, on the other hand, we stimulate the O system selectively and powerfully, we would succeed in producing analgesia. While NO's tonic activity may be decreased, the large increase in O would be overpowering and PT would be decreased. Obviously such activation of the O system would be reversible by naloxone. Furthermore, if the animal had been previously made tolerant to opiates, the opiate receptor sensitivity would be decreased and the activation of O would be less effective in blocking pain transmission. Thus, a direct activation of the O system would exhibit both naloxone blockade and cross tolerance with morphine. There are, of course, many possible ways of activating the O system. Pharmacological administration of opiates would do so directly by binding to the opiate receptors. Electrical stimulation of endorphinergic neurons would release endorphins. Environmental and/or physiological events would engage the system directly or activate pathways pre-synaptic to the opioid link which result in increasing the activity of O.

Other events would activate the NO system and produce analgesia which should be resistant to the effects of naloxone. If, however, the O system is still active, and is contributing to the analgesia, then the administration of naloxone would eliminate this component and result in a partial or subtle blockade of analgesia by the opiate antagonist.

If both O and NO are simultaneously activated, naloxone would, again, have partial effects. The oscillations between the two systems and the feedback from the comparator circuit are complex enough to make it quite a difficult situation to predict. The effects of naloxone may vary with time after the induction of analgesia, and may be easily modifiable by other variables which determine the delicate balance between the three components, P, O, and NO.

Finally, analgesia can be brought about by interfering with pain input, decreasing its sensitivity or efficacy (i.e., decreasing the P component). In this case, O and NO are *relatively* more active, though they have not been directly activated. Naloxone would block the O component, and thus restore some of the sensitivity to pain. Here again, a reversal of analgesia by naloxone would occur, although the O system had not been activated above resting levels. This effect of naloxone is similar to the balance hypothesis of striatal function. There, the balance is thought to occur between dopamine and acetylcholine. When dopaminergic transmission is decreased—as is the case in Parkinson's disease—one can restore the balance either by increasing dopamine (administering L-Dopa) or by decreasing acetylcholine (administering Cogentin). The latter treatment, while implicating ACh in the critical balance, does not mean that Parkinson's disease is due to an excess production of ACh. Similarly, a naloxone reversal of analgesia as depicted above would not mean that opiate mechanisms caused the analgesia in the first place—but only that opiate systems are critical in the balance which determines pain transmission and responsiveness.

Conclusions on the Significance of Naloxone Blockade

In sum, the following conclusions and caveats can be drawn about using naloxone to implicate endorphins in analgesic events:

1. The lack of a naloxone effect in a normal, non-analgesic animal does not mean endorphins are unimportant in pain transmission. It does not even mean that they are tonically inactive. Rather, it may mean that they are involved in a tightly regulated multicomponent circuit which is difficult to disrupt under some testing conditions.
2. If an analgesic phenomenon is entirely mediated by an endorphinergic mechanism, it should be completely naloxone reversible. Furthermore, the analgesia should be decreased in a morphine-tolerant animal.
3. Partial reversal by naloxone can occur under three conditions: the first is a situation where both opioid and non-opioid mechanisms are activated. The second is when only non-opioid mechanisms are enhanced but the opioid mechanisms remain tonically active until naloxone removes their influence. The last is when pain transmission is somewhat impaired and the critical balance determining PT is disrupted. Naloxone may, in part, restore this balance. A blocker of the NO system would have a similar effect.
4. It follows from (3.) that, if naloxone reverses an analgesic event, we cannot automatically conclude that the analgesia is mediated by an increase in the activity of endorphins, but only that endorphins are tonically important in the regulation of pain. The analgesia itself could be due to activation of other pain inhibitory mechanisms or to a decrease in pain transmission.

Criteria for the Endorphinergic Nature of an Analgesic Phenomenon

What is, then, a reasonable set of criteria for implicating endorphins in an analgesic phenomenon? While naloxone is necessary, it is obviously not sufficient. Even if the above model is totally wrong, one could evolve many others which at least point to the pitfalls of equating naloxone-reversibility with endorphin activation. We should therefore strive for a convergence of evidence before we can state that an analgesic phenomenon—such as SPA, stress-induced analgesia, placebo, congenital insensitivity to pain, or acupuncture—is due to the activation of endorphins.

The criterion of cross tolerance with morphine is a second and obvious one. While activation of the O system would be clearly less effective in a tolerant animal, what would be the effect of tolerance if NO is being activated? If we assume that tolerance results in a decrease of affinity, capacity, or efficacy of opiate receptors, then the role of the O system may be minimized. However, the NO system could still be activated, and because of the tolerance could escape the inhibitory control by O. Therefore, one could produce analgesia via a non-opiate mechanism which would be enhanced rather than diminished in a morphine-tolerant animal. Such a phenomenon has been observed with stress-induced analgesia (Akil et al., 1978c) and with acupuncture analgesia (Cheng et al., 1979). Interestingly, these phenomena are partially or totally reversible by naloxone. In the case of stress-induced analgesia, another group using mice has shown cross-tolerance with morphine (Chesher and Chan, 1977). It is likely that some of these treatments activate both opiate and non-opiate mechanisms of pain inhibition; that, in a tolerant animal, the non-opiate mechanisms exhibit compensatory increases which more than make up for the loss of the opiate component, particularly due to the loss of the inhibition via OR on them.

Still, it appears that both naloxone and cross-tolerance to morphine would be criteria for stating that an analgesia is primarily endorphinergic. Are these two criteria, taken together, sufficient? Not if we consider the balance hypothesis. Here, P would be decreased, thus producing analgesia. Pain responsiveness could be restored if the OR at PT is made less effective by a history of tolerance. The phenomenon could therefore appear cross-tolerant to morphine. On the other hand, NO may be more active in that tolerant animal, and no effect or a paradoxical effect of morphine tolerance would be observed.

Thus, the complexities of the checks and balances proposed above would point to the need for multiple criteria for stating that an analgesic phenomenon is caused by activation of opioids. These would include:

1) Naloxone reversibility of the analgesia
2) Loss of the analgesia in a morphine-tolerant subject
3) A demonstration of release of enkephalin, endorphin, or other opioids prior to or during the analgesia
4) A reasonable correlation between the time course of endorphin levels, release and/or turnover, and the time course of pain responsiveness
5) A loss of the analgesia if one or several opioid pathways are destroyed
6) An enhancement of the analgesia if the breakdown or metabolism of the opioid in question is decreased

Some of these criteria need to await our better understanding of brain opioid systems, their anatomy, regulation, turnover, and metabolism.

Nonetheless, they should be kept in mind prior to attributing causation to an analgesic event. More criteria will undoubtedly emerge as we gain a better understanding of the endogenous opioids and non-opiate pain control mechanisms, and as we acquire more tools for altering the responsiveness of these systems in a more specific fashion.

Some Limitations and Predictions of the Model

As I stated earlier, this is merely a working model aimed at directing attention to the complexity of pain control and the involvement of endorphins in it. Its major weaknesses arise from the fact that it is too general. It would be better if we could write Substance P instead of Pain Input, 5HT of NE instead of NO, enkephalin or β-endorphin instead of O, m or k instead of OR. All this would be highly premature and probably oversimplified. We will probably have to evolve many such circuits for different levels of the CNS, with different interactions. Whereas the tail flick response may go through two or three such way-stations, a learned escape response would be processed through many more.

The other problem is that we have no understanding as to the conditions which engage O versus NO, versus both. These are likely to be determined by the environmental and physiological variables impinging on the animal, as well as the particularly pain response being measured. It is conceivable that different individuals would exhibit their own profile, favoring one mode of pain control over the other. After all, our autonomic nervous systems have their unique patterns of responsiveness to an activating stimulus, with one individual exhibiting dramatic changes in heart rate while another would exhibit primarily changes in galvanic skin response (GSR). Such differences in coping with pain may be due to genetic factors, to sensory and autonomic events associated with the noxious input, as well as to the history of the organism. Such individual differences would render our study of pain control even more difficult. One would hope, nonetheless, that we could elaborate behavioral models which bias pain regulation in one direction or the other, allowing us to evolve testable hypotheses.

If the model described in this paper represents some realistic aspects of pain control, some prediction would follow as to the interactions between opioid and non-opioid mechanisms. For example, if the O system really inhibits the NO system, then one could find a condition where a non-opiate analgesia may be somewhat enhanced rather than inhibited by naloxone. Interestingly, a recent report has shown that low doses of naloxone enhance rather than block placebo-induced analgesia (Levine et al., 1979), although higher doses resulted in a blockade. If NO inhibits O, then a non-opiate analgesia may result in a decrease in turnover, tone, or release of some endorphins. Furthermore, when pain transmission is decreased (e.g., blockade of substance P in some circuits?), then not only should it be naloxone-reversible, but, under the balance hypothesis, it should be blocked by agents which would decrease NO but do not ordinarily affect analgesia mediated by the endorphinergic systems.

In sum, this model, in spite of its weaknesses, allows us to point to the problems in using naloxone as the only indicator of endorphinergic role in pain regulation. It permits us to define some criteria for implicating endorphins in analgesic phenomena. Finally, it gives us some framework in which to evolve and refine hypotheses as to the interactions between pain input and endorphinergic and non-endorphinergic pain inhibition.

SOME FUTURE DIRECTIONS

The foregoing discussion about the complexity of pain control does not detract from the fact that we have made great progress toward a better understanding of analgesic mechanisms. The endogenous opioids, their anatomy, their relationship to other active substances in brain and pituitary open up new avenues for basic science and clinical studies. The following are some directions which derive directly from recent findings, which may have important implications both theoretically and clinically.

The presence of ACTH or α-MSH in β-endorphin neurons suggests that these peptides may interact with β-endorphin and its receptor. While the exact mechanisms of interactions remain to be elucidated, it is possible to foresee the possibility of modulating the β-endorphin system by interacting with ACTH and related peptides.

While analgesia has been produced by direct activation of the opiate receptors or by electrical stimulation of endorphin pathways, it may be useful to find pharmacological tools to activate and release brain endorphins. We have reported on some peptides which appear capable of releasing brain β-endorphin (Akil et al., 1978b). Their analgesic potencies remain to be determined. However, such an approach would have great potential for human clinical pain. While being non-invasive, it offers the possibility of minimizing the problem of tolerance and dependence, by allowing the endogenous regulation of the neuronal system to prevent extensive activation. For example, it may be possible for the endorphinergic system to limit the releasable amount of transmitters by decreasing its synthesis. This would be determined via the natural feedback mechanisms of the system, and allow enough waxing and waning of transmitter levels at the synapse to prevent full-blown tolerance. In fact, even electrical stimulation of the systems appears to offer this advantage, since we observe little tolerance with this latter technique (Richardson and Akil, 1977b).

Finally, another way to potentiate endorphinergic effects without direct receptor activation resides in inhibiting endorphin breakdown. We and others have been studying a specific enzyme which metabolizes enkephalin, termed enkephalinase (Sullivan et al., 1978). We have described various inhibitors of this enzyme. Here again, it is conceivable that some of these substances would prove highly valuable in amplifying enkephalinergic pathways and bringing about analgesia.

As our understanding of endogenous opioid systems evolves, as we know more about their anatomy, synthesis, metabolism, and receptors, we can hope to devise new and rational methods for pain relief. However, these advances have to progress hand in hand with advances in our understanding of pain mechanisms in general and the role of both endorphinergic and non-endorphinergic mechanisms in pain control in particular.

ACKNOWLEDGEMENTS

This work was supported in part by the Mental Health Research Institute, University of Michigan and by National Institute of Drug Abuse Grant DA02265-01 and a grant from the Scottish Rite Schizophrenia Research Foundation. The author gratefully acknowledges the assistance of Ms. Carol Criss in the manuscript preparation.

REFERENCES

Akil, H., and Liebeskind, J.C. Monoaminergic mechanisms of stimulation-produced analgesia. *Brain Res.* 94, 279–296 (1975).

Akil, H., and Mayer, D.J. Antagonism of stimulation-produced analgesia by P-CPA, a serotonin synthesis inhibitor. *Brain Res.* 44, 692–697 (1972).

Akil, H., Hewlett, W., Barchas, J.D., and Li, C.H. Binding of ^{3}H-β-endorphin to rat brain membrane: characterization of opiate properties and interaction with ACTH. *Eur. J. Pharmacol.* 64, 1–8 (1980).

Akil, H., Madden, J., Patrick, R., and Barchas, J.D. Stress-induced increase in endogenous opiate peptides: concurrent analgesia and its partial reversal by naloxone, in *Opiates and Endogenous Opioid Peptides*. H.W. Kosterlitz, ed. Elsevier/North Holland, Amsterdam (1976a), pp. 63–70.

Akil, H., Mayer, D.J., and Liebeskind, J.C. Antagonism of stimulation-produced analgesia by naloxone, a narcotic antagonist. *Science* 191, 961–962 (1976b).

Akil, H., Mayer, D.J., and Liebeskind, J.C. Comparaison chez le rat de l'analgesie induite par stimulation de la substance grise et l'analgesie morphinique. *C.R. Acad. Sci.* Ser. D. 274, 3603–3605 (1972).

Akil, H., Richardson, D.E., and Barchas, J.D. Pain control by focal brain stimulation in man in relation to enkephalins and endorphins, in *Mechanism of Pain and Analgesic Compounds*. 11th Miles Int. Symposium, Raven Press, New York (1979), pp. 239–247.

Akil, H., Richardson, D.E., Barchas, J.D., and Li, C.H. Appearance of β-endorphin-like immunoreactivity in human ventricular cerebrospinal fluid upon analgesic electrical stimulation. *Proc. Natl. Acad. Sci. USA* 75, 5170–5172 (1978a).

Akil, H., Richardson, D.E., Hughes, J., and Barchas, J.D Enkephalin-like material elevated in ventricular cerebrospinal fluid of pain patients after analgesic focal stimulation. *Science* 201, 463–465 (1978b).

Akil, H., Watson, S.J., Barchas, J.D., and Li, C.H. β-Endorphin immunoreactivity in rat and human blood: Radioimmunoassay, comparitive levels and physiological alterations *Life Sci.* 24, 1659–1666 (1979).

Akil, H., Watson, S.J., Berger, P.A., and Barchas, J.D. Endorphins, β-LPH, and ACTH: biochemical, pharmacological and anatomical studies, in *The Endorphins: Advances in Biochemical Psychopharmacology*. Vol. 18. E. Costa and E.M. Trabucchi, eds. Raven Press, New York (1978c), pp. 125–139.

Akil, H., Watson, S.J., Levy, R., and Barchas, J.D. β-Endorphin and other 31K fragments: pituitary and brain systems, in *Developments in Neuroscience*. Vol. 4, *Characteristics and Function of Opioids*. J.M. VanRee and L. Terenius, eds. Elsevier/North Holland, Amsterdam (1978d), pp. 123–134.

Beecher, H.K. *Measurement of subjective responses*. Oxford U. Press, New York (1959).

Beluzzi, J.D., Grant, N., Garsky, V., Sarantakis, D., Wise, C.D., and Stein, L. Analgesia induced *in vivo* by central administration of enkephalin in rat. *Nature* 260, 625–626 (1976).

Bernston, G.G., and Walker, J.M. Effect of opiate receptor blockade on pain sensitivity in the rat. *Brain Res. Bull.* 2, 157–159 (1977).

Bloom, F.E., Rossier, J., Battenberg, E.L.F., Bayon, A., French, E., Henricksen, S.J., Siggins, G.R., Segal, D., Browne, R., Ling, N., and Guillemin, R. β-Endorphin: cellular localization, electrophysiological and behavioral effects, in *The Endorphins: Advances in Biochemical Psychopharmacology*. Vol. 18. E. Costa and M. Trabucchi, eds. Raven Press, New York (1978), pp. 89–109.

Bodnar, R.J., Kelly, D.D., Spiagga, A., Ehrenberg, C., and Glusman, M. Dose-dependent reductions by naloxone of analgesia induced by cold-water stress. *Pharmacol. Biochem. Behav.* 8, 667–672 (1978a).

Bodnar, R.J., Kelly, D.D., Steiner, S.S., and Glusman, M. Stress-produced analgesia and morphine-produced analgesia: Lack of cross tolerance. *Pharmacol. Biochem. Behav.* 8, 661–666 (1978b).

Bradbury, A.F., Feldberg, W.F., Smyth, D.G., and Snell, C. Liptotropin C-fragment: An endogenous peptide with potent analgesic activity, in *Opiates and Endogenous Opioid Peptides*. H.W. Kosterlitz, ed. Elsevier/North Holland Publishing Co., Amsterdam (1976), pp. 9–17.

Buchsbaum, M.S., Davis, G.C., and Bunney, W.E. Naloxone alters pain perception and somatosensory evolved potentials in normal subjects. *Nature* 270, 620–622 (1977).

Cheng, R., Pomeranz, B., and Yu, G. Electro-acupuncture reduces signs of withdrawal in morphine dependent mice and shows no cross-tolerance with morphine. Paper presented at the Meeting of the International Narcotic Research Conf., June 1979.

Chesher, G.B., and Chan, B. Footshock-induced analgesia in mice: its reversal by naloxone and cross-tolerance with morphine. *Life Sci.* 21, 1569–1574 (1977).

Cox, B.M., Goldstein, A., and Li, C.H. Opioid activity of peptide (β-LPH 61-91), derived from β-lipotropin. *Proc. Natl. Acad. Sci. USA* 73, 1821–1823 (1976).

Dehen, H., Willer, J.C., Prier, S., Bouran, F., and Cambier, J. Congenital insensitivity to pain and the "morphine-like" analgesic system. *Pain* 5, 351–358 (1978).

Elde, R., Hokfelt, T., Johansson, O., and Terenius, L. Immunohistochemical studies using antibodies to leucine-enkephalin: initial observations on the nervous system of the rat. *Neuroscience* 1, 349–351 (1976).

Frederickson, R.C.A., Burgis, V., and Edwards, J.D. Hyperalgesia induced by naloxone follows diurnal rhythm in responsivity to painful stimuli. *Science* 198, 756–758 (1977).

Frederickson, R.C.A., Wesche, D.L., and Richter, J.A. Mouse brain enkephalins: study of diurnal changes correlated with changes in nociceptive sensitivity, in *Developments in Neuroscience*. Vol. 4, *Characteristics and Function of Opioids*. J.M. VanRee and L. Terenius, eds. Elsevier/North Holland, Amsterdam (1978), pp. 169–172.

Goldstein, A., and Hilgard, E.R. Failure of opiate antagonist naloxone to modify hypnotic analgesia. *Proc. Natl. Acad. Sci. USA* 72, 2041–2043 (1975).

Goldstein, A., Lowney, L.I., and Pal, B.K. Stereospecific and non-specific interactions of the morphine congener levorphanol in subcellular fractions of mouse brain. *Proc. Natl. Acad. Sci. USA* 68, 1742–1747 (1971).

Goldstein, A., Pryor, G.T., Otis, L.S., and Larsen, F. On the role of endogenous opioid peptides: Failure of naloxone to influence shock escape threshold in the rat. *Life Sci.* 18, 599–604 (1976).

Grevert, P., and Goldstein, A. Effects of naloxone on experimentally induced ischemic pain and on mood in human subjects. *Proc. Natl. Acad. Sci. USA* 74, 1291–1294 (1977).

Hadfield, J.A. The influence of hypnotic suggestion on inflammatory conditions. *Lancet* 2, 678–679 (1917).

Hayes, R., Bennett, G.J., Newlon, P.G., and Mayer, D.J. Behavioral and physiological studies of non-narcotic analgesia in the rat, elicited by certain environmental stimuli. *Brain Res.* 155, 69 (1978).

Henderson, G.J., Hughes, J., and Kosterlitz, H.W. A new example-sensitive neuro-effector junction: Adrenergic transmission in the mouse vas deferens. *Brit. J. Pharmacol.* 46, 764–766 (1972).

Hilgard, E.R. A quantitative study of pain and its reduction through hypnotic suggestion. *Proc. Natl. Acad. Sci. USA* 57, 1581–1586 (1967).

Hosobuchi, Y., Adams, J.E., and Linchitz, R. Pain relief by electrical stimulation of the central gray matter in humans and its reversal by naloxone. *Science* 197, 183–186 (1977).

Hosobuchi, Y., Rossier, J., Bloom, F., and Guillemin, R. Electrical stimulation of periaqueductal grey for pain relief in humans is accompanied by elevation of immunoreactive β-endorphin in ventricular fluid. *Science* 203, 279–281 (1979).

Hughes, J., Smith, T.W., Kosterlitz, H.W., Fothergill, L.A., Morgan, B.A., and Morris, H.R. Identification of two related pentapeptides from the brain with potent opiate agonist activity. *Nature* 258, 577–579 (1975).

Jacob, J.J., Tremblay, E.C., and Colombel, M.C. Facilitation de reactions nociceptives par la naloxone chez la souris et chez le rat. *Psychopharmacologia* 37, 217–233 (1974).

Jacquet, Y.F., and Lajtha, A. Morphine action at central nervous system sites in rat: analgesia and hyperalgesia depending on site and dose. *Science* 182, 490–491 (1973).

Kangawa, K., Matsuo, H., and Igarashi, M. α-neo-endorphine: a "big" leu-enkephalin with potent opiate activity from porcine hypothalami. *Biochem. Biophys. Res. Comm.* 86, 153–160 (1979).

Kelly, D.O., and Glusman, M. Aversive thresholds following midbrain lesions. *J. Comp. Physiol. Psych.* 66, 25–34 (1968).

Levine, J.D., Gordon, N.C., and Fields, H.L. Naloxone dose dependently produces analgesia and hyperalgesia in postoperative pain. *Nature* 278, 740–741 (1979).

Levine, J.D., Gordon, N.C., Jones, R.T., and Fields, H.L. The narcotic antagonist naloxone enhances clinical pain. *Nature* 272, 826–827 (1978).

Liebeskind, J.C., Guilbaud, G., Benson, J-M., and Oliveras, J-L. Analgesia from electrical stimulation of the periacqueductal gray matter in the cat. *Brain Res.* 50, 441–446 (1973).

Liebeskind, J.C., Mayer, D.J., and Akil, H. Central mechanisms of pain inhibition: studies of analgesia from focal brain stimulation, in *Recent Advances in Pain Research and Therapy*. J.T. Bonica and D. Albe-Fenard, eds. Raven Press, New York (1976), pp. 261–268.

Liebman, J.M., Mayer, D.J., and Liebeskind, J.C. Mesencephalic central gray lesions and fear-motivated behavior in rats. *Brain Res.* 23, 353–370 (1970).

Li, C.H., Barnafi, L., Chretien, M., and Chung, D. Isolation and structure of β-LPH from sheep pituitary glands. *Excerpta Medica* 3, 111–112 (1965–66).

Li, C.H., and Chung, D. Isolation and structure of an untriakontapeptide with opiate activity from camel pituitary glands. *Proc. Natl. Acad. Sci. USA* 73, 1145–1148 (1976).

Madden, J., Akil, H., Patrick, R.L., and Barchas, J.D. Stress-induced parallel changes in central opioid levels and pain responsiveness in the rat. *Nature* 266, 1358–1360 (1977).

Mains, R.E., Eipper, B.A., and Ling, N. Common precursor to corticotropins and endorphins. *Proc. Natl. Acad. Sci. USA* 74, 3014–3018 (1977).

Mau, P.L., and Chen, C.H. Mechanism of acupunctural anesthesia. *Dis. Nerv. Syst.* 33 (11), 730–735 (1972).

Mayer, D.J., and Hayes, R. Stimulation-produced analgesia: development of tolerance and cross-tolerance to morphine. *Science* 188, 941–943 (1975).

Mayer, D.J., and Price, D.D. Central nervous system mechanisms of analgesia. *Pain* 2, 379–404 (1976).

Mayer, D.J., Price, D.D., and Raffi, A. Antagonism of acupuncture analgesia in man by the narcotic antagonist naloxone. *Brain Res.* 121, 368–372 (1977).

Mayer, D.J., Wolfe, T.L., Akil, H., Carder, B., and Liebeskind, J.C. Analgesia resulting from electrical stimulation in the brainstem of the rat. *Science* 174, 1351–1354 (1971).

Melzack, R., and Wall, P.D. Pain mechanisms: a new theory. *Science* 150, 971–979 (1965).

Moon, H.D., Li, C.H., and Jennings, B.M. Immunohistochemical and histochemical studies of pituitary β-lipotropin. *Anat. Rec.* 175, 524–538 (1973).

Pert, C.B., and Snyder, S.H. Opiate receptor: demonstration in nervous tissue. *Science* 179, 1011–1014 (1973).

Pomeranz, B., and Chiu, D. Naloxone blockade of acupuncture analgesia: endorphin implicated. *Life Sci.* 19, 1757–1762 (1976).

Prieto, G.J., Giesler, J.G., and Cannon, T.T. Evidence for site specificity in naloxone's antagonism of SPA in the rat. *Soc. Neurosci, Abstr*, 5,614 (1979).

Proudfit, H.K., and Anderson, E.G. Blockade of morphine analgesia by destruction of a bulbospinal serotonergic pathway. *Pharmacologist* 16, 203 (1974).

Reynolds, D.V. Surgery in the rat during electrical analgesia induced by focal brain stimulation. *Science* 164, 444–445 (1969).

Richardson, D.E., and Akil, H. Pain reduction by electrical brain stimulation in man: Part 1: Acute administration in periaqueductal and periventricular sites. J. Neurosurg. 47, 178–183 (1977a).

Richardson, D.E., and Akil, H. Pain reduction by electrical brain stimulation in man: Part 2: Chronic self-administration in the periventricular gray matter. *J. Neurosurg.* 47, 184–194 (1977b).

Rossier, J., French, E.D., Rivier, C., Ling, N., Guillemin, R., and Bloom, F.E. Footshock induced stress increases β-endorphin levels in blood but not brain. *Nature* 270, 618–620 (1977).

Simantov, R., Kuhar, M.J., Uhl, G.R., and Snyder, S.H. Opioid peptide enkaphalin: immunohistochemical mapping in rat CNS. *Proc. Natl. Acad. Sci. USA* 74, 2167–2171 (1977).

Simon, E.J., Hiller, J.M., and Edelman, I. Stereospecific binding of the potent narcotic analgesic (^{3}H) etorphine to rat-brain homogenate. *Proc. Natl. Acad. Sci. USA* 70, 1947–1949 (1973).

Sullivan, S., Akil, H., and Barchas, J.D. *In Vitro* degredation of enkephalin: evidence for cleavage at the Gly-Phe bond. *Commun. Psychopharm.* 2, 525–531 (1978).

Sullivan, S., Akil, H., Blacker, D., and Barchas, J.D. Preliminary characterization and comparison with angiotensin converting enzyme. *Life Sci.* (in press).

Terenius, L. Characteristics of the "receptor" for narcotic analgesics in synaptic plasma membrane fraction from the rat brain. *Acta Pharmacol. Toxicol.* 33, 377–384 (1973).

Terenius, L., and Wahlstrom, A. Morphine-like ligand for opiate receptors in human CSF. *Life Sci.* 16, 1759–1764 (1975).

Verri, R.A., Graeff, F.G., and Corrado, A.P. Effect of reserpine and AMPT on morphine analgesia. *Int. J. Neuropharmacol.* 7, 283–292 (1968).

Vogt, M. The effect of lowering 5HT content of the rat spinal cord on analgesia produced by morphine. *J. Physiol.* 194, 236, 483 (1974).

Von Knorring, L., Alamay, B.G.L., Johansson, F., and Terenius, L. Pain perception and endorphin levels in cerebrospinal fluid. *Pain* 5, 359–366 (1978).

Watson, S.J., and Akil, H. α-MSH in rat brain: occurrence within and outside brain β-endorphin neurons. *Brain Res.* 182, 217–223 (1980).

Watson, S.J., and Akil, H. The presence of two α-MSH positive cell groups in rat hypothalamus. *Eur. J. Pharmacol.* 58, 101–103 (1979).

Watson, S.J., Akil, H., Berger, P.A., and Barchas, J.D. Some observations on the opiate peptides in schizophrenia. *Arch. Gen. Psychiat.* 36, 35–41 (1979).

Watson, S.J., Akil, H., Richard, C.W., and Barchas, J.D. Evidence for two separate opiate peptide neuronal systems and the coexistence of β-lipotropin, β-endorphin, and ACTH immunoreactivities in the same hypothalamic neurons. *Nature* 275, 226–228 (1978a).

Watson, S.J., Akil, H., Sullivan, S.O., and Barchas, J.D. Immunocytochemical localization of methionine-enkephalin: preliminary observations. *Life Sci.* 25, 733–738 (1977).

Watson, S.J., Richard, C.W., and Barchas, J.D. Adrenocorticotropin in rat brain: immunocytochemical localization in cells and axons. *Science* 200, 1180–1182 (1978b).

Wei, E., and Loh, H. Physical dependence on opiate-like peptides. *Science* 195, 1262–1263 (1976).

Yaksh, T.L., Yeung, J.C., and Rudy, T.A. An inability to antagonize with naloxone the elevated nociceptive thresholds resulting from electrical stimulation of the central gray. *Life Sci.* 18, 1193–1198 (1976).

Index

GPSR Compliance

The European Union's (EU) General Product Safety Regulation (GPSR) is a set of rules that requires consumer products to be safe and our obligations to ensure this.

If you have any concerns about our products, you can contact us on ProductSafety@springernature.com

In case Publisher is established outside the EU, the EU authorized representative is:

Springer Nature Customer Service Center GmbH
Europaplatz 3
69115 Heidelberg, Germany

Batch number: 10607212

Printed by Printforce, the Netherlands